MW01061970

NEUROPSYCHOLOGY OF COGNITIVE DECLINE

Neuropsychology
of Cognitive Decline

A Developmental Approach to Assessment and Intervention

Holly A. Tuokko
Colette M. Smart

THE GUILFORD PRESS
New York   London

Printed in the United States of America

This book is printed on acid-free paper.

Last digit is print number: 9   8   7   6   5   4   3   2   1

The authors have checked with sources believed to be reliable in their efforts to
provide information that is complete and generally in accord with the standards
of practice that are accepted at the time of publication. However, in view of the
possibility of human error or changes in behavioral, mental health, or medical
sciences, neither the authors, nor the editors and publisher, nor any other party
who has been involved in the preparation or publication of this work warrants
that the information contained herein is in every respect accurate or complete,
and they are not responsible for any errors or omissions or the results obtained
from the use of such information. Readers are encouraged to confirm the
information contained in this book with other sources.

Library of Congress Cataloging-in-Publication

Names: Tuokko, Holly, author. | Smart, Colette M., author.
Title: Neuropsychology of cognitive decline : a developmental approach to
    assessment and intervention / Holly A. Tuokko, Colette M. Smart.
Description: New York : The Guilford Press, [2018] | Includes bibliographical
    references and index.
Identifiers: LCCN 2018014986 | ISBN 9781462535392 (hardback : alk. paper)
Subjects: | MESH: Cognitive Dysfunction—diagnosis | Aged | Geriatric
    Assessment—methods | Cognitive Dysfunction—therapy | Risk Factors
Classification: LCC RC524 | NLM WT 150 | DDC 618.97/689—dc23
LC record available at *https://lccn.loc.gov/2018014986*

About the Authors

Holly A. Tuokko, PhD, a clinical neuropsychologist, is Professor of Psychology and a member of the graduate faculty in the Clinical Psychology Training Program at the University of Victoria, British Columbia, Canada, where she is also a research affiliate of the Institute on Aging and Lifelong Health. Prior to joining the University of Victoria, Dr. Tuokko was Supervising Psychologist at the Clinic for Alzheimer Disease and Related Disorders at UBC Hospital and worked on a geriatric mental health outreach team. She coordinated the neuropsychological component of the Canadian Study of Health and Aging and was awarded Senior Investigator status by the Canadian Institutes of Health Research from 2002 to 2007 for a program of research on mental health and aging, including the evolution of cognitive disorders. Dr. Tuokko was the Psychological Health theme leader for the Canadian Longitudinal Study of Aging from its inception until 2017.

Colette M. Smart, PhD, a clinical neuropsychologist, is Associate Professor of Psychology and a member of the graduate faculty in the Clinical Psychology Training Program at the University of Victoria, British Columbia, Canada, where she is also a research affiliate of the Institute on Aging and Lifelong Health. Previously, Dr. Smart was a staff neuropsychologist and clinician–researcher at the Johnson Rehabilitation Institute and the Neuroscience Institute, both affiliates of JFK Medical Center in Edison, New Jersey. Her current research integrates her knowledge of aging and dementia with principles and practices of neurorehabilitation. Dr. Smart is a core member of the Subjective Cognitive Decline Initiative, an international working group of clinician–researchers, in which she focuses on the role of cognitive-experimental tests in detecting subjective cognitive decline, as well as nonpharmacological interventions such as mindfulness training.

Acknowledgments

Looking back over a long career, I can identify a few key people who influenced its trajectory. Drs. Otfried Spreen and Louis Costa were academic mentors within the field of neuropsychology but oh so much more in terms of career coaches. Little did I know during my graduate training that I would follow the career path of a true scientist–practitioner. My interdisciplinary experiences at the Clinic for Alzheimer Disease and Related Disorders under the guidance of Dr. B. Lynn Beattie and my community outreach experiences opened my eyes to the different subsets of clientele with which a clinical neuropsychologist may come into contact. Together with active leadership engagement in large, epidemiological research projects like the Canadian Study of Health and Aging and the Canadian Longitudinal Study on Aging, these experiences have reinforced for me the many different ways we learn about our subject matter, and how these influence our thinking about research and clinical practice. Throughout my career, I have maintained a passion for understanding the older adult experience that began with my grandparents and served me well when caring for my own parents. To all of these people who came before, and to Holly Williams, who assisted in the preparation of the manuscript, I am eternally grateful.

—H. A. T.

In the spirit of acknowledging one's elders, I am grateful for many mentors and collaborators who have been part of my own developmental trajectory, particularly Drs. Joseph Giacino, Laura Rabin, and Sid Segalowitz—I say with sincerity that my career would not be what it is today without your support. Thank you to my wonderful clinical neuropsychology colleagues at the University of Victoria—and particularly Holly, for your mentorship and friendship—without whom the opportunity to collaborate on this book would not have been possible. I also wish to acknowledge the members of my research team, SMARTLab. Your curiosity, enthusiasm, and humor have been a true source of inspiration, and it has been a joy to support you on your own academic journeys. Writing a book can be a stressful and time-intensive endeavor. I thank Kayla and Barb for hosting my writing trips to Moontide Farm, providing much needed peace and solitude to work. Thanks also to JaBig, who provided the musical soundtrack to the many writing marathons needed to complete the work. I also benefited from the reliable support of family and friends, too many to mention— you know who you are. And last but not least, I thank my grandmother, Catherine, something of an outlier on the trajectories of cognitive decline. You are the person who in many ways first piqued my interest in studying aging and working professionally with older adults, instilling in me an appreciation of the many benefits of intergenerational relationships, which remain a cornerstone of my life today.

—C. M. S.

Together, we wish to thank the many older adults and their families whom we have had the pleasure to serve over the years. Experiences with you not only have fueled our pursuit of knowledge but have shaped the way we live and love. We also thank the many undergraduate and graduate students we have taught and mentored over the years who have kept us on our toes and made our respective journeys memorable and rewarding.

Contents

Part III. Interventions for Late-Life Cognitive Decline

PART I

An Overview of Cognitive Decline in Later Life

CHAPTER 1

Introduction to the Study of Cognitive Decline

Cognitive functioning and changes in cognitive functioning associated with age have been of interest to clinicians and researchers alike for over a century. In the latter half of the 19th century, early explorers of "the science of mental life," or psychology, identified aspects of cognition, including memory and reasoning, and pursued new methods for understanding their structure and functions (James, 1890). This led to subsequent investigations into how cognitive functions differ across ages and as people age.

In the same era, an association between advanced age and disorders affecting cognition was recognized, and in early 1910, Gaetano Perusini, a colleague of Alois Alzheimer, published a paper concerning "Clinically and Histologically Peculiar Mental Disorders of Old Age" (Perusini, 1910). Since that time, there has been intense interest in understanding the nature and development of cognition by researchers studying healthy aging and by clinicians seeking ways to identify, manage, and ultimately remediate disorders of cognition associated with aging. It has only been within the last quarter century that these previously distinct lines of inquiry have come together as connections among biological, psychological, and sociological processes at play in relation to aging have been clearly articulated. From the biological perspective, it has become increasingly clear, particularly with the advent of neuroimaging techniques and gene mapping techniques, that age-associated changes in cognitive functions and age-associated disorders of cognition can be linked to changes in health status, which, in turn, can be linked to changes in brain function. Similarly, it has also become increasingly clear that age-associated changes in cognitive functions and age-associated disorders of cognition influence the everyday behaviors and

3

social functions required to engage in and adapt to changes in one's living environment. These realizations, taken in conjunction with what is now recognized as worldwide population aging (United Nations, 2013), contribute to the importance of understanding influences on trajectories of cognitive decline.

The structure of the population in developed countries is changing as people are living longer than ever before and birth rates are dropping. It is estimated that by 2050, the proportion of older adults in the population of developed countries will exceed 25% and that children under 15 years of age will make up only 16% of the population (Cohen, 2003). Many older adults will benefit from, and be able to take advantage of, the opportunities available to them as the structure of society changes. However, the prevalence of disorders that affect cognitive functions rises sharply with age, such that approximately 65% of people age 85 and over will experience some form of cognitive impairment (Graham et al., 1997). Half of these people will show marked impairment in cognitive functions that significantly interferes with their daily living (i.e., diagnosis of dementia or major neurocognitive disorder [NCD]) at a very high cost to the affected individuals, their families, and society.

Based on our current understanding of Alzheimer's disease (AD), the most prevalent form of dementia, the underlying neurodegenerative process may be present for years, if not decades, before the cognitive and behavioral manifestations are apparent (Bookheimer et al., 2000; Braak & Braak, 1998). While features of mild cognitive impairment (MCI) can be identified, a variety of different trajectories for those with MCI have been observed that appear to be influenced by protective or exacerbating factors. Moreover, it is generally agreed that some degree of cognitive decline occurs because of the aging process, making elusive the early identification of cognitive decline associated with underlying pathological processes and the prediction of the trajectories and rates of decline.

In this book, we articulate an applied neuropsychological approach that integrates principles and practices of clinical neuropsychology with research from basic and cognitive neuroscience and lifespan development. We identify and summarize research addressing the many factors affecting trajectories of cognitive decline and provide practical guidance for those working in a clinical or research capacity with older adults. The aim of this first section of the book is to provide an examination of the approaches to the study of cognitive decline in later life and examine those factors that appear to be protective or exacerbating of decline. In so doing, those factors that have been shown to be, or have promise of being, modifiable will be identified. In this chapter in particular, we describe the approaches taken to the study of later-life cognitive decline, including a focus on changes in cognition typically associated with the aging process (i.e., cognitive aging) and changes in cognition reflective of age-associated disorders (i.e., NCDs).

First, we briefly describe the information concerning the concept of cognitive aging studied in well-functioning older adults distinguishable from those experiencing cognitive impairment. We then introduce and review the concepts relevant to the detection and evolution of disorders affecting cognitive functions in older adulthood.

Approaches to the Study of Cognitive Decline in Well-Functioning Older Adults

Cognitive Aging

Many decades of research have focused on the relations between different aspects of cognition (e.g., memory, intelligence) and aging. In so doing, distinctions are made within different types of cognitive processes and the manner in which changes in these processes seen with age have been investigated. For example, multiple forms of memory have been distinguished: memory systems (declarative vs. nondeclarative; episodic vs. semantic) and memory tasks (explicit vs. implicit). Similarly, distinctions are often made between two components of intelligence: crystallized (or knowledge) and fluid (or problem solving).

Investigations of cognitive aging have identified a number of factors that influence the interpretation of the findings from this research and make simple conclusions about the associations between age and various aspects of cognition challenging. These include characteristics of the research methods used to conduct the studies, such as research design (i.e., cross-sectional vs. longitudinal) and sample selection (i.e., the characteristics of the people included in the study) (Campbell & Stanley, 1963). Cross-sectional studies compare groups of individuals of different ages at one point in time and may be vulnerable to cohort effects. That is, observed differences among age groups may be related to the point in history at which the person was born and may not be indicative of age-related differences per se. Conversely, longitudinal studies, those that follow a single group over time to measure age-related change, are particularly susceptible to practice effects (i.e., the effects of repeated exposure to the measures being used to assess cognitive functions over time) and selective dropout. Selective dropout refers to the possibility that people who withdraw from the study or are lost to follow-up may be those who perform poorly on the cognitive tasks because of such things as poor motivation or illness. The remaining sample, then, has different characteristics from the original sample, and this may limit the interpretation of findings. Sample selection may also affect the observed findings in that certain populations (e.g., those in better health; those of higher socioeconomic status; or those who live an active lifestyle) may perform better on measures of cognitive function. This could affect the findings of cross-sectional studies, if the groups of different ages differ in other ways as well. That said, more sophisticated research designs and data analytic techniques that take these concerns into consideration are being employed more frequently; converging evidence suggests that declines in a variety of cognitive tasks, such as specific aspects of memory functioning, speed of processing, and executive functions, typify older adults. The exact timing of when decline begins and the nature of conditions that accelerate or mitigate the rate of decline continue to be topics of debate.

Theoretical Approaches to the Study of Cognitive Aging

A number of theories that differ in emphasis have been proposed to account for observed changes over time in cognitive performance (e.g., see Craik & Salthouse, 2008, or Park & Schwarz, 2000, for reviews). Here we will briefly highlight some foundational perspectives, and then we will introduce more recent work moving toward a coherent integrated account of cognitive aging.

Information-Processing Approaches

Much of the early work in the field of cognitive aging emerged from the information-processing approach that emphasizes the types of processing involved in completing a cognitive task. This model uses a computer metaphor, where information enters the system, is transformed, then stored in various ways, and is later retrieved. For example, a number of processes influence the ability to recall a specific piece of information. How well the information was initially encoded or picked up, how well it was stored or retained, and how effectively it is retrieved are viewed as separate components of the recall process. Tasks can be designed in such a way that performance on each component can be examined and the source of recall problems can be ascertained. Decades of research on cognitive aging from this perspective have yielded important distinctions concerning whether and how aging affects component cognitive processes (e.g., attention, memory, visuospatial processing, and executive functions). In addition, other, more generalized cognitive processes have been proposed to account for, or explain, the observed relationship between age and performance on these cognitive component processes. Perhaps the most prominent proposal in this regard is that generalized slowing in processing speed can account for the observed areas of age-related declines (Salthouse, 1992, 1996, 1997). From this perspective, basic cognitive operations are processed too slowly to permit higher-level processes to take place efficiently. However, it is also clear from accumulated research findings that different domains of cognition may change differentially within and across individuals (Mungas et al., 2010; Van Petten et al., 2004).

Intraindividual Differences

While much of the research in the field of cognitive aging has examined the interindividual differences and similarities between people of different ages, the study of variations in cognitive functioning within individuals across occasions (or intraindividual variability) has gained much attention in recent years. There is now considerable evidence that intraindividual cognitive variability can be viewed as a systematic source of individual differences and is of important predictive value for aging-relevant outcomes (Martin & Hofer, 2004). For example, Hultsch, Strauss, Hunter, and Mac-Donald (2008) note that intraindividual variability, or inconsistencies in performance over relatively short periods of time, is characteristically seen most prominently in children and older adults. In addition, they note that intraindividual variability is a good indicator of cognitive aging, that this variability seems to be accentuated in older adults with a cognitive disorder such as dementia, and that it may be predictive of multiple outcomes, not all of which are maladaptive.

Contextual Approaches

These approaches suggest that age differences in cognitive functioning can be determined, or significantly influenced, by other characteristics of the individual such as attitudes, interests, and social context. These approaches emphasize aging as a dynamic process of adaptation that takes into consideration both gains (e.g., experience) and losses (e.g., slowing of processing speed) experienced through the aging process. One example of a contextual approach is the selective optimization and compensation model proposed by Baltes and Baltes (1990). This model proposes that, as people age, they selectively restrict activities in which they engage, based on personal importance and relevance, to maintain optimal functioning. In addition, they may employ compensation strategies to overcome any limitations or challenges experienced. This approach situates cognitive performance within the broader context of personal choice and motivation, recognizing that individuals actively adapt to changing circumstances, including changes in physical/biological functioning.

Another theoretical approach that features personal motivation as central to understanding cognitive decline associated with aging is Carstensen's (1993) socioemotional selectivity theory. This theory proposes that, as people age, their motivations shift from the pursuit of knowledge (i.e., youth) to the pursuit of emotional satisfaction (i.e., older adults). This shift is proposed to occur in response to the perceived change in temporal horizon (i.e., time is perceived as constrained). People become less interested in the acquisition of knowledge and skills but more invested in the emotional aspects of life. This motivational shift is proposed to have consequences for cognitive performance in that cognitive resources (e.g., attention and memory capacity) are selectively devoted to seeking information that will enhance individuals' current mood and satisfaction with life.

Biological Approaches

These approaches maintain that cognitive decline occurs because of biological changes experienced by all living things as they age. Specifically, with the increased availability of neuroimaging techniques such as computed tomography (CT), magnetic resonance imaging (MRI), single photon emission computed tomography (SPECT), positron emission tomography (PET), functional magnetic resonance imaging (fMRI), magnetocephalography, and near-infrared spectroscopic imaging (NIRSI), decline in cognitive abilities has been clearly linked to structural (e.g., plaque and tangle formation, cell death and atrophy), biochemical (e.g., decreasing levels of neurotransmitters such as acetylcholine), and functional (e.g., areas of activation) changes occurring within the brain. Suffice to say that many theories have been proposed to explain the biological changes typical of the aging process (e.g., rate of living theories, cellular theories, programmed cell death theories), though none provides a comprehensive explanation of all observed age-associated changes. Instead, here we focus on a few biologically based theories relevant to our goals in examining trajectories of cognitive decline in later life.

While aging has been associated with changes in many aspects of brain function, particular attention has been focused on the frontal lobes as they seem most vulnerable to advancing age (Raz & Rodrigue, 2006; Raz, Rodrigue, Kennedy, & Acker, 2007; West, 1996). The frontal lobes are associated with executive functions, or those processes associated with the management, regulation, and control of other complex cognitive processes (Elliott, 2003), including working memory, reasoning, task flexibility, and problem solving (Monsell, 2003), as well as task planning and execution (Chan, Shum, Toulopoulou, & Chen, 2008).

The frontal aging hypothesis proposes that selective reduction in frontal lobe function underlies the decline in cognitive processes associated with aging (e.g., Dempster, 1992; Hartley, 1993; West, 1996). While there is support for this position, nonfrontal regions undergo similar reductions in function, and numerous studies link specific age-related cognitive changes (e.g., memory) with structural changes in a variety of brain regions. In addition, younger and older adults show differences in regional brain activation patterns in response to cognitive tasks. For example, older adults may show bilateral frontal activation in response to tasks that prompt unilateral activation in younger adults (e.g., Grady, 2012; Grady, McIntosh, Rajah, Beig, & Craik, 1999). Although initially this contralateral activation was thought to undermine cognitive function and to be the source of some of the cognitive deficits seen with aging, more recent findings suggest that this contralateral recruitment is supportive of cognitive functions and serves a compensatory function.

Brain reserve capacity (BRC) is a model that proposes that functional impairment will occur when an absolute cutoff or threshold of neural damage is reached. Individual differences in BRC explain why clinical symptoms are expressed earlier in some people than in others. The same amount of neural damage, then, may result in clinical symptoms being manifest in someone with low BRC but not in someone with more BRC. This model has received substantial support, and factors that may enhance BRC, thereby exerting a "protective effect" against the expression of cognitive impairment, have been proposed. We will address some of these factors in the next chapter.

The BRC model has limitations. Stern (2002) therefore proposed the cognitive reserve model, which views differences in how effectively cognitive paradigms are used to approach a problem as paramount to the expression of clinical symptoms. There is no single absolute threshold of neural damage beyond which impairment occurs. Instead, brain structures or networks not typically invoked are activated to compensate for neural disruptions. Those people with greater cognitive reserve are more effective in invoking these alternate neural pathways to accomplish the cognitive or functional task at hand.

These compensatory processes indicate that there is plasticity in both brain changes and behavior throughout the aging process. This neuroplasticity, or structural and functional changes of the brain, occurs as a result of interactions between the brain and behavior. In addition, it is now known that neural stem cells persist in the adult brain and that new neurons can be generated throughout the lifespan. These emerging findings concerning the capability of the brain to change and adapt support the contention that behavioral compensation is possible and may even alter the underlying structure and function of brain regions.

Integrative Approaches

The biopsychosocial model (Engel, 2012), originally proposed in 1977, provides a broad holistic framework for conceptualizing the multiple determinants of complex conditions or situations (e.g., clinical presentation of cognitive decline). This model proposes that biological (e.g., genetics, physical functioning, and medical conditions), psychological (e.g., thoughts, emotions, and behaviors), and social (e.g., socioeconomical, socioenvironmental, and cultural) factors interact and influence the development and behavior of each individual. While this model is generally accepted and has been applied in many contexts, it is pervasive in the study of adult development and aging (Whitbourne, Whitbourne, & Konnert, 2015). The relative influences of biological, psychological, and social factors are taken into consideration, and it is acknowledged that aging is complex and not manifest as a simple, linear trajectory across the lifespan. This emphasis on development takes a lifespan perspective, acknowledging that development is (1) multidirectional (involving both growth and decline); (2) plastic, in that new learning can occur at any point in the lifespan; and (3) influenced by a wide variety of forces (e.g., the historical time and culture within which a person is aging) (Baltes, 1987).

More recently, particularly in response to the availability of neuroimaging techniques that can detail how brain functions and structures change with age, the need for integrative approaches specific to the study of cognitive aging has been recognized (e.g., Hofer & Alwin, 2008). Linking this information with the decades of research that has characterized the nature of, and factors influencing, cognitive aging is the complex challenge facing the growing area of cognitive neuroscience. These emerging theories are necessarily interdisciplinary and incorporate an array of biological and neurophysiological factors with other information derived from earlier work concerning compensatory processes within the brain and through cognitive engagement that influences brain aging.

The scaffolding theory of aging and cognition aging (STAC; e.g., Park & Reuter-Lorenz, 2009; Reuter-Lorenz & Park, 2014) is one such integrative model. It takes into consideration the following observations emerging from cognitive neuroscience and aging research: cognitive functions and neural structures show significant declines with advanced aging; functional activity of the brain increases with age, particularly in the frontal cortex, and may be indicative of the recruitment of alternate neural pathways to compensate for age-related accumulation of neural disruptions (i.e., compensatory scaffolding); scaffolding is the brain's dynamic, normal response to challenge, at any age, and may be entirely limited by significant pathology (e.g., pathological sequelae of AD); and cognitive activity such as engaging in stimulating experiences promotes scaffolding.

The STAC was revised (STAC-r) in 2014 to take into consideration life-course (i.e., accumulation of experiences) and lifespan factors (i.e., states an individual has experienced from birth to death) that enhance or deplete neural resources. This allows for the influences of positive (e.g., educational attainment, intellectual engagement) and negative (e.g., emotional or environmental stress) factors extraneous to the brain to contribute to the neural scaffolding process. These protective and risk factors will be addressed later in this section. By including these factors within STAC-r, brain structure and functions may change in either direction (i.e., gains or losses) as a function of plasticity, development, and life-course influences.

Evolution of Disorders Affecting Cognitive Functions in Older Adulthood

While some degree of cognitive decline may be an integral part of the aging process, the identification of, and intervention for, disorders of cognition have been the focus for many clinicians (e.g., clinical neuropsychologists, geriatricians, and geriatric psychiatrists) providing care to older adults. The biopsychosocial model (described above) has been adopted widely within clinical practice and provides the framework for obtaining the essential information required for accurate diagnosis and identification of avenues for effective interventions. The emphasis on the biopsychosocial and lifespan perspectives in the study of adult development and aging (Whitbourne et al., 2015) extends to the clinical practice of geriatric neuropsychological assessment and intervention (Clare & Woods, 2004; Puente & McCaffrey, 1992). As many factors beyond the presence of biological pathological processes can affect cognitive functioning, it is imperative that researchers and clinicians alike are knowledgeable about the complex characteristics of the aging process and age-related vulnerabilities that may influence the assessment process (American Psychological Association, 2012).

Inherent in the process of identifying cognitive impairment is a reliance on understanding what typifies normal cognitive decline. The many factors that can influence cognitive decline are addressed in Chapter 5. As is shown here, clinicians have benefited from and adopted methods derived from theories of cognitive aging to apply in a clinical context. The application of these methods and techniques in the clinical setting has provided both clarity and controversy concerning the manner in which cognitive functioning and pathology are related. Certainly, descriptive distinctions in the patterns and progress of cognitive change related to different underlying pathologies have been the focus of much research that, in turn, has resulted in improved clinical practice. Yet, there is not always a close correspondence between underlying pathology and cognitive symptoms (Riley, Snowdon, Desrosiers, & Markesbery, 2005). This speaks to the complexity of the aging process and the need for ongoing research and theory development to clarify the factors at play. That is, we need to continue our quest to understand the factors that place individuals at greater risk for cognitive decline (see Chapter 3) or are protective against cognitive decline (see Chapter 2). How these factors relate to, or perhaps modify, the underlying pathological process has yet to be fully determined.

For over half a century, researchers and clinicians have been proposing and evaluating ways to classify cognitive impairment emerging in later life. Cognitive and behavioral changes may be the first indications of an underlying pathological process, and the pathological process itself may not be easily identified premortem. By necessity, then, these classifications are often based on constellations of acquired cognitive and behavioral deficits (i.e., they represent a decline from a previously attained level of functioning) that are presumed to be linked to a specific underlying etiology. For example, the 2015 *International Classification of Diseases—10th edition—Clinical Modification* (2015 ICD-10-CM; World Health Organization, 2015) contains diagnostic codes for various forms of dementia within diseases of the nervous system (e.g., dementia with Lewy bodies

[DLB], AD) or within mental, behavioral, and neurodevelopmental disorders (e.g., unspecified dementia, dementia not classified elsewhere).

The fifth edition of the *Diagnostic and Statistical Manual of Mental Disorders* (DSM-5; American Psychiatric Association, 2013) identifies twelve different etiological subtypes of major (including disorders previously referred to as dementias) and mild NCDs and takes into consideration that other etiological subtypes may exist. The most common etiological subtypes include AD, frontotemporal lobar degeneration (FTLD), DLB, and vascular dementia (VaD). Of note, FTLD has been characterized as a spectrum of diseases that includes disorders of behavior and language and may include disorders primarily affecting movement such as amyotrophic lateral sclerosis (ALS), corticobasal degeneration syndrome (CBDS), and progressive supranuclear palsy (PSP), where cognitive impairment may occur to varying degrees (*www.theaftd.org/understandingftd/ftd-overview*). The developmental course and patterns of cognitive and behavioral deficits associated with these etiological subtypes may be useful for distinguishing among them, particularly with respect to major NCDs and will be addressed in Chapter 8.

The distinction between major and mild forms of NCD is inherently arbitrary and based primarily on the severity of cognitive deficits and the extent to which the cognitive deficits interfere with capacity for independence in everyday activities. That is, major and mild NCDs are viewed as existing on a spectrum of cognitive and functional impairment. The identification of mild NCDs, as distinct from typical age-associated cognitive decline and the classification of mild NCDs into etiological subtypes, both may prove quite challenging. Earlier efforts to develop ways to classify mild forms of cognitive impairment that are insufficient to warrant a diagnosis of dementia (see Tuokko & Hultsch, 2006a), yet predictive of continued decline to dementia, have been met with limited success to date. However, interest in classifications that capture milder forms of cognitive impairment remains. These milder forms of cognitive impairment may or may not be predictive of continued cognitive decline reflective of specific forms of underlying pathology and eventual poor outcomes. When the identification of milder forms of cognitive impairment is considered to be descriptive (as opposed to prescriptive of future decline), the focus of assessment and intervention strategies can be on specific functional, social, and care needs for the individual (Tuokko & Hultsch, 2006b). The importance of providing interventions intended to optimize the functioning and well-being of the individual and to minimize risk associated with existing disability is self-evident, and the evidence base has been building over the last decade. Guidance for clinicians concerning assessment and intervention issues will be addressed in detail in Chapters 6 (on subjective cognitive decline [SCD]) and 7 (on MCI). Intervention strategies of relevance across the trajectories of cognitive decline (i.e., normal aging, SCD, MCI, dementia) are addressed in Chapters 9–12.

The Current Context

At this point in the developmental trajectory of knowledge concerning cognitive decline in later life, we are challenged with bringing together information obtained through various lines of inquiry for application in a clinical context. Certainly in recent years, particularly with the advent of neuroimaging techniques, the links among age-associated changes in cognitive functions, age-associated disorders of cognition, changes in health status, and changes in brain are becoming more clearly articulated. Similarly, our understanding of the interactions of age-associated changes in cognitive functions and disorders of cognition with everyday behaviors and social functions required to engage in and adapt to changes in one's living environment is growing and influencing how and when we intervene to enhance or improve a person's current level of cognitive, emotional, and behavioral functioning.

Our overarching goals in this book are to provide a summary of the research to date that addresses the many factors affecting trajectories of cognitive decline and to also provide practical guidance for those working in a clinical or research capacity with older adults to enhance or improve their current level of cognitive, emotional, and behavioral functioning. In keeping with this applied approach, we present appendices that include exemplars of tools for use by clinicians and students for collecting relevant information. We acknowledge that the focus and nature of assessment and intervention strategies may differ for those showing typical cognitive decline from those who already manifest some form of cognitive impairment. We also acknowledge that subjective concern regarding cognitive decline and mild forms of cognitive impairment may or may not be indicative of a trajectory of increasing severity of cognitive impairment reflective of an underlying progressive pathological process. That is, there is not one trajectory of cognitive decline in later life but many. Myriad factors influence these trajectories—some that enhance the likelihood of further decline and others that appear to be protective against it. The importance of these factors may occur at various points in, or across, the lifespan and may vary depending on the historical and cultural context.

Figure 1.1 illustrates the structure we have adopted in this book for examining trajectories of cognitive decline in later life. A hypothetical trajectory of cognitive decline from cognitive decline that typifies age-related cognitive decline through SCD, MCI, to dementia (thick descending curve) is depicted at the top of the figure. While this indeed may be the trajectory traveled by some, others may show relatively little ongoing decline or even improvement in cognitive functions over time (thin lines). An individual's trajectory of cognitive decline takes place across time within a historical and cultural context (background in top section). The historical context refers to the historical time in which a person lives as well as the historical background of the individual (e.g., medical, social, educational history).

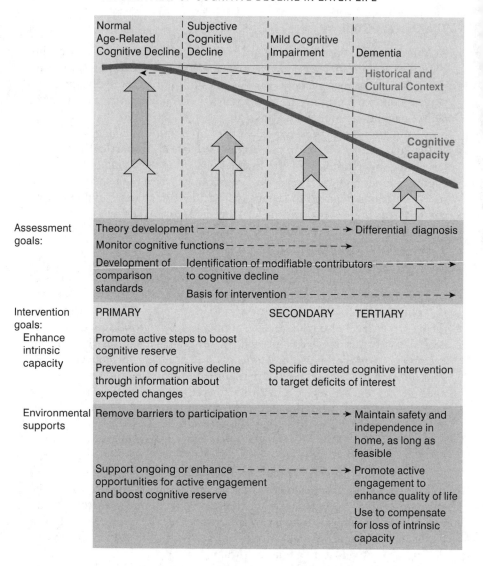

FIGURE 1.1. Trajectories of cognitive decline.

In the first section of this book, we examine factors that are predictive of or protective against cognitive decline that have been observed at various points in the hypothetical trajectory of cognitive decline. The goals and methods for assessment (first shaded horizontal band), intervention (second lighter horizontal band) and suitable environmental supports (bottom horizontal band) may or may not be similar at different points in the trajectory. In the latter part of the book, assessment goals and methods as well as intervention strategies are articulated in relation to identifiable conditions along the trajectory of cognitive decline. The intense study of age-related cognitive decline contributes to theory development and to the characterization of age-related cognitive decline as a comparison standard for use in identifying cognitive impairment. Ongoing assessment becomes crucial for monitoring change once impairment is evident for diagnostic purposes and for identifying opportunities for intervention or modification of factors that may be contributing to ongoing decline. We demonstrate that interventions and environmental supports may be beneficial for enhancing current cognitive function and/or preventing further decline or at least slowing its rate (vertical arrows providing resistance against cognitive decline). These interventions and supports pertain to healthy older adults and to those with SCD where the primary goal is to prevent the manifestation of disease (primary prevention). They also pertain to persons who already have manifest cognitive impairment (i.e., MCI), where the focus is on slowing the rate of further decline (secondary prevention), or to persons with significant cognitive impairment such as dementia (tertiary prevention), where the primary objective is to minimize functional disability and, again, slow the rate of further decline.

Summary and Conclusions

In this chapter, we have reviewed some of the seminal approaches to the study of cognitive aging as experienced by well-functioning older adults and provided a framework for an integrated approach to examining age-related cognitive changes observed over decades of research. We have noted some of the caveats associated with this body of work in terms of the evolution of concepts and methods that may influence how typical these observed changes may be. We have introduced the concept of cognitive impairment in the context of underlying age-associated pathological processes that may present with differing cognitive profiles. And yet, we have noted that, on an individual basis, the identification and prediction of those who will invariably be diagnosed with a disorder of cognition is far from simple. We have alluded to factors that may influence the manifestation of cognitive changes, whether or not an assumption of underlying pathology is made. These will be addressed in detail in the following two chapters.

CHAPTER 2

Factors Protective against Cognitive Decline

Through the study of cognitive aging and neurocognitive disorders, a number of factors or situations have been identified that appear to positively influence or preserve cognitive functions. Initially, associations were observed between level of cognitive functioning and lifestyle activities suggestive of a protective effect on cognition. More recently, the positive influence of these factors has been attributed to their impact on the brain either directly, through altered brain structure or functions, or indirectly by increasing capacity for engaging in compensatory processes (Reuter-Lorenz & Park, 2014). Moreover, it has become increasingly clear that many of these factors are modifiable through intervention. Some interventions will be addressed later in this book. In this chapter, we will examine some of the factors that have been associated with better cognitive functioning or less cognitive decline: educational attainment, multilingualism, social interaction, complex cognitive activities, physical activity, and nutrition. Where possible, we will comment on these associations in relation to cognitive aging in the context of healthy aging and within the context of NCDs. For the purpose of these discussions, the concept of cognitive decline refers to the rate, or speed, of change in cognitive functions that takes place over time. We will discuss these proposed lifestyle protective factors with the understanding that behaviors people engage in are likely to have biological consequences and vice versa. We will highlight these proposed biological mechanisms prior to summarizing the chapter.

Education

Associations between educational attainment and cognitive functions have been documented within samples of nondemented older adults as well as those with dementia. Specifically, within nondemented samples, well-educated older adults appear to live longer and demonstrate less cognitive decline as they age. In addition, people with higher educational attainment are less likely to develop dementia, particularly AD and VaD (Meng & D'Arcy, 2012). There are substantial bodies of research examining each of these observed associations, and we will address them here briefly.

Cognitive Aging

The association between higher educational attainment and reduced cognitive decline has been noted in several studies using a variety of measures of cognitive function, including measures that provide an omnibus or global score to reflect cognitive status (e.g., the Mini-Mental State Examination [MMSE]; Farmer, Kittner, Rae, Bartko, & Regier, 1995) or measures of more specific domains such as verbal recall, recognition memory (Colsher & Wallace, 1991), or nonverbal memory (Le Carret, Lafont, Mayo, & Fabrigoule, 2003). Typically, these studies follow participants over a number of years and categorize their educational attainment (e.g., less than 12 years of education versus 12 or more years or education—White et al., 1994; less than 6 years of education vs. those with 6 or more years of education—Le Carret et al., 2003). Some studies have also examined highly educated samples (e.g., those with graduate degrees) demonstrating that those with the highest educational attainment experienced slower rates of cognitive decline (Lee, Buring, Cook, & Grodstein, 2006).

Yet, not all studies find an association between educational attainment and cognitive decline. It has been proposed that most of the literature demonstrating this association has been conducted using two points in time (i.e., baseline and second point in time). When research has been conducted using multiple time points, this association has not been observed as frequently as when two time points were used (Wilson et al., 2009). That is not to say that there is no association between educational attainment and level of cognitive functioning, as this robust relationship has been repeatedly demonstrated in cross-sectional studies. Instead, the multipoint longitudinal data suggest that education has little or no association with rate of change in cognition (i.e., steepness of cognitive decline; e.g., Christensen et al., 2001). It must be noted that the measures of cognitive functions used in different studies may influence these findings and that educational attainment may be more related to decline on some measures or domains of cognition than others. Similarly, the ways in which educational attainment are measured (e.g., years of schooling) assumes equivalence of educational quality across people which is unlikely to be true. Incorporating some measure of educational quality might provide additional insights into whether and how education may positively influence cognitive decline (e.g., Manly, Byrd, Touradji, Sanchez, & Stern, 2004).

Cognitive Impairment

An association between education and MCI has also been noted by Sattler, Toro, Schönknecht, and Schröder (2012), with control participants in their prospective study on adult development and aging showing higher educational attainment than patients with either MCI or AD. However, in a systematic review of predictors of dementia in MCI, educational attainment did not seem to predict those who will decline to dementia in most studies that examined this relationship (Cooper, Sommerlad, Lyketsos, & Livingston, 2015).

Support for the observation that people with higher educational attainment are less likely to develop dementia has come from many epidemiological studies conducted worldwide (e.g., Meng & D'Arcy, 2012; Sharp & Gatz, 2011). As in the cognitive aging literature, these studies have typically categorized educational attainment and demonstrated an association between level of education and a diagnosis of dementia in very large, population-based samples. Those with higher educational attainment were found to receive a diagnosis of dementia less frequently. Those with a lower education level were found to be at higher risk for being diagnosed with dementia, and the magnitude of this increased risk varied depending on the study (e.g., Sharp & Gatz, 2011). For example, a fourfold increase in risk of a diagnosis of AD was observed for individuals with less than 7 years of education in the Canadian Study of Health and Aging (Canadian Study of Health and Aging Working Group, 1994). To obtain this estimate, 258 clinically confirmed cases of AD were contrasted with 535 cases that were clinically determined to be cognitively intact and matched with the AD cases on age, geographic region of residence, and institutionalization.

As with the cognitive aging literature, not all studies have shown an association between educational attainment and diagnosis of dementia (Fratiglioni, 1993; Sharp & Gatz, 2011). Sharp and Gatz (2011) note that support for an education–dementia relationship was found more consistently in studies conducted in developed regions of the world than in those conducted in developing regions. Overall, they conclude that the education–dementia relationship is most consistent where "educational attainment is reflective of intellectual ability rather than privilege" (p. 300).

The association between educational attainment and the trajectory of cognitive decline within those diagnosed with dementia has also been investigated. Perhaps surprisingly, many studies have observed an accelerated rate of cognitive decline to be associated with higher educational attainment (Andel, Vigen, Mack, Clark, & Gatz, 2006; Meng & D'Arcy, 2012; Stern, Albert, Tang, & Tsai, 1999; Teri, McCurry, Edland, Kukull, & Larson, 1995; Wilson et al., 2004). It was this accelerated decline post-diagnosis of AD, taken in conjunction with the observed "protective" effect of educational attainment for initial diagnosis of dementia, that prompted the propositions that individuals with higher cognitive reserve (with educational attainment being a proxy for or source of) can tolerate greater brain pathology and that cognitive deficits will be detected later in these individuals than in those with lower cognitive reserve. That is, those with higher cognitive reserve will manifest severe brain pathology at diagnosis and behavioral functioning cannot be maintained. Hence, decline postdiagnosis will be rapid (Stern, 2002). Subsequent research employing neuroimaging techniques generally support this position (Stern, 2012), though much concerning the underlying neural mechanisms has yet to be determined.

Multilingualism

As with the research on educational attainment, associations have been documented between language practices (monolingual, bilingual, or multilingual) and cognitive functions within samples of nondemented older adults as well as those with cognitive impairment, including dementia. Specifically, it has been shown in nondemented samples that older adults who speak more than one language outperform their monolingual counterparts on cognitive tasks. In addition, in relation to monolingual people, those who speak two or more languages have been shown to be less likely to develop cognitive impairment without dementia (Bialystok, Craik, Binns, Ossher, & Freedman, 2014; Ossher, Bialystok, Craik, Murphy, & Troyer, 2013; Perquin et al., 2013; Zahodne, Schofield, Farrell, Stern, & Manly, 2014) or dementia (Alladi et al., 2013; Bialystok, Craik, & Freedman, 2007; Freedman et al., 2014; Liu, Yip, Fan, & Meguro, 2012), particularly AD. There are growing bodies of research examining each of these observed associations that we will address here briefly. It must be stated that not all studies find these associations (e.g., Clare et al., 2014); clearly, this area is still under intense scrutiny.

Cognitive Aging

The association between multilingualism and cognitive function has been observed in only a few studies to date. In a cross-sectional, representative sample of Israeli older adults, Kave, Eyal, Shorek, and Cohen-Mansfield

(2008) noted that performance on two cognitive screening instruments differed depending on whether two, three, or more than three languages were spoken. These effects were observed even when age, education, gender, place of birth, and age at immigration were taken into consideration. Moreover, these results held true for a subsample of older adults who had acquired no formal education at all. Subsequently, the effect of multilingualism on later-life cognitive performance was examined in the Lothian birth cohort (Deary et al., 2007) where it was possible to control for initial differences in childhood intelligence (Bak, Nissan, Allerhand, & Deary, 2014). An effect of bilingualism, independent of childhood intelligence, gender, socioeconomic status, and immigration, was most notable for measures of reading, verbal fluency, and general intelligence. As shown in the study by Kave et al. (2008), knowing three or more languages produced stronger effects than knowing two. Those with higher childhood IQ seemed to benefit more from early acquisition of a second language, whereas those with lower childhood IQ benefited more from later acquisition. Few differences were observed between bilingual people who actively used both languages and those who rarely used their second language, possibly because of the low frequency of second language use overall. The authors speculated that acquisition of a second language may leave lasting cognitive traces independent of subsequent use.

Cognitive Impairment

Support for the observation that people who speak more languages are less likely to develop cognitive impairment, without dementia, has come from studies conducted in countries where multiple languages are commonly used. In a Canadian study, Ossher and colleagues (2013) examined the effect of bilingualism on age of diagnosis for people categorized with single (n = 29 monolingual, 19 bilingual) or multiple domain (n = 22 monolingual, 21 bilingual) amnestic MCI using the following criteria: new memory complaint, objective memory impairment for age, normal general cognitive function, normal daily activities, and absence of dementia or other significant medical or psychiatric condition that could account for memory impairment (Petersen, 2004). They also questioned them about their language practices. An interaction effect was observed where later age at diagnosis for bilinguals was only evident for those categorized with single-domain amnestic mild cognitive impairment.

In another study by this Canadian research team, Bialystok et al. (2014) reported that bilingual people (n = 36) with a diagnosis of MCI according to the Albert et al. (2011) criteria were older than comparable monolinguals (n = 38) both at age of onset and date of first clinic visit. This finding could not be attributed to other lifestyle variables such as diet, social activities, or physical activity, smoking, or alcohol consumption. The bilingual participants in their study had been speaking two or more languages fluently since early adulthood at least weekly. All participants were proficient in English but spoke a variety of other languages (and so did not represent any specific sociocultural group). On measures of cognitive functioning, the monolingual and bilingual samples did not differ, despite differing by age, indicating that bilinguals were not waiting longer to seek diagnosis. These researchers did not note any differences in rate of cognitive decline between monolinguals and bilinguals on three occasions over a period of approximately 1 year.

Luxembourg has three official languages, and its people frequently switch from one language to another. As part of the MemoVie prospective cohort study on cognitive aging and dementia in Luxembourg (Perquin et al., 2012), a retrospective, nested, case–control design was used to examine the relations between cognitive impairment and multilingualism. Nondemented volunteers aged 65 years and older were classified as exhibiting cognitive impairment (n = 44) or as being cognitively intact (n = 188) and were questioned about their language practices. After adjusting for education and age, a lower risk for cognitive impairment was observed for those who practiced more than two languages. Speaking three or more languages was associated with a sevenfold increase in this protective effect. In this study, the effects of concomitant practice of several languages on cognition were examined, but greater concomitant practice did not show greater protection in relation to number of languages spoken over the lifespan. Acquisition of more than two languages earlier in life resulted in a more pronounced protective effect on cognition later in life.

In 2007, Bialystok et al. reported that Canadian bilingual dementia patients (n = 93) showed a delay in the age at onset of 4 years 1 month, in relation to monolinguals (n = 91) after controlling for gender, educational attainment, and employment status. Comparable levels of cognitive impairment were evident at initial visit. The bilingual participants in this study had been speaking two or more languages regularly and proficiently most of their adult lives. The vast majority of these patients were diagnosed with AD (132/184).

This same Canadian group of researchers later published similar results indicating that bilingual patients with probable AD reported the onset of symptoms 5 years, 1 month, later and were diagnosed 4 years, 3 months, later than monolinguals (Craik, Bialystok, & Freedman, 2010). This was further replicated by this group in 2014 (Bialystok et al., 2014). In both of these latter studies, the language groups were equivalent on measures of cognitive functions (e.g., measures of executive functions) and the observed delays were not due to other possible confounds such as differences in educational attainment, immigration status, occupational level, or gender. Another Canadian group of researchers first examined age of onset and age at diagnosis of AD for monolingual versus multilingual patients attending a memory clinic in Montreal, and then examined those who were nonimmigrant English–French bilinguals (Chertkow et al., 2010). A small but significant protective effect was seen for those who spoke more than two languages. However, the nonimmigrant bilingual group showed no benefit in relation to age of onset or age of diagnosis. When an immigrant bilingual subgroup was examined, they showed a delay in diagnosis of AD of 5 years.

In a large study (n = 648) of case records of people with dementia in India, Alladi et al. (2013) observed that bilingual patients developed dementia 4 years, 5 months, later than monolingual patients, independent of education, occupation, gender, and urban versus rural residence. This effect was observed for various forms of dementia including AD, frontotemporal lobar disease, and VaD and was also observed for illiterate patients. No additional benefit was observed for speaking more than two languages.

Few longitudinal investigations have been conducted to date to determine whether the rate of decline of bilinguals will differ from that of monolinguals. Bialystok et al. (2014) did not note any differences in rate of cognitive decline on measures of executive functions between Canadian monolinguals and bilinguals with AD over three occasions during a period of approximately 1 year.

Cognitive Leisure Activities

Over the past decade, there has been growing evidence that participation in a range of activities that involve cognitive stimulation can reduce the risk of cognitive impairment, including dementia. For example, it has been suggested that complex leisure and work environments facilitate the maintenance of cognition into older age (Andel, Kåreholt, Parker, Thorslund, & Gatz, 2007; Schooler, Mulatu, & Oates, 2004). Some studies have noted that higher work demands are associated with lower risk for cognitive impairment (e.g., Bosma et al., 2003). Similarly, some studies have reported that complexity of primary lifetime occupation appears to reduce the risk or delay the onset of AD (Andel et al., 2005; Stern et al., 1995), after which accelerated cognitive decline may be seen (Andel, Vigen, Mack, Clark, & Gatz, 2006) in keeping with Stern's (2002) cognitive reserve hypothesis. In addition, it has been shown that more frequent cognitive leisure activity is associated with reduced cognitive decline in nondemented older adults (e.g., Bosma et al., 2002; Hultsch, Hertzog, Small, & Dixon, 1999). In addition, people who engage in more cognitive leisure activity are less likely to develop MCI or dementia, particularly AD (e.g., Leung & Lam, 2007; Sattler et al., 2012). There is a substantial body of research examining these observed associations that we will address here briefly.

Cognitive Aging

As early as 1999, Hultsch and colleagues described a relationship between changes in intellectually related activities (e.g., hobbies) and changes in cognitive functioning in a sample of 250 middle-aged and older adults who were assessed three times over 6 years. Similarly, Bosma and colleagues (2002) followed 830 middle-aged to older adults over 3 years and noted that those participating in more mental activities were less likely to show cognitive decline. Moreover, those with the best baseline performance on cognitive measures were more likely to increase the number of activities they engaged in over this same time period. Other studies have taken sensory functions into account when examining the relations among general lifestyle activities and cognitive functioning in specific domains (e.g., processing speed, verbal fluency) and have shown that lifestyle activities are related to specific cognitive domains (Ghisletta, Bickel, & Lovden, 2006; Newson & Kemps, 2005). More recently, Wilson and colleagues (2013) reported an association between more frequent cognitive activity (e.g., reading books, visiting the library, writing letters) across the lifespan and slower later-life cognitive decline. This association continued to be evident independent of common neuropathic conditions experienced by healthy older adults.

Cognitive Impairment

An association between cognitive leisure activity and MCI has also been observed, with people who were highly cognitively active showing a reduced risk of being identified with MCI (Sattler et al., 2012; Schroder et al., 1998; Verghese et al., 2006; Wang et al., 2006). In a prospective cohort of 437 people older than age 75 years living in the community, Verghese et al. (2006) observed that a lower risk of development of amnestic MCI was associated with high and moderate levels of cognitive activity participation. The types of cognitive leisure activities reported by participants in this study included reading, writing, crossword puzzles, board or card games, group discussion, or playing music. The observed association remained robust even after controlling for age, sex, education, chronic illness, depression, and baseline cognitive status.

In a large prospective study of older adults in communities within Chongqing, China, an association between the development of cognitive impairment in people aged 55 years and older and 13 cognitive leisure activities was investigated over a 5-year time period (Wang et al., 2006). Reading and playing board games such as mah-jong or chess or card games such as poker were associated with a reduced risk of being identified with cognitive impairment. Moreover, watching television was associated with an increased risk of cognitive impairment.

In another investigation, Sattler et al. (2012) examined 321 people at baseline and 12 years later when the participants were in their early 70s. The types of cognitive leisure activities examined in this study included reading books, reading magazines/newspapers, solving crossword puzzles, participating in courses, and participating in professional training. The association between high levels of cognitive leisure activities and reduced risk of MCI, as defined by the aging-associated cognitive decline criteria (Schroder et al., 1998), was observed and remained robust even after controlling for educational attainment and socioeconomic status (SES).

An association between engagement in cognitive leisure activity and a decreased risk for developing dementia has been observed repeatedly in large-scale epidemiological studies and cohort and case–control studies (Karp et al., 2006; Leung & Lam, 2007; Scarmeas, Levy, Tang, Manly, & Stern, 2001; Stern & Munn, 2010; Verghese et al., 2003; Wang, Karp, Winblad, & Fratiglioni, 2002; Wilson et al., 2002). Cognitive leisure activities have been defined in a number of ways, and most report that only high levels of engagement in cognitive leisure activities were found to be associated with a reduced risk for dementia. Some have reported that the greatest benefit is observed for participants who, in addition to engaging in high levels of cognitive leisure activities, also engage in high levels of physical and social activities (Karp et al., 2006). Stern and Munn (2010) noted that when cognitive leisure activities were engaged in during middle or late adulthood, a reduced risk for AD and other dementias was observed. In addition, they noted that some activities (e.g., reading) may be more protective than others.

Social Interaction

As is evident in the preceding section, many cognitive leisure activities may include a social component (i.e., involve interactions with others), and there is substantial research to support a positive impact of social engagement/participation on a number of health-related phenomena, including healthy cognitive aging. In addition, it has been observed that people who engage more socially are less likely to develop cognitive impairment or dementia (e.g., Amieva et al., 2010; Leung & Lam, 2007; Sattler et al., 2012). Here, we will briefly address some of the research examining the association between social environmental factors and cognitive health.

Cognitive Aging

Social networks, social engagement, social support, social contact, and social activities are all terms used in the study of social environment (Pillai & Verghese, 2009). Marital status, number and frequency of social contacts, satisfaction with relationships, and perceptions of quality of support are all ways of characterizing a person's social environment. An association between high frequency of emotional support and better cognitive function has been observed in healthy older adults (Seeman, Lusignolo, Albert, & Berkman, 2001). In addition, a positive association between social ties and maintenance of cognitive function was observed in a longitudinal study of older adults in Spain (Zunzunegui, Alvarado, Del Ser, & Otero, 2003). When examining the conjoint trajectories of cognitive function, social ties, and social engagement in this longitudinal study, it was observed that higher levels of family ties and engagement were associated with better cognitive functions until about 80 years of age (Beland, Zunzunegui, Alvarado, Otero, & Del Ser, 2005). Better cognitive functioning was also noted in women with friends than in those without friends.

Cognitive Impairment

A number of studies have examined the relations between social environmental factors and cognitive impairment, including dementia (Pillai & Verghese, 2009). For example, in a large prospective cohort of older women, larger social networks were associated with lower risk of incident dementia over a 4-year period (Crooks, Lubben, Petitti, Little, & Chiu, 2008). In another large prospective epidemiological study, it was shown that older adults who felt very satisfied with their social network had a reduced risk of developing dementia 5–15 years later (Amieva et al., 2010).

Physical Activity

Over the past two decades, it has become increasingly clear that engaging in physical activity and/or exercise has many health-related benefits. Physical activity is one area where the research has moved from the observation of associations to interventions where the impact of increased physical activity on cognitive and brain functions has been studied. Here we will briefly summarize this large body of literature and comment on some of the observed associations to date.

Cognitive Aging

Associations between physical activity and cognitive functioning have been observed through cross-sectional and longitudinal studies of healthy older adults (Denkinger, Nikolaus, Denkinger, & Lukas, 2012; Leung & Lam, 2007). Long-term high levels of physical activity (i.e., 10–15 years) have been shown to reduce the risk of cognitive decline by 20% (Weuve et al., 2004). In a prospective sample of rural-dwelling older adults, more self-reported exercise was protective against cognitive decline over 2 years. Over a 10-year period, associations between exercise duration and intensity were shown to have independent effects on amount of cognitive decline observed in healthy older men (van Gelder et al., 2004). Moreover, it has been shown that early life (ages 15–25) physical activity rates are associated with better cognitive function in older men (though not women) (Dik, Deeg, Visser, & Jonker, 2003).

Cognitive Impairment

Physical activity also has been shown repeatedly to reduce the risk of cognitive impairment or dementia (Denkinger et al., 2012; Leung & Lam, 2007). Data from the Canadian Longitudinal Study on Aging, a large epidemiological study of dementia prevalence, linked both self-reported exercise (Lindsay et al., 2002) and physical activity (Laurin, Verreault, Lindsay, MacPherson, & Rockwood, 2001) to a reduced risk for cognitive impairment without dementia and dementia. Other support for the apparent protective effect of physical activity for cognitive impairment, including dementia, comes from the Honolulu Asia Aging Study (Abbott et al., 2004), the Mayo Clinic Study of Aging (Geda et al., 2010), and many other prospective epidemiological studies included in a meta-analysis by Hamer and Chida (2009). From their meta-analysis, Hamer and Chida (2009) report that high levels of physical activity reduce the risk of AD by 45% and, more generally, dementia by 28%. No associated reduction in the risk of Parkinson's disease (PD) was observed. In addition to the associations between physical activity and dementia seen in later life, self-reported physical activity levels in teenage, early, and midlife have also been shown to be inversely related to dementia in later life (Fritsch et al., 2005; Middleton, Barnes, Lui, & Yaffe, 2010; Rovio et al., 2005).

Nutrition

For decades, the association of dietary supplements with cognitive aging has been studied, with a more recent shift to examining the synergistic effects of foods and nutrients consumed together in healthy dietary patterns. Like research on physical activity and cognitive functions, research on nutritional supplements and dietary patterns has moved from observation of associations with cognitive functions to intervention studies. Here we will briefly summarize and comment on some of the observed associations to date.

Cognitive Aging and Impairment

Many studies have examined the associations of cognitive functions with individual nutrients such as folate (Araujo, Martel, Borges, Araujo,

& Keating, 2015), omega-3 fatty acids (Jiao et al., 2014; Kroger et al., 2009), and various antioxidants such as vitamin C, vitamin E, betacarotene, lutein, flavoids, and lignans (Nooyens et al., 2015). Similarly, associations among blood glucose levels, diet-based glycemic load, and cognitive performance have been observed (Seetharaman et al., 2015). While some support for associations between higher levels of these nutrients and better cognitive function or reduced risk for cognitive impairment or dementia (Roberts et al., 2010; Shea & Remington, 2015) has been shown, greater support is emerging for combined effects such as healthy dietary patterns (Shea & Remington, 2015; van de Rest, Berendsen, Haveman-Nies, & de Groot, 2015). Specifically, the dietary pattern known as the Mediterranean diet (MeDi) has been under scrutiny because of its many health benefits (Sofi, Abbate, Gensini, & Casini, 2010). This dietary pattern is typical of populations living in the Mediterranean basin and has remained relatively constant over time. It consists of high intake of olive oil as the main source of fat, high consumption of plant foods such as fresh or dried fruits and vegetables, legumes, and cereals, moderate intake of fish, low-to moderate intake of dairy products, and low intake of meat and poultry. The use of many condiments and spices and regular but low-to-moderate intake of wine during meals is also typical of this dietary pattern. Many of the nutrients that have been studied individually are present in this diet.

Evidence derived from epidemiological studies indicates that greater adherence to the MeDi is associated with less cognitive decline and/or a reduced risk of dementia, including AD (Feart, Samieri, & Barberger-Gateau, 2015; Hardman, Kennedy, Macpherson, Scholey, & Pipingas, 2016; Lourida et al., 2013; Shea & Remington, 2015; van de Rest et al., 2015). However, it also appears that the benefits may not be as apparent in some populations as in others (Feart et al., 2015). It may be that long-term adherence to such a dietary pattern may be necessary for protective effects to be seen or that adherence to MeDi is part of a healthier lifestyle, in general, and may be associated with higher education or socioeconomic status (Feart et al., 2015).

Other dietary patterns, such as the Dietary Approach to Stop Hypertension (DASH), have been shown to have many health benefits (Tangney, 2014). Like the MeDi, DASH consists of high consumption of fruits, vegetables, nuts/seeds/legumes, low or nonfat dairy, in addition to intake of lean meats/fish/poultry, low consumption of sweets, saturated fats, and sodium. The main difference between DASH and MeDi is the almost exclusive use of olive oil and regular use of wine with meals in the MeDi (Tangney, 2014). In addition, the DASH focus on low- or nonfat dairy stems from differences in the types of dairy practices undertaken in different parts of the world (Hoffman & Gerber, 2013). In large-scale observational studies, an association between adherence to DASH and reduced rates of change in cognition has been observed (Norton et al., 2012; Tangney, 2014; Wengreen et al., 2013).

Evaluation of the Available Literature

While there is growing evidence in support of the protective effects for each of these activities, some concerns have been raised about the way these factors have been studied. Most of these studies are observational in nature and are subject to biases such as selection bias and survival bias (Stern & Munn, 2010). In each area, measurement issues have been identified as a cause for concern. For example, most of this research relies on self-report of engagement in the activities and may not be accurate, particularly when people are being asked to recall activities from the distant past (Miller, Taler, Davidson, & Messier, 2012). Moreover, the number and types of activities included in the evaluation of factors such as physical or leisure activities are restricted and may underestimate level of engagement for some (Leung & Lam, 2007; Miller et al., 2012). Another measurement issue is that factors controlled for in the analyses differ between the studies, and some potentially important factors, such as sensory functioning, are rarely considered. The manner in which the factors in question have been operationalized has also been identified as a cause for concern. As a case in point, studies differ in how they define education, and level or years of educational attainment may mean different things in different cultures or cohorts (Sharp & Gatz, 2011). Nutrition studies differ in terms of how adherence to the dietary pattern in question has been quantified, the duration of adherence to the dietary patterns, and at what point in the lifespan these associations are measured. Similarly, measurement of complexity of work, leisure activity, or social engagement is difficult to quantify, and most of these activities involve multiple factors (i.e., cognitive, social, and physical). While some investigators have tried to parse these elements apart (e.g., Karp et al., 2006; McDowell, Xi, Lindsay, & Tierney, 2007; Reed et al., 2011), they may, in fact, be inextricably interwoven and highly interdependent.

The common element among these activities seems to be engagement in complex ongoing, learning resulting in an enriched intellectual and/or social environment. Engaging in stimulating activities may also be associated with feelings of mastery and self-efficacy, which, in turn, serve to motivate continued engagement. Certainly, in childhood, educational attainment is known to be influenced by many factors such as parental SES and socioemotional influences as well as biological and health-related factors (e.g., genes, ante-, peri-, and postnatal environments) (Sharp & Gatz, 2011). In adulthood, educational attainment predicts occupation, SES, living environment, and the likelihood of engaging in stimulating leisure activities. Those with higher educational attainment, higher socioeconomic status, or greater social participation are more likely to engage in healthy behaviors such as regular exercise and nutritious diets. Perhaps there are underlying personal characteristics or traits associated with pursuit of heightened engagement in complex ongoing learning. In a systematic review examining the role of personality in relation to dementia in later life across fifteen studies, it was concluded that conscientiousness was associated with reduced risk and that neuroticism was associated with increased risk. The findings for openness were tentative (Low, Harrison, & Lackersteen, 2013). Other personality domains examined in this review, such as extraversion and introversion, did not appear to be associated with dementia in later life.

The most frequently proposed explanation for the observed association between these lifestyle factors and cognitive function in later life emerging from these studies is the cognitive reserve hypothesis (Stern, 2002, 2012). This hypothesis proposes that brain structures or networks actively compensate for neural disruptions by invoking cognitive processes or compensatory cognitive strategies that are related to overall level of cognitive functioning. Engagement in the complex ongoing learning associated with a variety of lifestyle factors or life experiences leads to greater cognitive reserve. Individuals with high cognitive reserve can employ these compensatory strategies to maintain their functioning, in spite of possible underlying disruptions in neural functioning within the brain. That is, people with high cognitive reserve can tolerate more neural damage before there is an impact on their performance on tasks or everyday activities. In this way, symptoms indicative of underlying brain pathology will emerge later in people with high cognitive reserve than in those with low cognitive reserve. While the nature of the neural mechanisms that underlie this cognitive reserve is, as yet, unknown (Stern, 2012), this is the focus of much present neurocognitive research (Gold, Johnson, & Powell, 2013; Gold, Kim, Johnson, Kryscio, & Smith, 2013; Schweizer, Ware, Fischer, Craik, & Bialystok, 2012).

Numerous biological mechanisms may be associated with the protective effects observed through some of these lifestyle factors that affect overall general and cognitive health. These mechanisms include vascular, antioxidant, and anti-inflammatory pathways known to be associated with neural damage (Frisardi et al., 2010). For example, physical activity improves cerebral blood flow and oxygen delivery, while decreasing the accumulation of free radical oxidative proteins (Hamer & Chida, 2009; Leung & Lam, 2007). Similarly, foods central to MeDi and DASH are rich in antioxidants and anti-inflammatory agents and are associated with reduced cholesterol and low-density lipoproteins (Feart et al., 2015).

The factors protective for cognitive decline typically have been identified through cross-sectional, correlational studies. Findings from studies of the impact of education, multilingualism, cognitive leisure activities, social interaction, physical activity, and nutrition on cognitive functioning suggest that these interrelationships are complex and that cognitive functioning in later life can be influenced by experiences that occur throughout the life course. Trajectories of cognitive decline, then, are influenced by the intrinsic biological make-up of the individual and by interactions with environmental exposures across the life course. These interactions may be synergistic or antagonistic. The resulting trajectories of cognitive decline in later life are likely to vary widely by individual and may be at least partially dependent on the person's cognitive developmental trajectory prior to the onset of decline.

With the recognition that active engagement in lifestyle behaviors may protect against cognitive decline, longitudinal intervention studies are currently underway. These studies will examine the extent to which modifiable factors such as physical activity and nutritional intake can alter cognitive aging. Many of these studies (e.g., Morris et al., 2015) are directed toward healthy older adults and are of relatively short duration. This research will yield important information concerning the feasibility of modifying cognition in later life. In addition, it will be important to determine the impact of interventions differing in type, duration, and intensity on various aspects of cognitive functioning. Randomized designs or case–control studies will provide additional information on the causal connections among protective factors and cognitive functioning.

The selection of reliable methods to assess cognitive change over relatively short intervals will be important in this context. Reliance on self-report of engagement in cognitively stimulating activities or brief screening measures of cognition may not yield sufficient information about the possible beneficial impact that interventions may have on cognitive functions. Advances in technology may make the collection of reliable comprehensive cognitive data more feasible than it has been in the past.

It may be of equal, if not more, importance to determine the cognitive consequences of long-term behaviors or interventions undertaken during early and middle adulthood, or even childhood. The observation that modifiable factors such as education attainment and multilingual proficiency appear to be protective against cognitive decline in later life may prompt social policy changes to promote these or other beneficial activities. However, as yet the associations remain as observations and remain to be fully understood.

Implications for Clinical Practice

Perhaps one of the most important messages for clinical practice emerging from this brief review of factors protective of cognitive health is to consider the role that cognitive reserve may play in the clinical case picture. Inquiring about indicators of cognitive reserve (e.g., educational or occupational attainment) that may influence the interpretation of cognitive test performance is essential. One must be mindful that the detection of cognitive decline in people with high cognitive reserve may be challenging (Stern,

2012). In addition, cognitive reserve may affect the rate of cognitive decline after diagnosis and how effective interventions may be. Another important message is that lifestyle factors can affect cognitive health, and although we cannot be prescriptive about exactly what each person needs to maintain his or her cognitive health, it is relatively clear that engaging in exercise, eating a healthy diet, and keeping cognitively and socially active will be of benefit.

Summary and Conclusions

This brief overview shows that various lifestyle activities are associated with better cognitive functions in later life. From a developmental perspective, it appears that experiences engaged in throughout the life course can benefit cognitive functions in later life. Even in later life, benefits from engaging in physical and cognitively stimulating leisure activities have been observed. This suggests that the influence of these, and possibly other, lifestyle factors is not static but may change across a person's life depending on exposures and pursuits.

Despite the challenges associated with studying the protective effects of long-term lifestyle behaviors on cognitive functions in later life, there is growing support for this position from multiple sectors and across disciplines. What remains to be fully understood are how strongly these factors can modify cognitive aging and how the timing of exposure to these factors (i.e., when in the life course) affects their impact on cognitive functions in later life. For example, associations between the behaviors engaged in during early and middle adulthood and cognitive status in late adulthood have been observed but are not yet fully understood (Borghesani et al., 2012; Ihle et al., 2015). Over the past decade, there has been a move from observation of associations toward intervention research where the types, duration, and intensity of exposures can be more clearly defined. It is hoped that under these more controlled conditions, the difficulties in studying the interrelationships of these lifestyle factors and cognitive health will be overcome.

CHAPTER 3

Factors Predictive
of Cognitive Decline

A number of factors, identified through study of cognitive aging and neurocognitive disorders, negatively influence or deplete cognitive resources and present as risk factors for accelerated cognitive decline or the development of cognitive impairment, including dementia. As noted in Chapter 2, the identification of risk factors has emerged from observational studies where healthy older adults or those with some evidence of cognitive impairment are followed over time. Underlying biological mechanisms have been proposed that impact brain function either directly, through altered brain structure or functions, or indirectly, through decreasing capacity for engaging in compensatory processes. As was shown in the previous chapter, at least some of these risk factors are modifiable and at least some of the identified risk factors are also protective factors. Here we will examine some of the most notable factors that have been associated with cognitive decline or the development of cognitive impairment, including dementia.

Cognitive functioning may be negatively influenced by many medical conditions and treatments for underlying medical concerns (Armstrong & Morrow, 2010; Tarter, Butters, & Beers, 2001). For example, cognitive impairment may occur in conjunction with cancer treatments such as radiation therapy, chemotherapy, or hormone therapy (Janelsins, Kesler, Ahles, & Morrow, 2014). It may also occur in conjunction with other neurological conditions such as multiple sclerosis (Amato, Zipoli, & Portaccio, 2006) or neuropsychiatric conditions such as schizophrenia (Irani, Kalkstein, Moberg, & Moberg, 2011; Rajji, Miranda, & Mulsant, 2014; Rajji & Mulsant, 2008; Rajji et al., 2013; Shah, Qureshi, Jawaid, & Schulz, 2012). These types of disorders are typically excluded in dementia research.

It is possible that the cognitive impairment associated with at least some of these medical disorders will predispose individuals to later cognitive decline or to the development of a neurodegenerative condition such as AD. This distinction between cognitive impairment associated with a specific medical condition and cognitive impairment in the context of underlying neurodegenerative pathology, such as that seen in AD, is important when we consider risk factors for cognitive decline. While many studies focus on one form of dementia as the outcome of interest (e.g., AD), others consider all causes of dementia that may be reflective of differing underlying pathological processes.

At the outset of this chapter, we will briefly comment on a few notable situations in relation to the protective factors discussed in Chapter 2 where the negative side of the factor has been clearly characterized as posing an increased risk for cognitive decline: low educational attainment and social isolation. In the remainder of this chapter, we will focus primarily on biomedical factors associated with the development of degenerative neurocognitive disorders. For the purpose of these discussions, the concept of cognitive decline refers to changes in cognitive functions that take place over time, and cognitive impairment refers to any neurocognitive disorder including degenerative dementias.

Education

While high levels of educational attainment have been shown to have a protective effect with respect to cognitive decline and the development of cognitive impairment, some researchers have stressed the importance of low levels of educational attainment as a risk factor for cognitive decline and impairment. This finding, across studies, has been demonstrated in a meta-analysis conducted by Caamano-Isorna, Corral, Montes-Martinez, and Takkouche (2006), who noted that education as a risk factor for AD met the Bradford-Hill criteria for causality. According to these criteria, the risk of an AD diagnosis is higher in individuals with low education relative to those with higher education, and risk increases when educational attainment decreases. This observation has been documented longitudinally, using different methods and studying many different international populations.

Social Isolation

In contrast to the studies showing that people who engage more socially are less likely to have cognitive impairment or dementia, others have stressed the importance of the association between lack of social ties or social isolation and risk of accelerated cognitive decline or cognitive impairment (Bassuk, Glass, & Berkman, 1999; Berkman, Glass, Brissette, & Seeman, 2000; Fratiglioni, Wang, Ericsson, Maytan, & Winblad, 2000; Kuiper et al., 2015; Saczynski et al., 2006). For example, in the large Kungsholmen Project, a community-based cohort followed over 3 years, Fratiglioni et al. (2000) observed that individuals living alone and those who had no friends or family were at increased risk for developing dementia. When three different social network variables (i.e., being married and living with someone; having children with daily to weekly satisfying contacts; having relatives/friends with daily to weekly satisfying contact) were combined, a limited social network increased the risk of being diagnosed with dementia by 60%. In a recent meta-analysis, people with less frequent social contact, those who participated less in social activities, and those who reported feelings of loneliness were more likely to develop dementia (Kuiper et al., 2015). In addition, the results of this review conclude that low levels of social interaction are most closely associated with developing dementia rather than size or satisfaction with social networks. Interestingly, the relationship between social isolation and dementia risk may be bidirectional. For example, it has been hypothesized that, given the long course of cognitive decline that is apparent prior to a diagnosis of dementia, social withdrawal could be a behavioral consequence of the underlying disease process (Amieva et al., 2010). In fact, a decrease in social engagement from midlife to late life has been associated with dementia risk (Saczynski et al., 2006).

Health and Medical Factors

A number of medical conditions have been shown to be associated with an increased risk for cognitive decline or development of cognitive impairment. Many of these conditions are also risk factors for cerebrovascular diseases that may be associated with VaD and AD (Collins & Kenny, 2007).

Smoking

Findings from early case-controlled and prospective cohort studies of the relationship between smoking and risk for dementia have been contradictory (Almeida, Hulse, Lawrence, & Flicker, 2002). It has been proposed that these conflicting findings may be the result of competing mortality: smokers may be at greater risk for developing dementia but die before they do (Cooper et al., 2015). However, most recent studies have found that current smokers are at an increased risk for developing dementia (Deckers et al., 2015), and a meta-analysis of prospective studies found that current smoking was associated with a 59% increased risk for developing AD (Peters et al., 2008). Moreover, it has been suggested that medicinal nicotine use may be harmful for older adults at risk for neurological disorders (Swan & Lessov-Schlaggar, 2007). While smoking emerged as a risk factor for people with dementia onset by age 87, this was not the case for those over 87 years of age (Ganguli et al., 2015). Similarly, current smoking did not appear to increase the risk of developing dementia in people with MCI (Cooper et al., 2015), and smoking did not appear to be associated with cognitive decline in people diagnosed with dementia (Blom, Emmelot-Vonk, & Koek, 2013). Little evidence is available to support an association between past smoking and risk for cognitive decline or dementia. It has been proposed that current smoking may have effects through vascular or inflammatory processes or increased oxidative stress, all of which may negatively affect cognitive functioning (Swan & Lessov-Schlaggar, 2007).

Diabetes

Support for a link between diabetes mellitus (insulin and noninsulin dependent) and subsequent development of dementia has been observed in numerous studies (Chatterjee et al., 2016; Cooper et al., 2015; Patterson, Feightner, Garcia, & MacKnight, 2007; Tschanz, Norton, Zandi, & Lyketsos, 2013). This increased risk was noted in the Canadian Study of Health and Aging, a large, national, longitudinal epidemiological study of dementia in Canada, where type 2 diabetes mellitus at baseline was associated with an increased risk of vascular cognitive impairment (VCI; without dementia) and VaD 5 years later (MacKnight, Rockwood, Awalt, & McDowell, 2002). In more recent studies, people with diabetes and MCI were at an increased risk for developing dementia (AD or any-cause dementia) over time (Li et al., 2011, 2012; Xu et al., 2010). Moreover, people with impaired glycemia (i.e., impaired fasting glucose), whether or not they were diagnosed with diabetes, were more likely to be diagnosed with dementia after 2 years than those people with MCI and normal glycemic levels (Morris, Vidoni, Honea, & Burns, 2014). It has also been shown that people treated for diabetes are less likely to develop dementia than those not treated (Li et al., 2011).

Blood Pressure

The relationship between blood pressure and change in cognitive functions has been studied for many years and appears to be quite complex. Both hyper- and hypotension have been associated with the development of cognitive impairment and dementia. Long-standing hypertension or high blood pressure measured in midlife (i.e., age 40–64 years) has been shown to be related to cognitive decline and an increased risk of dementia in later life (Collins & Kenny, 2007; Power et al., 2011; Qiu, Winblad, & Fratiglioni, 2005; Whitmer, Sidney, Selby, Johnston, & Yaffe, 2005).

However, no clear relationship has been shown between hypertension and development of dementia from MCI (Cooper et al., 2015). Management in midlife with antihypertensive medications can attenuate any increased risk for dementia in later life, and certain compounds may have neuroprotective properties beyond their influence on blood pressure (Kennelly & Collins, 2012). In later life, hypertension has been observed to be associated with increased risk for dementia in some (Deckers et al., 2015) but not in most longitudinal studies (Kennelly & Collins, 2012; Power et al., 2011). However, hypotension or low blood pressure (Collins & Kenny, 2007; Kennelly & Collins, 2012; Power et al., 2011; Qiu, von Strauss, Fastbom, Winblad, & Fratiglioni, 2003) may be a risk factor in later life for dementia and AD. It appears that blood pressure values decrease in the years preceding the onset of AD and continue to change as the disease progresses (Razay, Williams, King, Smith, & Wilcock, 2009). In addition, high and low blood pressure values appear to be related to faster cognitive decline in people with AD (Razay et al., 2009). Orthostatic hypotension, or a sudden drop in blood pressure on standing, has also been associated with cognitive decline and dementia (Kennelly & Collins, 2012), and is prevalent in people with dementia, particularly those with DLB and PD (Collins & Kenny, 2007). However, there is considerable controversy concerning these findings (Sambati, Calandra-Buonaura, Poda, Guaraldi, & Cortelli, 2014). High blood pressure starting in midlife may be related to white matter lesions and risk for stroke, and both hypertension and hypotension may be related to poor cerebral perfusion (i.e., poor blood flow with the brain) that triggers brain changes detrimental to brain health (Collins & Kenny, 2007; Kennelly & Collins, 2012).

Obesity

A number of studies have examined obesity as a risk factor for the development of dementia. While findings vary across studies, in a meta-analysis, it was concluded that midlife obesity increased the risk of dementia by 60% (Barnes & Yaffe, 2011). The effects of obesity are likely to be interrelated with other cerebrovascular risk factors such as hypertension and diabetes (Deckers et al., 2015).

Cholesterol/Hyperlipidemia

Findings from a number of studies link high cholesterol levels with an increased risk for developing all-cause dementia and AD (Deckers et al., 2015; Patterson et al., 2007; Toro et al., 2014). Meta-analyses for findings from prospective studies concluded that high midlife serum cholesterol increases the risk for dementia (Anstey, Lipnicki, & Low, 2008), with a 54% increased risk in older adults with high serum cholesterol (Anstey,

Cherbuin, & Herath, 2013). Moreover, an association has been observed between low-density lipid proteins and a faster rate of cognitive decline in people with dementia (Blom et al., 2013).

Neuropsychiatric Symptoms or Disorders

Examination of neuropsychiatric disorders as risk factors for cognitive impairment, including dementia, has focused primarily on depression as increasing the risk of developing AD. Systematic reviews and meta-analyses examining multiple studies have consistently concluded that a history of depression increases the risk for developing all-cause dementia or AD later in life (da Silva, Gonçalves-Pereira, Xavier, & Mukaetova-Ladinska, 2013; Deckers et al., 2015; Diniz, Butters, Albert, Dew, & Reynolds, 2013; Jorm, 2001; Ownby, Crocco, Acevedo, John, & Loewenstein, 2006). In addition, there is strong evidence that more depressive symptoms are predictive of developing all-cause dementia in people with any type of MCI (Cooper et al., 2015). Two hypotheses have been proposed to explain this association: either the association of depression with development of dementia is a reflection of an emotional response to the dementia diagnosis, or depression is itself a prodromal phase of dementia. Support for the first hypothesis is limited, given that depression has been observed many years prior to the onset of dementia (da Silva et al., 2013). While both disorders have been linked to common etiological factors such as inflammation and vascular changes (da Silva et al., 2013), it is still unclear whether they are manifestations of the same underlying disease process. Even in the absence of dementia, abnormalities in brain structure and function are apparent in people with a history of depression. These alterations in brain function may negatively affect the cognitive reserve of people with depression, thereby increasing susceptibility to the manifestation of dementia symptoms (da Silva et al., 2013). Similarly, disruptions in social contact or other lifestyle alterations that may occur in concert with depression may also contribute to the complex interactions between these disorders. A multiple pathways model has been proposed (Butters et al., 2008) that addresses how the brain changes seen in depression may interact with AD pathology promoting the clinical manifestation of AD.

While some other neuropsychiatric conditions have been examined as risk factors for dementia, the evidence to date is sparse. Of five studies included in the systematic review by da Silva et al. (2013), all found a higher risk of developing dementia or AD for those with bipolar disorder. There is some evidence to support the presence of neuropsychiatric symptoms in people with any type of MCI as predictive of progression to all-cause dementia (Cooper et al., 2015; Edwards, Spira, Barnes, & Yaffe, 2009). It has been reported, in a predominantly male veterans cohort, that post-traumatic stress disorder was associated with a twofold increase in the risk of developing dementia, even after those with a history of head injury, substance abuse, or clinical depression were excluded from the analyses (Yaffe et al., 2010). However, studies examining apathy and anxiety symptoms in people with MCI as predictors of incident dementia have shown inconsistent findings (Cooper et al., 2015).

Potentially Reversible Causes of Cognitive Impairment

A great variety of acute conditions can result in transient or more persistent changes in cognitive function in older adults, including but not limited to various vitamin deficiencies (e.g., B12), hormonal imbalances (e.g., reduced testosterone), and thyroid disturbances (Simmons, Hartmann, & DeJoseph, 2011). Many of these conditions are treatable and could secondarily reduce an older adult's cognitive complaints (and any associated cognitive impairment). A comprehensive reversible dementia work-up may also reveal more malignant causes for cognitive disturbance, such as HIV/ AIDS or neurosyphillis (Simmons et al., 2011). Urinary tract infections are a common cause of cognitive deterioration in older adults; however, this often gives rise to more florid cognitive and neurobehavioral symptoms (i.e., delirium), which would bring an individual to urgent medical attention rather than to a typical outpatient setting (McConnell, 2014).

Increasing age also brings an increased likelihood of chronic medical conditions, which may account at least in part for the relatively high endorsement of cognitive complaints in typical population-based samples of older adults (Cooper et al., 2011; Jonker, Geerlings, & Schmand, 2000; Slavin et al., 2010). Some conditions of which the clinician should be particularly mindful are chronic pain (Allaz & Cedraschi, 2015; Gibson, 2015; Goesling, Clauw, & Hassett, 2013), sleep and metabolic disturbances such as blood sugar dysregulation (McConnell, 2014), and unmanaged vascular risk factors such as hypertension and hypercholesteremia (Sahathevan, Brodtmann, & Donnan, 2011). Appropriate management of these conditions could all improve an older adult's perceived (and actual) current cognitive status. In addition, certain conditions such as chronic pain may involve the use of medication that, while alleviating the pain symptoms, may have iatrogenic effects on cognition.

Other Identified Medical Risk Factors

Evidence is continuing to build for a number of other potential risk factors for the development of dementia, but, as yet, the findings are mixed or contradictory. While head trauma has been found to be associated with an increased risk for developing dementia in some studies (Gardner et al., 2014; Perry et al., 2016; Plassman et al., 2000), no association has been found in other studies (Lindsay et al., 2002). Head injury studies differ with respect to how the injuries are characterized (e.g., severity, location of damage, and age of onset), and how diagnoses of dementia are made. Certainly, head injuries of significant severity are likely to be associated with some degree of cognitive impairment, whereas a dementia diagnosis typically implies a progressive course of decline. Exposure to neurotoxins can also negatively impact brain function, and some studies have noted an increased risk for developing AD after exposure to defoliants and fumigants (Hayden et al., 2010; Tyas, Manfreda, Strain, & Montgomery, 2001). While a systematic review of the effect of benzodiazepine use and the development of dementia revealed mixed results (Verdoux, Lagnaoui, & Begaud, 2005), more recent research has identified an increased risk that is stronger for long-term benzodiazepine use (Billioti de Gage et al., 2014). Levels of sex hormones (e.g., estrogen, progesterone, androgen) show complex relations with cognitive functions (Carcaillon et al., 2014; Hsu et al., 2015; Maki, 2012; Xing, Qin, Li, Jia, & Jia, 2013), and no firm conclusions have emerged to date. Renal dysfunction has emerged as a new possible risk factor (Bugnicourt, Godefroy, Chillon, Choukroun, & Massy, 2013; Murray et al., 2016; Seliger, Wendell, Waldstein, Ferrucci, & Zonderman, 2015), with the results of a meta-analysis indicating that renal dysfunction is associated with a 39% increase in the risk for cognitive impairment (Etgen, Chonchol, Forstl, & Sander, 2012). Several forms of heart disease have been related to cognitive decline and increased risk for dementia (Deckers et al., 2015), with a 36% increased risk for dementia in people with atrial fibrillation (Kalantarian, Stern, Mansour, & Ruskin, 2013). As noted previously, the effects of heart disease are likely to be interrelated with other vascular risk factors such as hypertension, obesity, and diabetes (Deckers et al., 2015; Jefferson et al., 2015).

Genetic Factors

A number of dementia-associated genes have been identified (see Table 3.1), and much research is ongoing to identify additional risk factor genes or disease-causing genes (Gatz, Jang, Karlsson, & Pedersen, 2014; Padilla & Isaacson, 2011). Most of this research has been focused on AD, but the genetic influences on other forms of dementia are also being studied. Here we will briefly mention some of this work, acknowledging that this field is relatively new and continues to grow rapidly. Recent updates can be found at *www.alzforum.org* or through the U.S. National Human Genome Research Institute.

The three genes associated with early onset familial AD (see Table 3.1) are causative and share a common pathogenic pathway that leads to the abnormal production of beta-amyloid protein. Numerous mutations have been identified in these genes and are linked to AD. In late onset AD, the

TABLE 3.1. Genes Associated with Dementia

Neurodegenerative disorder	Identified genes	% cases accounted for
AD		
Early onset (before age 65 years)	• Amyloid precursor protein (APP)[a]	60% familial; 13% autosomal dominant; 10–15% of familial early onset
	• Presenilin 1	30–70% of familial early onset
	• Presenilin 2	1% of familial early onset
Late onset (after age 65 years)	• ApoE • Sortilin-related receptor L • Clusterin	20–50% of late onset
FTLD	• Microtubule-associated protein tau • Granulin • Chromatin-modifying protein 2B gene • Vasosin-containing protein gene	5–10% of familial
Human prion disease (e.g., Creutzfeldt–Jakob disease; Gerstmann–Straüssler–Scheinker syndrome)	• Prion protein gene	15% (familial autosomal dominant)

[a]Important in all forms of AD.

genetic contribution is in terms of genetic susceptibility, and the strongest association has been with the ε4 allele of the apolipoprotein E (*APOE*) gene (Gatz et al., 2014). Individuals homozygous (have two) for ε4 alleles have a 5- to 15-fold risk for AD, whereas individuals heterozygous (have only one) for ε4 alleles have a two- to threefold increased risk for developing AD (Matthews, 2010). In addition, having one or more ε4 alleles seems to predispose those people sustaining head injuries to an increased risk for developing AD pathology (Mauri et al., 2006; Padilla & Isaacson, 2011). While the association between *APOE* ε4 and AD has been replicated many times, the exact pathologic mechanism is still not fully understood.

Other genes continue to be identified as potential modifiers of susceptibility to AD or age of onset for AD, but none have shown associations with AD as strong as those seen for age, sex, family history, and *APOE* status (Gatz et al., 2014). This suggests that considerable genetic heterogeneity is involved in AD and has led researchers to consider the additive and interactive effects of multiple genes. In addition, the interaction between genetic status and environmental influences is emerging as an important line of inquiry with respect to AD. Epigenetic mechanisms are biological regulators of gene expression. Links have been made between epigenetic alterations and a number of pathological processes including neurodegenerative diseases such as AD. It has been proposed that many epigenetic mechanisms are triggered by environmental lifestyle factors (Nicolia, Lucarelli, & Fuso, 2015). It has also been proposed that environmental factors (e.g., heavy metals, cytokines, or dietary factors) experienced in early life can lead to changes in gene expression either immediately or much later in life in response to a secondary trigger (Lahiri, Maloney, Basha, Ge, & Zawia, 2007). How these biological and lifestyle factors interact in influencing cognitive health in later life is the topic of much current biomedical research.

In FTLD, an autosomal dominant pattern of inheritance has been identified for approximately 10% of cases, while another 30–40% of cases present with a family history of a related diagnosis without a clear genetic connection (Padilla & Isaacson, 2011). Variants of FTLD seem to differ with respect to genetic influence, with the behavioral variant showing the strongest familial association and the semantic variant showing the least (Rohrer et al., 2009). At least four gene mutations have been identified (see Table 3.1) (Padilla & Isaacson, 2011; Rabinovici & Miller, 2010) in relation to FTLD.

Some other rarer forms of dementias have also been identified as being due to prion protein gene mutations (e.g., Creutzfeldt–Jakob disease; Qina et al., 2014). Prion diseases may manifest in a variety of ways such as rapidly progressive dementia with myoclonus in Creutzfeldt–Jakob or slowly progressive ataxia followed by later onset of dementia in Gerstmann–Sträussler–Scheinker syndrome.

While the search for genetic links to various forms of dementia is ongoing, these relationships are not straightforward, and testing for genetic susceptibility currently has only limited diagnostic value and so is typically discouraged (Padilla & Isaacson, 2011). Some research suggests that response to pharmacological agents may vary depending on the presence of specific genes. To date, most of this work is being conducted in relation to *APOE* ε4 (e.g., ε4-positive or ε4-negative carriers); the goal of these pharmacogenetic studies is to identify those patients who may respond best to particular therapies (e.g., cholinesterase inhibitors, insulin sensitizing agents). In addition, some studies have found that differences in *APOE* ε4 presence (i.e., positive or negative) may also influence the effectiveness of pharmacological interventions to prevent incident dementia. For example, in those who were taking statins, the risk for developing dementia was reduced by up to 56%, even in people with the high-risk ε4 allele (Haag, Hofman, Koudstaal, Stricker, & Breteler, 2009).

Bioage and Biomarkers

Bioage is a concept that refers to the functioning of physiological systems and processes within the body as an indicator of developmental status that can be related to health decrements and cognitive decline (DeCarlo, Tuokko, Williams, Dixon, & MacDonald, 2014). In addition to the multiple medical conditions we have already identified as risk factors for cognitive decline, overall health as measured by the accumulation of health deficits is related to neurodegenerative risk (Song, Mitnitski, & Rockwood, 2010, 2011). Compromised physiological functioning (e.g., weakened strength, sensory deficits, body mass) has been shown to be associated with cognitive decline over time (MacDonald, DeCarlo, & Dixon, 2011; MacDonald, Dixon, Cohen, & Hazlitt, 2004). While it is important to take these indirect markers into consideration, markers reflecting the key underlying biological processes involved in the evolution of cognitive decline are also being identified. In particular, biological markers have been identified that may appear early in the developmental course of neurocognitive disorders and are being targeted as keys to understanding and potentially preventing neurodegeneration. A multitude of such markers are emerging in the field. However, only two influential processes that have been shown to be linked to many age-related disorders, including those affecting cognition, will be mentioned briefly here: inflammation and oxidative stress. The important roles played by other biological factors, most notably vascular health and genetics, were identified earlier in this chapter.

Inflammation—the response of the immune system to harmful stimuli—is an adaptive and health-promoting process. This adaptive process may be impaired during aging, resulting in chronic inflammation that can lead to tissue degeneration and be detrimental (Franceschi & Campisi, 2014). This "inflammaging" is a significant risk factor for many different aging-related disorders, including the neurodegenerative processes. While the etiology of inflammation remains largely unknown, interventions that alter the dynamics of chronic inflammation hold promise for managing or preventing many conditions. Low-dose aspirins and statins are already being used in this way.

The oxidative stress theory of aging is based on the premise that molecules within cells react to oxygen, causing deleterious effects on cell functioning. The level of oxidative stress is the balance between oxidant generation and oxidant defense. Oxidative stress has been linked to many age-related disorders such as diabetes and neurodegenerative disorders. Moreover, oxidative stress may be involved in the initiation or propagation of inflammatory responses associated with cognitive decline or neurodegeneration (DeCarlo et al., 2014).

Evaluation of the Available Literature

As is true of any area of research, the studies included in this review are limited in various ways. Where possible, we included meta-analyses or systematic reviews that combine study findings to provide comprehensive overviews of an area. Most of these reviews included case–control studies as well as prospective cohort studies. However, in some cases, we were unable to locate reviews, and so the findings reported may relate to the outcomes of a single study. This evidence remains inconclusive, and contradictory findings may emerge in the literature. Across the studies reviewed, the manner in which cognitive decline, cognitive impairment, or dementia status was operationalized differed. These differences, as well as the samples studied and the manner in which the risk factors were measured, may contribute to the lack of movement toward consensus for some risk factors.

Although numerous individual risk factors have been identified, it has also been observed that a diverse array of health deficits, when combined, may exert an effect on cognitive functions (Song et al., 2010, 2011). For example, obesity, diabetes, and dyslipidemia clustering together are known as metabolic syndrome (MetS), which is associated with increased risk for cognitive impairment and dementia (Kim & Feldman, 2015). Risk factors may, in fact, be cumulative, as proposed by Song and colleagues (Mitnitski, Song, & Rockwood, 2012, 2013; Song et al., 2011), or they may interact in synergistic or antagonistic ways (Deckers et al., 2015). Certainly, it appears that the ε4 allele of the ApoE gene may influence the response to other risk factors (e.g., head injury) (Padilla & Isaacson, 2011). In addition, multiple genes appear to be implicated in AD and other dementias and may interact. Moreover, the interaction between genetic status and environmental influences in the expression of cognitive decline and impairment is an emerging area of study within epigenetics.

A number of other promising biomarkers, in addition to genes, are emerging that, when combined with other information, may lead to new avenues for early identification of conditions before the impact on cognitive functioning is apparent (DeCarlo et al., 2014). Certainly, there is evidence that the onset of some neurocognitive disorders can be 10 or more years prior to the first clinical signs (Thorvaldsson et al., 2011). Some of these biomarkers may link to pathways underlying multiple disorders (e.g., vascular health, inflammation, oxidative stress). Once these biomarkers are available, it may be possible to recruit participants for study based on stage of disease process rather than clinical presentation (Cooper et al., 2015).

To date, the longitudinal research on cognitive change over time has been pursued through large-scale observational studies, with some being focused primarily on evolution of cognition over time, others on the impact of disease processes on cognition, while still others examine changes across a broad spectrum of health-related domains including cognition. By necessity, the depth of measurement within the cognitive domain differs among these types of longitudinal studies. Efforts are underway (Piccinin & Hofer, 2008) to facilitate the integration and to synthesize the information available within different studies and across domains (e.g., cognition, health, lifestyle exposures). This type of research necessarily involves interdisciplinary collaboration and the application of statistical methods and procedures that facilitate comparative analyses across datasets. In particular, it will be important to unravel the relative magnitudes of impact that disease processes, social factors, and activities engaged in by individuals have on trajectories of cognitive decline. Smaller scale longitudinal research on the relations between cognitive functions and underlying physiological structures and functions is also emerging and is contributing information vital to the neuropsychology of aging. Conceptualizing aging as a biological process that can be identified through biomarkers rather than chronology (e.g., bioage) suggests that paradigm shifts may be taking place. Once reliable biomarkers are available, it may be possible to recruit participants for study based on biological function rather than chronological age and clinical presentation. The emerging area of epigenetics has also illuminated the ways in which interactions between genes and environmental influences can manifest in the expression of cognitive decline and impairment.

These studies are pointing to the development of theories (e.g., cognitive reserve; scaffolding theory of cognitive aging) that will explain or predict the relations among these domains. In addition, there is a growing recognition that methods to identify and monitor intraindividual (i.e., within person) change in cognitive functioning are becoming available. Information derived from the application of these methods will complement existing evidence derived from the study of between-person (e.g., age groups) differences. While providing valuable insights into change over time, much of this research continues to be correlational in nature. Demonstration that changes in cognitive functioning are temporally related to changes in health status or brain function will provide much needed evidence to support integrated theory development.

Implications for Clinical Practice

The most important message for clinical practice emerging from this review is that a variety of medical conditions can increase the risk for cognitive decline and the development of NCDs. A number of different research groups are in the process of developing tools to assess the risk for developing AD (Anstey et al., 2013; Barnes, Cenzer, Yaffe, Ritchie, & Lee, 2014; Barnes et al., 2009; Lee, Ritchie, Yaffe, Stijacic Cenzer, & Barnes, 2014; Mitnitski et al., 2013; Song et al., 2011) or dementia based on risk factors. The underlying biological mechanisms are not currently well understood, and testing for genetic and other biomarkers is not generally recommended for routine clinical practice. However, many of the identified risk factors are modifiable through appropriate medical management (e.g., hypertension) or lifestyle change (e.g., smoking).

It is important to inquire about these risk factors and determine how well they are being managed. Adherence to medications can reduce the risk for later cognitive decline (e.g., hypertension). It is also important to note that seemingly unrelated medical conditions may interact or have cumulative effects over time. Moreover, it appears that midlife health status is very important to later-life cognitive health. It has been proposed that this may be when preventive intervention will be most effective (Deckers et al., 2015), and some projects have begun to target modifiable risk factors in midlife (*www.inmindd.eu*).

Summary and Conclusions

This review shows that many factors may increase the risk for cognitive decline or cognitive impairment in later life. While we have focused on some of the medical disorders and proposed biological mechanisms underlying their impact on cognition through brain changes, it is also clear that these biological processes influence and are influenced by the environment. Moreover, it appears that the impact of these risks may be cumulative across the lifespan and may interact to present as cognitive decline or as a neurocognitive disorder emerging in later life.

PART II

Assessment Strategies for Late-Life Cognitive Decline

CHAPTER 4

An Integrative, Developmental Approach to Assessment

This part of the book focuses on assessment of cognitive decline in older adults. Each chapter addresses issues of concern for the characterization of cognitive functioning at different points or stages in a developmental trajectory (see Table 4.1)—specifically, normal cognitive decline (Chapter 5), SCD (Chapter 6), MCI (Chapter 7), and dementia (Chapter 8). These clinical presentations are addressed separately for clarity and convenience, and to recognize that changes in cognitive functioning may or may not be predictive of increasing cognitive decline. That said, many forms of dementia characterized by relatively severe cognitive impairment are progressive in nature and show increasing cognitive difficulties prior to a diagnosis of dementia. Certainly, much of the focus on SCD and MCI has been on the prodromal conditions thought to herald the onset of neurodegenerative conditions such as AD. While in many instances this developmental trajectory is evident, less clear is the issue of how, early in the trajectory, to distinguish between those cases that will or will not show progressive cognitive changes over time.

Each chapter in Part II provides specific information relevant to the assessment of cognitive functioning at a particular stage of cognitive decline. In each instance, however, a comprehensive, integrative process of assessing for cognitive decline is fundamental in an applied neuropsychological approach (Potter & Attix, 2006). This is true when the assessment is being made primarily for diagnostic purposes, or when the focus is on intervention. The current chapter presents a general overview of this assessment process, and specific issues may be revisited in individual chapters that follow. We address a number of special ethical considerations when

TABLE 4.1. Features Relevant to the Trajectory/Stage of Cognitive Decline/Impairment

Stage of cognitive decline/impairment	Characteristics
Normal aging	Minor cognitive lapses (e.g., word-finding) within the scope and severity of other older adults of similar demographic background
SCD	Significant concern about the meaning of minor cognitive lapses
MCI	Cognitive impairment that is beyond normal aging (e.g., >1.5 SD below performance of peers with similar demographics), yet instrumental activities of daily living remain intact; includes the prodromes for AD and other dementias (e.g., VCI)
Dementia (various types)	Cognitive impairment substantially below normal aging (i.e., >2 SD below peers) with impairment in one or more instrumental activities of daily living

assessing older adults, and these, too, may be revisited within the context of individual chapters. We also explore the expanding role of technology in cognitive assessment and describe the use of these technologies in monitoring typical cognitive decline or identifying and monitoring cognitive impairment in later life.

Our approach to assessment is commensurate with the American Psychological Association (2012) guidelines for the evaluation of age-related cognitive change. These guidelines recommend fourteen specific professional behaviors to promote proficiency and expertise in assessing age-related cognitive change:

1. Psychologists performing evaluations of dementia and age-related cognitive change are familiar with the prevailing diagnostic nomenclature and specific diagnostic criteria.
2. Psychologists gain specialized competence in assessment and intervention with older adults.
3. Psychologists are aware of the special issues surrounding informed consent in cognitively compromised populations.
4. Psychologists seek and provide appropriate consultation in the course of performing dementia and age-related cognitive change evaluations.
5. Psychologists are aware of cultural perspectives and of personal and societal biases and engage in nondiscriminatory practice.

6. Psychologists strive to obtain all appropriate information for conducting an evaluation of dementia and age-related cognitive change, including pertinent medical history and communication with relevant health providers.
7. Psychologists conduct a clinical interview as part of the evaluation.
8. Psychologists are aware that standardized psychological and neuropsychological tests are important tools in the assessment of dementia and age-related cognitive change.
9. When evaluating for cognitive and behavioral changes in individuals, psychologists attempt to estimate premorbid abilities.
10. Psychologists are sensitive to the limitations and sources of variability and error in psychometric performance and to the sources of error in diagnostic decision making.
11. Psychologists make an appropriate use of longitudinal data.
12. Psychologists recognize that providing constructive feedback, support, and education as well as maintaining a therapeutic alliance can be important parts of the evaluation process.
13. As part of the evaluation process, psychologists appropriately recommend interventions available to persons with cognitive impairment and their caregivers.
14. Psychologists are aware that the full evaluation of possible dementia is an interdisciplinary, holistic process involving other health care providers. Psychologists respect other professional perspectives and approaches. They communicate fully and refer appropriately to support integration of the full range of information for making decisions regarding diagnosis, level of severity, and elements of the treatment plan.

To provide context for the following discussion, we begin with an illustrative case study.

Deborah is a 66-year-old, Caucasian, right-handed woman with a master's degree in library science who has been referred by her family physician for assessment with respect to some behavioral change noted by family members. Deborah herself is willing to "go along" with the assessment but feels she is no different from any of her friends.

Deborah worked as a university librarian until her retirement at age 65. She reported that she was "ready to retire" because she was finding the ever-changing technological demands in the workplace to be extremely stressful and tiring. Her husband of 35 years had died 3 years earlier of a massive heart attack after a protracted period of disability during which Deborah provided substantial amounts of physical and emotional support for him on a daily basis. Her daughter, Sandra, accompanied her to the assessment and reported that her mother had become increasingly forgetful and moody over the past 1–2 years. She was concerned that her mother seemed to fatigue easily and had lost interest in her hobbies (e.g., painting, yoga, and socializing with her friends at coffee shops and recreation center classes).

Deborah has a history of postpartum depression. She took part in some form of "talk therapy" at the time (30 years ago) but has not received any other form of therapy or treatment for depression. She is taking medications for high blood pressure and arthritis pain. She has fallen repeatedly over the past 4 months. This has resulted in bruising and embarrassment but no bones were broken and, despite intensive investigations, there has been no identified cause for the frequent falls. She reported being far less physically active than in the past and finds this somewhat disturbing, as her daily 3-mile walks were something she really enjoyed.

Deborah reports feeling lonely since her daughter moved across the country, and she looks forward to her daughter's visits (once every 4–6 months). Deborah was the child of a single mother and grew up in relative poverty. Her mother was very young when Deborah was born, and their home life was unstable, with frequent moves made to new towns in search of employment opportunities. Deborah and her mother lost contact many years ago, and she has since passed away. Deborah says she feels guilty that she did not try harder to get along with her mother. She feels she has been a good mother to her own daughter, and she states that she would like to be more involved in her daughter's life than is currently possible.

This case study illustrates the richness and complexity of working with older adults. Although this book focuses on trajectories of cognitive decline within late life, we see that, in reality, older adults' current function is influenced by trajectories that go back in time to birth and early development. While they may come to the attention of a neuropsychologist with concerns about cognitive decline, older adults bring a lifetime of experiences that can affect their current presentation, including early attachments, interpersonal relationships, occupational functioning, and core values and beliefs. An older adult is a constellation of many forces moving through developmental time, exerting influence over and likewise being affected by his or her environment.

An Applied Neuropsychological Approach to Assessment

Neuropsychological assessment is a holistic and integrative process whereby test results are collected and interpreted within a biopsychosocial framework. As is evident in this case study, many factors both intrinsic and extrinsic to the person may be contributing to the clinical presentation of an older adult. Early life experiences, interpersonal relationships, and environmental exposures at various points in the lifespan all influence a person's developmental trajectory, and these multiple determinants of cognitive function must be taken into consideration in the assessment process. The nature and content of the assessment are likely to vary depending on the primary purpose of the assessment (e.g., diagnostic, monitoring or intervention) and the degree of cognitive impairment present. However, in most instances, a comprehensive evaluation is warranted.

Collection of Contextual Information

Just as cognitive function is multiply determined, information will be collected through a number of different methods (e.g., interviews, testing, observation) and possibly from a number of different sources (e.g., the person being assessed, family members, or friends of the person). It will be important to determine the reason for referral from the perspective of the referring agent, the person being assessed, and a collaborative informant (e.g., family members or friends of the person), if available. As we will see in later chapters (e.g., Chapter 6), the perception of type and progression of cognitive changes may provide useful information for distinguishing between conditions. Requisite information will be gathered about the person's prior level of functioning (i.e., cognitive, social, occupational, medical), current sensory functioning (e.g., vision, hearing, motor functions), and the presence of any comorbid diseases and disorders. Gathering this information is important because dysfunction in many different body systems (e.g., pulmonary, renal, hepatic) can adversely influence cognitive functioning (Armstrong & Morrow, 2010; Tarter et al., 2001; see Appendix 4.1 for sample interview domains and interview questions).

For older adults, the impact of physical health on cognition is complex and multifactorial. There are various pathways through which physical health can relate to cognitive functioning. First, perturbations in certain medical conditions (e.g., diabetes, chronic pain, insomnia) can cause transient fluctuations in cognitive performance (e.g., Zhou et al., 2014). Second, so-called vascular risk factors (e.g., hypertension, hypercholesteremia, type II diabetes) can be a major source of cognitive impairment in the elderly. Evidence suggests that vascular disease is rapidly becoming the second major etiological factor in dementia following AD (Alzheimer's Association, n.d.; Skrobot et al., 2017). Given that these vascular risk factors are modifiable, maintenance of vascular health is critical. Third, medications for certain medical conditions can create iatrogenic effects on cognitive function, such as drowsiness or fatigue. Fourth, chronic stress has been shown to create *immunosenescence,* or accelerated aging of the immune system. Early work in the field of psychoneuroimmunology demonstrated that older adults who were caregivers continued to show immunosenescence for months and even years after the person being cared for was deceased (Graham, Christian, &

Kiecolt-Glaser, 2006). Finally, coping with chronic health issues at any age can take a psychological toll, including depression and anxiety. Particularly for older adults, such psychological symptoms can adversely affect cognition, as well as overall quality of life (Lockwood, Alexopoulos, Kakuma, & Van Gorp, 2000).

Whenever possible, medical records including the results of medical laboratory tests and imaging studies will be obtained. This contextual information is essential for interpretation of the profile of strengths and weaknesses obtained through the administration of standardized measures of cognitive functioning. The application of the best available normative standards will help determine whether there are any identifiable areas of impairment. (This topic will be addressed in greater detail in Chapter 5.) All of this information is then integrated by an individual who possesses specialized knowledge of adult development and the aging process, including medical aspects of aging, psychopathology, and neuropathology in older adults (i.e., a comprehensive neuropsychological evaluation) (Attix & Welsh-Bohmer, 2006; American Psychological Association, 2014; McGuire, 2009; Russo, Bush, & Rasin-Waters, 2013b).

Much historical and contextual information can be obtained through a clinical interview with the individual and corroboration from a knowledgeable informant whenever possible (American Psychological Association, 2012). The interview with the person taking part in the evaluation gives clinicians the opportunity to observe behaviors and become familiar with the person's characteristics. Interviewing a knowledge informant can provide insight into the individual's daily functioning and can provide information concerning the onset and course of cognitive and behavioral changes. A number of structured, clinical tools are available to assist in collecting this historical and contextual information. See Appendix 4.1 for sample interview domains and questions.

If we were to interview Deborah and her daughter separately, we might see that their reports differ. Although Deborah is reported to show little concern about her cognitive functioning, on closer questioning she may share additional information about changes in her cognitive functioning and daily activities. She may also reveal some reasons for the change in physical activity levels (e.g., residual pain from falls, fear of reinjury, effects of medications). Deborah's daughter may be able to clearly articulate the types of cognitive changes she has noticed in her mother and describe the sequence of emergence of these changes. Additional information about Deborah's mood and behavioral changes may also be forthcoming. For example, it may be that because of her unstable childhood, she has always been quite anxious and fearful and that this apprehensiveness has been heightened by the cascade of age-associated changes she has experienced (e.g., prolonged caregiving for her husband, retirement, physical distance from her daughter).

Direct Measurement of Cognition

A number of factors should be considered when selecting measures to assess the most important cognitive domains. It may be necessary to assess across a broad range of cognitive domains (see Appendix 4.2 for sample domains and an interpretation grid), and, depending on the situation, to assess deeply within one or more domains. For example, multiple forms of memory can be assessed and may be affected to greater or lesser degrees. Similarly, executive functions are numerous and can be assessed in a variety of ways. While many measures are available (Lezak, Howieson, Loring, Hannay, & Fischer, 2004; Strauss, Sherman, & Spreen, 2006), it is important to select those that are age and culturally appropriate, and that have acceptable psychometric properties and normative data relevant for the individual being assessed. Only with an appropriate comparison standard can a clinician reliably determine levels of impairment. Whenever possible, it is also important to select measures without floor or ceiling effects and those sensitive to change, as serial assessments may be warranted to monitor for change over time.

Traditionally, neuropsychological assessments have involved the face-to-face administration of measures designed to be reflective of specific components of cognitive functioning. These measures have their basis in theory and have been shown to be sensitive to brain function in neurological populations. These measures were often initially developed to address a specific area of interest for use with a specific neurological population. Individual measures can be combined to create a battery of measures to address multiple domains of interest. This approach provides flexibility and allows the clinician to put together unique combinations of measures to address specific clinical questions. One limitation of this approach is that the normative data for each measure may come from populations that differ markedly from one another. This can lead to challenges when making interpretations and comparisons concerning levels of impairment among measures. In some cases, selected measures have been combined into a fixed battery, and normative data have been collected (co-normed), thereby permitting direct comparisons across measures within the battery. Such batteries may be quite comprehensive, whereas other simplified batteries have been designed as tools to screen for cognitive impairment. Some of these simplified measures briefly assess multiple domains so that direct co-normed comparisons across domains can be accomplished relatively quickly. However, few screening tools are sufficiently comprehensive or sensitive to detect subtle cognitive impairments and therefore should not be the only measures of cognition used in the context of diagnostic decision making.

If the profile of cognitive functioning depicted in Appendix 4.2 was Deborah's, she would be demonstrating a relatively circumscribed memory impairment. If this pattern of impairment were evident across a number of similar measures of memory, this might increase our conviction that this as an area of weakness for Deborah. We would examine how she performed the tasks (e.g., was she fully engaged, or was she disinclined to exert much effort on the tasks?). Our next task would be to determine why she might be experiencing these difficulties (e.g., in relation to a change in medications or subsequent to a fall). Here information about the speed of onset and the duration of symptoms will be crucial to making a determination. If there is no identifiable medical reason for this change, social and situational circumstances as well as issues related to mood will need to be addressed.

In addition to measures of cognition, it is important to assess for a range of conditions that may affect cognitive functioning. Measures of mood (see Appendix 4.2 for sample domains) and personality may be relevant in many cases. Selection of instruments relevant for older adults will be important, as many personality measures provide little normative data for older adults. Some specific measures of depression (e.g., Geriatric Depression Scale; Brink et al., 1982) and anxiety (e.g., Geriatric Anxiety Scale; Segal, June, Payne, Coolidge, & Yochim, 2010) have been developed for use with older adults, as the manner in which symptoms are expressed in older adults may differ from their expression in younger adults. As noted in relation to Deborah, throughout the assessment, much can be gained by observing how the individual performs a task or responds to the testing situation. This information, too, can be integrated into the overall evaluative process.

Diversity Issues

Other practical considerations in the assessment process include the diversity of the clients who are taking part in the assessment process. Issues such as linguistic and cultural diversity, as well as differences in educational background, are common concerns in the assessment process, and clinicians need to be mindful of how best to address them. There is a vibrant literature on these issues in neuropsychology (e.g., Ardila, 2005; Pedraza & Mungas, 2008). Because educational, linguistic, and cultural biases can lead to misidentification of NCDs (McCurry et al., 2001), we need to be aware of cultural nuances and the sociocultural influences that may affect the cognitive assessment. Certainly, in the current cohort of very old individuals, the type and quality of educational attainment may be quite distinctly different from that of younger cohorts of older adults; this may be particularly evident in relation to race or cultural context (Manly & Mungas, 2015).

Cross-cultural differences may be apparent in terms of differences in values, attitudes and beliefs, and/or interpersonal behavior (Ardila, 2005). This may include the manner in which the person is addressed and information is gathered during the assessment process, as well as the understanding that cognitive assessment is a culture-dependent activity (Ardila, 2003). One's culture is a way of being that includes shared beliefs and social norms that can be distinct from ethnicity and race. Adapting assessment methods and procedures that have been developed by and for use with people in Western countries may not be applicable or appropriate to people from all cultures (Ardlia, 2007). At least five different aspects of culture have been identified that may affect cognitive test performance: patterns of abilities, cultural values, familiarity, language, and educational attainment. Moreover, it may not be feasible or advisable to create normative information on standard measures for people of all languages and cultures. Pedraza and Mungas (2008) articulated a number of arguments against the proliferation of race- or ethnicity-based normative data, including the argument that race- or ethnicity-based normative data may be perceived as support for the inaccurate position that race reflects biological categories of people rather than socially constructed ones and may result in conformist attitudes toward differences in cognitive test performance between culturally diverse groups. Instead, it has been argued that equivalence of measures across cultures may be a more reasonable goal (Pedraza & Mungas, 2008). Various forms of equivalence such as procedural or metric equivalence, as well as equivalence in how measures are interpreted in the context of culture, have been identified. The scarcity of available cognitive measures for which these issues have been addressed affects their diagnostic validity for cross-cultural use. It is critically important, then, that clinicians understand that numerous factors can potentially affect cognitive test performance and that they seek ways to address these factors when making clinical judgments under less than ideal conditions.

The Expanding Role of Technology in Cognitive Assessment

With advances in technology, a variety of approaches have been taken to move cognitive assessment beyond the traditional paper-and-pencil tests administered and interpreted by professionals trained in neuropsychology. These approaches include adaptations that involve telephone, video, computerized, and online assessment protocols. It has been argued that the use of these technologies can result in savings of both costs and time, as well as in the increased accuracy of recording, scoring, and storing test results. Moreover, some of these technologies can be used to provide clinical services remotely, thereby facilitating access to a broader, larger, and often an underserved range of people than can engage in traditional face-to-face cognitive assessments. These technologies differ in terms of how similar the administration and response procedures are to traditional face-to-face test administration, and it is important that issues concerning the validity of these alternative modes of test administration be evaluated.

Video Teleconference-Based Cognitive Assessment

Video teleconference-based (VTC) cognitive assessments typically involve the administration of traditional cognitive measures using video teleconferencing equipment. Measures relying on verbal instructions and responses are particularly suited for this technique of administration, though drawing tasks can be accommodated with some additional instructions and procedures (Cullum, Hynan, Grosch, Parikh, & Weiner, 2014). To date, a variety of brief measures of cognition have been identified as suitable for VTC administration, and good agreement with face-to-face testing has been shown (Cullum et al., 2014; Hildebrand, Chow, Williams, Nelson, & Wass, 2004). However, it cannot be assumed that all cognitive measures could be validly administered in this way, and additional research is required with nonverbal tasks or tasks requiring additional equipment. Most studies to date have employed a limited number of measures with relatively small samples (Grosch, Weiner, Hynan, Shore, & Cullum, 2015; Harrell, Wilkins, Connor, & Chodosh, 2014). Typically, local staff members are required to seat the test taker in front of the VTC camera and introduce the remote examiner. These staff members remain available to the test taker but are not in the VTC testing room during the assessment. Tests are administered by experienced psychometrists in the standardized manner, with minor variations for some tasks (e.g., holding up drawings to the camera) (Cullum et al., 2014). Video teleconference-based cognitive assessment has been shown to be acceptable to both healthy older adults and those with mild forms of cognitive impairment (Parikh et al., 2013). However, it is possible that assessment via this technology may not be feasible for use with some test takers exhibiting behavioral issues (Cullum et al., 2014). Data security is an issue that can be addressed through the use of secure networks and with appropriate levels of data encryption and safeguards concerning privacy. Initial guidelines for implementation of VTC for clinical and research purposes are beginning to emerge (Turvey et al., 2013).

Telephone-Administered Cognitive Assessment

As with VTC-based measures, telephone-administered measures tend to be those that rely most heavily on verbal instructions and responses. Measures have been developed for telephone administration with different purposes. Most often, they are used for screening purposes to identify older adults with and without cognitive impairment (Wolfson et al., 2009). These tools have been derived from measures typically administered in person (e.g., the Mini-Mental State Examination or its extension, the

Modified Mini-Mental State Examination) or developed specifically for administration by telephone (see Table 4.2). Table 4.2 presents a summary of some available tools and should not be viewed as comprehensive. Additional information about these measures can be obtained by searching the names of the tests in library databases. When reported, these telephone-administered tools show strong correlations (.80–.90) with scores on cognitive measures administered in face-to-face sessions for those older adults with and without cognitive impairment (Wolfson et al., 2009). Administration time for most of these screening measures is reported to be between 10 and 20 minutes. While the sensitivity and specificity of these telephone screening tools tend to be reasonably good, not all of these tools may be sensitive enough to detect mild forms of cognitive impairment or reliably classify people with no cognitive impairment (Wolfson et al., 2009).

Some verbal measures included in longer, clinical cognitive test batteries have been administered over the telephone. These include measures of memory (e.g., Hopkins Verbal Learning Test; Carpenter, Strauss, & Ball, 1995), verbal fluency (e.g., Category Fluency Test; Lipton et al., 2003), and executive functions (e.g., Mental Alternation Test; McComb et al., 2011) or full batteries of cognitive tests (Mitsis et al., 2010). Typically, these tools have been shown to be interchangeable, with versions administered in person. However, measures of some domains are more resilient to the effects of mode of administration than others (McComb et al., 2011). These types of measures have some advantages over screening tools, particularly when administered to adults without cognitive impairment, as they (or at least some components within batteries) do not have ceiling effects. For this reason, they are also appropriate for use with a broader age range of adults. Batteries have also been specifically designed for use in assessing cognitive functions in adults of various ages (Rapp et al., 2012; Tun & Lachman, 2006) and have shown promise.

It has been shown, then, that a variety of cognitive measures can be reliably administered over the telephone and will yield comparable scores to in-person administration. In the case of screening for changes in cognitive functions, cognitive measures administered over the telephone may be a cost-effective way to determine whether more extensive, in-person assessment is warranted. The use of telephone administration has several advantages over in-person cognitive assessments in that administration costs are reduced, and those who, for reasons of distance or disability, do not have access to a testing facility can be included. In addition, biased responding may be more likely with in-person assessments, as perceived confidentiality may be decreased and the testing situation may inadvertently influence the respondent (Schwarz, Strack, Hippler, & Bishop, 1991). Particularly for research purposes in the case of large-scale epidemiological studies, telephone assessment may reduce burden and thereby reduce attrition in longitudinal studies. However, cognitive assessments conducted over the

TABLE 4.2. Telephone Cognitive Assessment Tools

Test name and studies	Notable features
Tools derived from the MMSE	
Telephone Modified Mini-Mental Status Exam (T3MS) (Norton et al., 1999)	Adapted version of the T3MS; discriminates between normal cognitive functioning and MCI
Adult Lifestyles Function Interview—Mini-Mental State Examination (ALFI-MMSE) (Roccaforte, Burke, Bayer, & Wengel, 1992)	Developed for use in patients with AD but has been used with a variety of clinical populations (Castanho et al., 2014)
Adult Lifestyles Function Interview—26-point Adaptation (Telephone Mini-Mental State Examination; TMMSE) (Newkirk et al., 2004)	26-point adaptation of the ALFI-MMSE; administered by a nurse clinician
Telephone Assessed Mental State (TAMS) (Lanska, Schmitt, Stewart, & Howe, 1993)	Four items; cannot detect subtle deficits; administered by a psychometrician
Telephone Interview of Cognitive Status (TICS) and Modified Telephone Interview of Cognitive Status (TICS-m) (Brandt, Spencer, & Folstein, 1988)	Used frequently in medium to large-scale studies (Herr & Ankri, 2013); translated in several languages; distinguishes reliably between normal cognition, MCI, and dementia (Knopman et al., 2010)
Mini-Mental State Examination Telephone (MMSET) (Kennedy, Williams, Sawyer, Allman, & Crowe, 2014)	Similar to TMMSE
Other tools	
Hopkins Verbal Learning Test (HVLT) (Carpenter et al., 1995)	12-item unique word lists (six different forms); used in patient populations
Category Fluency Test (CF-T) (Lipton et al., 2003)	Number of items generated in 1 minute for three different categories
Mental Alternation Test (MAT) (McComb et al., 2011)	Oral version of the Trail Making Test (TMT) that requires switching between tasks and typically takes less than 1 minute to administer; no ceiling effects like other oral versions of the TMT
Cognitive Assessment for Later Life Status (CALLS) (Crooks, Parsons, & Buckwalter, 2007)	Computer-assisted telephone-administered tool modeled on neuropsychological test batteries; takes approximately 30 minutes to administer; a technician records answers

(continued)

TABLE 4.2. (continued)

Test name and studies	Notable features
Telephone Cognitive Assessment Battery (TCAB) (Debanne et al., 1997)	Designed to discriminate between cognitively normal and mildly impaired individuals; administered by well-trained professionals
Telephonic Remote Evaluation of Neuropsychological Deficit (TREND) (Mundt, Kinoshita, Hsu, Yesavage, & Greist, 2007)	Computer automated telephone interactions initiated by participants using touch-tones or constrained verbal responses; takes 20 minutes to complete tasks; difficulty using this method may occur with severely impaired people
Short Portable Mental Status Questionnaire (telephone version) (SPMSQ) (Smith, Tremont, & Ott, 2009)	Adaptation of the 10-item SPMSQ (Roccaforte, Burke, Bayer, & Wengel, 1994)
Blessed Telephone Information–Memory–Concentration Test (TIMC) (Kawas, Karagiozis, Resau, Corrada, & Brookmeyer, 1995)	27-item adaptation of the TIMC Test; greater acceptance by participants than the face-to-face version; for use with patient populations
Telephone Screening Protocol (TELE) (Gatz et al., 1995; Gatz et al., 2002; Järvenpää et al., 2002)	Adaptation of the 10-item Mental Status Questionnaire with 11 additional items; designed for use with clinical populations
Structured Telephone Interview for Dementia Assessment (STIDA) (Go et al., 1997)	Designed to distinguish early AD from normal cognitive functioning; includes items from the MMSE and the TIMC Test; administered by skilled clinicians
Memory Impairment Screening—Telephone (MIS-T) (Smith et al., 2009)	Adaptation of the Memory Impairment Screening; more robust than the TICS for discriminating between dementia and normal cognitive functioning; outperformed CF-T and TICS when screening for dementia
Minnesota Cognitive Acuity Screen (MCAS) (Knopman, Knudson, Yoes, & Weiss, 2000)	Designed to discriminate among normal cognitive functioning, mild impairment, and AD
Brief Screen for Cognitive Impairment (BSCI) (Hill et al., 2005)	Three-item measure for distinguishing between normal cognitive functioning and dementia; administered by an experienced interviewer

(continued)

TABLE 4.2. (continued)

Test name and studies	Notable features
Brief Test of Adult Cognition by Telephone (BTACT) (Lachman, Agrigoroaei, Tun, & Weaver, 2014; Tun & Lachman, 2006)	Used as part of the Mid-Life in the United States study; applicable to well-functioning younger and middle-aged adults as well as older adults; recording the interview is recommended
Memory and Aging Telephone Screen (MATS) (Rabin et al., 2007)	Designed to screen for individuals with mild or significant cognitive impairment in longitudinal studies; contains subjective and objective cognitive items; no ceiling effects; administered by trained researchers/clinicians
Cognitive Telephone Screening Instrument (COGTEL) (Kliegel, Martin, & Jäger, 2007)	Designed to assess cognitive functioning across adulthood (e.g., large samples, cross-sectional, longitudinal, epidemiological)
Telephone Montreal Cognitive Assessment (T-MoCA and T-MoCA short) (Pendlebury et al., 2013)	Adapted from the Montreal Cognitive Assessment, originally designed to identify MCI

telephone have some limitations; for example, the examiner is unable to observe testing behavior; the assessment of verbal tasks has to be limited (i.e., there is no way to assess visuospatial and motor functions); and there is no control over the testing environment (e.g., preventing distractions or use of aids such as making note of materials to be recalled; see Mitsis et al., 2010). Assessments conducted over the telephone may be particularly difficult for people with severe cognitive impairment, those with poor telephone skills, or those with hearing loss (Castanho et al., 2014). Not all of the measures listed in Table 4.3 have been validated in relation to face-to-face administration of the same measures, and many of those that have been validated have inadequate sample sizes (Castanho et al., 2014). Few of these measures have been evaluated longitudinally, and there is no information concerning the sensitivity of these measures to change over time.

These measures were developed for different purposes, a fact that must be taken into consideration when selecting a specific tool. Castanho et al. (2014) provide an excellent summary of which tools are most appropriate for each goal: for those with normal cognitive functioning (e.g., BTACT, COGTEL, HVLT, MAT, MATS, TCAB, T3MS); for those with mild degrees of cognitive impairment (e.g., STIDA, TCAB, T-MoCA, T3MS), and for those with various forms of dementia (e.g., measures derived from the MMSE or SPMSQ, BSCI, MIS-T, STIDA, TELE, TIMC).

TABLE 4.3. Computerized Cognitive Assessment Tools

Test name and studies	Administered by	Device	Notable features
	Screening tools		
Cambridge Neuropsychological Test Automated Battery—Mobile(CANTAB Mobile)[a] (Zygouris & Tsolaki, 2015)	Self	iPad	Designed for assessing older adults worried about memory
Cognitive Function Test (CFT)[a] (Trustram Eve & de Jager, 2014)	Self	Web-based	Designed to detect subtle cognitive changes in adults 50–65 years of age
COGselftest[a] (Dougherty et al., 2010)	Self	Web-based	Patient receives feedback designed so no diagnosis can be inferred
MCI Screen[a] (Cho, Sugimura, Nakano, & Yamada, 2008; Rafii, Taylor, Coutinho, Kim, & Galasko, 2011; Shankle, Mangrola, Chan, & Hara, 2009; Trenkle, Shankle, & Azen, 2007)	Examiner	Web-based	Designed for screening older adults for cognitive impairment; Japanese version
CNS Vital Signs (CNSVS)[a] (Gualtieri & Johnson, 2005, 2006)	Self (initiated by assistant)	PC or Web-based	Available in 50+ languages, reports in English; not suitable for severe dementia
Cognitive Stability Index (CSI)[a] (Erlanger et al., 2002)	Testing technician	Web-based	All stimuli nonverbal; monitoring AD limited
CogState[a] (Darby et al., 2012; Falleti, Maruff, Collie, & Darby, 2006; Hammers et al., 2011, 2012; Lim et al., 2012, 2013)	Testing technician	Laptop	Numerous equivalent forms; can be used for frequent assessment (within hours); sensitive to mild degrees of cognitive impairment
Computer-Administered Neuropsychological Screen for Mild Cognitive Impairment (CANS-MCI)[b] (Ahmed, de Jager, & Wilcock, 2012; Tornatore, Hill, Laboff, & McGann, 2005)	Self with technician assistance	PC with touch screen	Specifically for screening for MCI; English, French, Spanish, Portuguese, and Dutch
Computer Assessment of Mild Cognitive Impairment (CAMCI)[b] (Saxton et al., 2009; Tierney & Lermer, 2010)	Self	Tablet PC	Designed for preclinical screening of abnormal cognitive decline

(continued)

63

TABLE 4.3. *(continued)*

Test name and studies	Administered by	Device	Notable features
MicroCog[a] (Elwood, 2001; Green, Green, Harrison, & Kutner, 1994; Gualtieri, 2004; Lopez et al., 2001)	Self	PC	Designed to screen older physicians for cognitive impairment and malpractice risk
		Assessment batteries	
Automatic Neuropsychological Assessment Metrics (ANAM)[a] (Jones, Loe, Krach, Rager, & Jones, 2008; Kane, Roebuck-Spencer, Short, Kabat, & Wilken, 2007; Levinson, Reeves, Watson, & Harrison, 2005; Roebuck-Spencer, Sun, Cernich, Farmer, & Bleiberg, 2007; Short, Cernich, Wilken, & Kane, 2007)	Testing technician	PC laptop (web-based available)	Originally developed to measure performance change in healthy people; modules including Dementia Battery
Cambridge Neuropsychological Test Automated Battery (CANTAB)[a] (Egerhazi, Berecz, Bartok, & Degrell, 2007; Lowe & Rabbitt, 1998; Sahakian & Owen, 1992)	Testing technician	PC with touch screen	Various batteries including detection of AD and MCI
Cognitive Drug Research Computerized Assessment System (COGDRAS)[a] (De Lepeleire, Heyrman, Baro, & Buntinx, 2005)	Examiner	PC with two-button response device	Adaption of the battery for use with patients with dementia (COGDRAS-D)
Computerized Neuropsychological Test Battery (CNTB)[a] (Cutler et al., 1993; Veroff, Bodick, Offen, Sramek, & Cutler, 1998; Veroff et al., 1991)	Examiner	PC	Not automated; designed for use with dementia
Mindstreams[a] (Doniger et al., 2006; Dwolatzky, Dimant, Simon, & Doniger, 2010; Dwolatzky et al., 2003; Fillit, Simon, Doniger, & Cummings, 2008)	Testing technician	PC	Available in different languages; adaptive tests
Touch Panel-type Dementia Assessment Scale (TDAS)[b] (Inoue, Jimbo, Taniguchi, & Urakami, 2011; Tsuboi et al., 2009)	Self	Combined computer with 14-inch touch screen	Designed for use with patients with dementia

[a]Designed for general application; [b] designed for specific application.

Computerized Cognitive Testing

With the growing availability and popularity of personal computers, adaptations of traditional cognitive measures and new measures of cognitive functions have been created for computerized applications. Various technological innovations have been incorporated into computerized cognitive assessments, including touch screens and web-based applications. Numerous computer-assisted instruments have been developed for screening purposes or for more thorough evaluation of a person's cognitive functioning (Zygouris & Tsolaki, 2015) (see Table 4.3). Table 4.3 presents a summary of some available tools and should not be viewed as comprehensive. Additional information about these measures can be obtained by searching the names of the tests in library databases. All tools on Table 4.3 are available in English, and some are available in other languages as well (see "Notable features" column of Table 4.3). New applications are being developed at a rapid pace, and information is not always available about normative data, length of administration, and other psychometric properties, making it difficult to comment on comparative effectiveness or suitability for specific purposes such as diagnosis, monitoring treatment, and follow-up (Wild, Howieson, Webbe, Seelye, & Kaye, 2008). Moreover, the available information tends to be provided only by the designer of the tool, and the potential for possible biases must be kept in mind. Many of these instruments include evaluations of a number of cognitive domains. Older instruments tended to be lengthier and assess cognitive domains more broadly, whereas some of the newer instruments are more targeted toward domains where early changes in function may be anticipated (Zygouris & Tsolaki, 2015). It is important to understand the purpose of the measure and its target audience when evaluating and selecting a suitable instrument for a specific use. Instruments designed to monitor healthy older adults for uncharacteristic changes in cognitive function may be distinctly different from those for use when monitoring change in people already identified with an NCD. It must also be noted that equivalence of the same measure administered in-person and via a computerized program cannot be assumed, as differences in stimulus presentation and response method may affect the test result. For example, latency of responses may differ between mechanical reaction time measurement and touch screens owing to the sensitivity of the touchscreen (Korczyn & Aharonson, 2007). In addition, it is possible that in some circumstances computer adaptation of a task may change the nature of the cognitive domains and processes being evaluated. For these reasons, it has been argued that determining the concurrent validity of a computerized tool by comparing it with its traditional counterpart may be less important than determining discriminant validity (i.e., how well the tool can discriminate between groups) (Zygouris & Tsolaki, 2015). Most of these measures have been designed to detect subtle or mild forms of cognitive impairment, while some were designed specifically for use with those already diagnosed with dementia.

The application of computerized cognitive assessment technology has many advantages over traditional in-person assessments, including the accurate recording of response information and automatic storage of data facilitating comparisons between people and across time. Some computerized programs are flexible enough to automatically adapt the testing protocol as levels of functioning change. Like other technologies (i.e., video and telephone applications), administration costs may be reduced; those who for reasons of distance or disability may not be able to access cognitive assessments can be accommodated; and the influence of an examiner can be minimized or eliminated. However, the use of computerized technologies is not without its own complexities. Test designers may not provide information concerning normative data and psychometric properties of their tools that would facilitate clinical interpretation of results. None of these instruments can be used to determine a final diagnosis as other factors in addition to cognitive test performance must be taken into consideration. While test designers are quick to adopt new technologies and seek out new applications, users (e.g., older adults, researchers, health care practitioners) may be less willing to embrace approaches that may be perceived as intimidating, as less personal, or even as a degradation of the patient–health professional relationship (Werner & Korczyn, 2012).

For some, lack of familiarity with technology and anxiety associated with computer use may influence their willingness to engage. For others, cost and the need to continually adapt to the ever-changing technological landscape may be perceived as deterrents. Understanding the factors that influence motivation and adherence to computerized assessment tools will be crucial for their acceptance and application. Motivational issues may be particularly important in the context of self-administered measures. As with other technological innovations, no well-defined guidelines are available to facilitate the implementation of such procedures into clinical practice. However, some studies—many of them emerging under the rubric of implementation science—are beginning to address the factors associated with adopting new technological innovations (Werner & Korczyn, 2012). This is important work, as the intensive effort and organizational, financial, and human investment involved in the integration of technological advances into clinical systems will succeed only if the targeted audiences are willing to engage.

Ethical Issues in the Assessment of Older Adults

When assessing older adults in the context of research or clinical practice, a number of special considerations need to be addressed to ensure that this work is conducted with high ethical standards. Specifically, it is important that researchers and clinicians are knowledgeable concerning the unique characteristics of the aging process and age-related vulnerabilities that may influence the assessment process. A variety of excellent resources are available to promote ethical practice and to facilitate ethical decision making (e.g., Russo, Bush, & Rasin-Waters, 2013a; see Table 4.4).

A number of principles form the foundation of human rights and ethical practice that are reflected, and must be addressed, within the assessment process (see Appendix 4.3 for a checklist of ethical issues to be addressed across the assessment process). Respect for autonomy refers to being able to make choices in the absence of interference and recognizes the basic human rights of competent adults to privacy, dignity and self-determination (Beauchamp & Childress, 2009; Koocher & Keith-Spiegel, 2008). Beneficence refers to the promotion of the person's welfare whereas nonmaleficence refers to the avoidance of harm. While these ethical considerations are relevant to research and clinical practice with all age groups, the prevalence and nature of the changes and disorders experienced by older adults make it particularly important to evaluate and address conditions that may impact the assessment process. As noted earlier, many factors can influence the assessment of a person's performance on measures of cognitive functioning including sensory and motor deficits, physical pain, underlying medical conditions, consumption of medications, or emotional and motivational states. In addition, response to the environmental demands of a testing session may differ based on prior experience or cultural factors. The physical, cognitive, and social changes associated with the aging process, both expected and pathological, increase the need to ensure that ethical issues are addressed at each step in the assessment process whether for research or for clinical purposes.

In addition, clinicians working with older adults need to consider a number of specific ethical issues. These issues revolve primarily around the need for specialized knowledge of adult development and the aging process, including medical aspects of aging, psychopathology and neuropathology in older adults, family and social systems, and cultural issues (American Psychological Association, 2014; McGuire, 2009; Russo et al., 2013a). Codes of conduct note that clinical service may only be provided by qualified personnel; qualifications are based on education, training, and supervised or professional experience (Russo et al., 2013a). Clinicians are expected to develop and maintain their knowledge base and skill sets to work with older adults (see Table 4.4 for resources).

Before the assessment process begins (see Appendix 4.3), it is imperative that information about the assessment process is provided to the older adult in a manner that is easily comprehended and that the older adult has the opportunity to ask questions and receive responses. The types of information to be provided include the nature and purpose of the assessment,

TABLE 4.4. Resources for Ethical Practice and Decision Making

Title	Description	Reference
General ethical resources		
Ethical principles of national professional bodies (psychological) and funding agencies and amendments		
American Psychological Association Ethical Principles and Code of Conduct	Goals to guide psychologists toward the highest ideals of psychology and are to be considered by psychologists in arriving at an ethical course of action. The following areas are addressed: clinical, counseling, and school practice of psychology; research; teaching; supervision of trainees; public service; policy development; social intervention; development of assessment instruments; conducting assessments; educational counselling; organizational consulting; forensic activities; program design and evaluation; and administration.	American Psychological Association (2002, 2010)
Canadian Psychological Association Code of Conduct	Ethical principles, values, and standards to guide psychological scientists, practitioners, or scientist–practitioners when engaging in a role related to research, direct service, teaching, learning (i.e., students, trainees), administration, management, supervision, consultation, employment (i.e., employer, employee), provision of expertise (e.g., peer review, expert witness testimony), development of social policy or any other discipline-related activity.	Canadian Psychological Association (2017)
Tri-council Policy Statement: Ethical Conduct for Research Involving Humans	Joint policy of Canada's three federal research agencies—the Canadian Institutes of Health Research (CIHR), the Natural Sciences and Engineering Research Council of Canada (NSERC), and the Social Sciences and Humanities Research Council of Canada (SSHRC)—to promote the ethical conduct of research involving humans.	Canadian Institutes of Health Research, Natural Sciences and Engineering Research Council of Canada, and Social Sciences and Humanities Research Council of Canada (2010)
Policy and Guidance	Policy and regulatory guidance materials to assist the research community in conducting ethical research that is in compliance with the U.S. Department of Health and Human Services regulations.	Office of Human Research Protections, U.S. Department of Health and Human Services (2018)

(continued)

TABLE 4.4. *(continued)*

Title	Description	Reference

State or provincial licensing and ethics boards

Local institutional ethics guidelines and committees

Books on ethics

Title	Description	Reference
Neuroethics in Practice: Medicine, Mind and Society	Overview of relevant scientific and bioethical perspectives with which to approach real-world ethical dilemmas.	Chatterjee & Farah (2013)
Ethical Issues in Clinical Neuropsychology	Discussion of ethical questions in neuropsychology and how to apply ethical guidelines to clinical interactions with specific patient populations including older adults.	Bush & Drexler (2002)
Ethical Decision-Making in Clinical Neuropsychology	Guide to ethical decision making in the daily practice of clinical neuropsychology that emphasizes positive ethics and models a decision-making process by which practitioners can successfully resolve common ethical challenges.	Bush (2007)

Specific ethical resources concerning older adults

Title	Description	Reference
American Psychological Association Guidelines for Psychological Practice with Older Adults	For self-assessment of knowledge, skills, and experience relevant to this area of practice; suggestions for seeking and using appropriate education and training to increase knowledge and skills.	American Psychological Association (2014)
Assessment of Older Adults with Diminished Capacity: A Handbook for Psychologists	Reviews psychological assessment in the context of capacities of particular importance when working with older adults (e.g., consent capacity, financial capacity, capacity to live independently, capacity to participate in research); provides a conceptual framework for conducting capacity assessments; provides practical guidance for clinicians, including an overview of assessment tools and worksheets.	American Bar Association Commission on Law and Aging & American Psychological Association (2008)

(continued)

TABLE 4.4. *(continued)*

Title	Description	Reference
Peak Model for Training in Professional Geropsychology	Provides comprehensive competencies in knowledge and skill areas including assessment, intervention, and consultation for self-evaluation by practitioners.	Karel, Molinari, Emery-Tiburcio, & Knight (2015); Knight, Karel, Hinrichsen, Qualls, & Duffy (2009)
Geriatric Mental Health Ethics: A Casebook	Presents a practical one-step model and, through a collection of case studies, demonstrates its implementation across a variety of therapeutic settings.	Bush (2009)

who will have access to the information, how the information may be used (and how this may impact the person's life), limits to confidentiality, involvement of third parties, and, in the case of clinical assessment, the fee (Russo et al., 2013b). Depending on the situation, particular care may need to be taken to ensure that all of this information has been understood (i.e., informed consent). It may be necessary to ensure that compensatory sensory aids are used (e.g., glasses or hearing aids; large print), the person is approached when most alert, supportive others are present (if desired by the person), or sufficient time for consideration is allowed.

In situations where there is concern about the older adult's ability to provide informed consent, for whatever reason, additional steps may need to be taken. The presence of cognitive impairment itself does not necessarily imply that a person is incapable of understanding and consenting. Whenever possible, the older adult should be involved in the decision-making process, and a surrogate decision-maker or guardian may be enlisted to support the person in providing a joint decision. In this case, the surrogate or guardian would be fully informed concerning the conditions of the assessment. Importantly, the exact requirements for obtaining consent for research or clinical assessment in this situation may differ by jurisdiction; therefore, familiarity with local state/provincial legal acts and regulations, as well as institutional ethics board guidelines, is essential (Bravo et al., 2010; McGuire, 2009).

In the consent process, the question of whether or not the obtained information will be shared with family members or third parties must be addressed. In some situations, this may be perceived as creating an ethical dilemma with conflict between the individual's autonomy and relational autonomy (autonomy supported and enhanced by others) (Russo et al., 2013a). For those becoming increasingly dependent on others, finding ways to encourage joint decision making and sharing of information with caring supporters will ultimately benefit the older adult. Also within the consent process, limits to confidentiality that must be declared include duties to report elder abuse (i.e., physical, psychological, verbal, material) (McGuire, 2009) or danger to self/others. The right to refuse service and the right to privacy (e.g., how much information to communicate to others) must be honored.

When preparing for the assessment (see Appendix 4.3), it is important that due diligence is done in selecting approaches and measures to address adequately the referral question and rule out alternative hypotheses (Russo et al., 2013a). This includes collecting information from a number of sources (e.g., interviews, testing, observation), selecting age-appropriate measures of an adequate sampling of relevant constructs (cognitive and noncognitive), applying appropriate normative data or considering factors that could influence normative data collected in a different decade (e.g., sample composition, Flynn effect, or cohort effects), and taking into consideration that many factors can influence the assessment of a person's performance on measures of cognitive functioning (e.g., sensory/motor deficits, pain, multimorbid medical conditions, medications, emotion, and motivation). Wherever possible, ways to mitigate the impact of these factors on the assessment should be employed.

The assessment needs to be conducted in a manner that supports the autonomy and dignity of the older adult and avoids harm. Using computerized assessment with an older adult who has had little or no exposure to computers or using a mouse and keyboard may require that the older person be given additional preparation and encouragement to feel comfortable with the test demands (Russo et al., 2013a). This may necessitate scheduling the assessment at a time when the person is able to perform at his or her best, conducting the assessment over several short sessions, or providing frequent rest breaks. Unintentionally, age-related stereotypes and biases (i.e., ageism) can be reinforced or elicited within the neuropsychological testing environment and can adversely affect cognitive test performance (Haslam et al., 2012; Kit, Tuokko, & Mateer, 2008). In such situations, self-efficacy and effort may be reduced and anxiety heightened, all of which negatively impact test performance and create a "self-fulfilling prophecy" (Suhr & Gunstad, 2002, 2005). While adequate training and experience may mitigate the pervasive ageism expressed in North American society, psychologists are not immune to ageism and must be aware of their own biases and the impact they may have on others (McGuire, 2009).

The older adult is to be given feedback (see Appendix 4.3) in accordance with the conditions addressed in the informed consent process (i.e., to whom information is disclosed). The manner in which the information is conveyed is as important as the information itself (Russo et al., 2013a). An approach to providing feedback (particularly when addressing loss of function) that is sensitive and supports the autonomy and dignity of the older adult will be of most benefit to all concerned. Providing negative feedback in the absence of sensitivity and support may lead the older adult to react with depression, despair, or withdrawal. The information should be provided clearly and at a level of detail that can be received by the older adult and his or her family members. Additional feedback sessions may be required to ensure complete understanding of the findings and their implications (McGuire, 2009). The feedback session is a dynamic, interactive process and represents an opportunity to provide education about the condition. In addition, available resources, support, and care options can be introduced, or guidance and support within a care system can be provided (Postal & Armstrong, 2013). When clients and their loved ones understand the condition, they may share information or concerns previously withheld. In addition, they may become more effective advocates for themselves and their loved ones (Postal & Armstrong, 2013). In their book *Feedback That Sticks,* Postal and Armstrong (2013) provide clinicians with practical strategies for approaching the feedback session. Key to providing feedback that sticks is making complex information accessible to the target audience. Drawing on communication theories, Postal and Armstrong identify the six key principles of effective communication: simplicity, unexpectedness, concreteness, credibility, emotions and stories. They also note that feedback begins during the clinical interview, which offers a time to build trust and enlist the client and family as collaborators in the assessment process. The assessment is framed to clarify an understanding of the condition and to address the goals of the client and family. It is important that information about poorly understood conditions be provided with great care. For example, the prognostic implications of MCI are uncertain, and this must be conveyed to the older adult. Before engaging in such discussion, the benefits of early diagnosis of a potentially degenerative process (i.e., respecting autonomy, relief of having a diagnosis, opportunity of engagement in decision making and planning) must be weighed with the risks (e.g., will the diagnosis precipitate fear and distress, reduce hope, induce depressive and/or suicidal ideation, stigma, and associated consequences?; Werner & Korczyn, 2008).

The key to ensuring that research and clinical practice with older adults is conducted with high ethical standards is to be familiar with the general ethical codes of conduct and specific considerations relevant to older adults and to apply these proactively at each step of the assessment process.

For research involving older adults, the ethical principles noted in Table 4.4 are typically explicitly addressed in the consent process, and familiarity with local institutional ethics board guidelines is essential (Bravo et al., 2010; McGuire, 2009). A situation that calls for additional consideration of the ethical implications is that of the clinician–researcher. Here, in accordance with codes of conduct, the clinician's primary duty is to provide optimal care, whereas the scientist must adhere to the procedures and methods described in the research protocol. There are different schools of thought on how to resolve this conflict: the fiduciary approach notes that the obligation to provide care should prevail, whereas the nonexploitation approach holds that the research being undertaken is to advance knowledge, not to benefit the participant. A third alternative described by Resnik (2009) is a contextual approach where the obligation to provide care varies by situation. Here, the clinical obligation to provide care increases with medical or psychological risk to the research participant, and special attention must be given to those most in need of help. For example, an incidental finding in a research study that carries little or no risk would not be pursued, whereas another incidental finding with immediate implications for the health status of the participant would be followed (Detre & Bockow, 2013), with further referral for evaluation and treatment. However, it is not reasonable to require someone to provide a clinical service that he or she cannot provide owing to lack of resources, expertise, or knowledge (Resnik, 2009).

Assessment of Trajectories of Cognitive Decline

As noted earlier, while longitudinal studies of cognitive decline have been able to demonstrate that many forms of dementia show developmental trajectories of increasing cognitive impairment, early indicators of those cases that will or will not show this progression remain elusive. That said, various constructs have emerged from this research that appear characteristic of cognitive functioning at different points or stages in the presumed developmental trajectory between normal aging, with subtle relatively innocuous cognitive decline, and the significant cognitive impairment impacting everyday functioning seen in dementia (see Table 4.1).

For decades, research has examined the effects of aging on cognition and other related psychological processes. Although changes in functioning clearly occur within individuals across the lifespan, it is also acknowledged that the effects of normal aging differ from the effects of age-associated disease processes. Distinctions between these processes are evident in the use of the terms *primary aging, secondary aging,* and *tertiary aging. Primary aging* denotes the normal, universally experienced, intrinsic changes that occur in concert with progressive alteration in the body's systems. *Secondary aging* refers to disease-related impairments in functioning that affect only a segment of the older population, whereas the rapid loss of multiple areas of function toward the end of life has been termed *tertiary aging* (Whitbourne, Whitbourne, & Konnert, 2015).

It must be reiterated that cognitive function is multiply determined, and we argue that the interpretation of assessment findings is from an integrative developmental perspective. Information about the many factors (e.g., medical, situation, relational) that may influence cognitive function is interpreted in the context of each individual's unique developmental presentation. Trying to address or conceptualize these problems in isolation might miss important links between them, as these problems may be mutually influential. We argue that an applied neuropsychological approach is necessarily an integrative one. This integrative process often reveals many possible contributors that then must be addressed systematically when formulating a diagnostic opinion or intervention plan. It is not an uncommon occurrence for an individual to present clinically with "a bit of this and a bit of that." This clinical reality, while disconcerting in the search of "pure" or "textbook" presentations of specific disorders, provides the comprehensive picture needed to ensure "best" clinical practice.

Summary and Conclusions

This chapter provides an overview of the integrative developmental approach to assessment. Here we explored the expanding role of technology (e.g., adaptations that involve telephone, video, computerized, and online assessment protocols) and ethical issues in the cognitive assessment of older adults. Technologically assisted assessments are frequently used in this context of normal cognitive aging, and the demands of these assessment methods may preclude their use where cognitive impairment may interfere with the assessment process itself. That is, in some cases, comprehension difficulties and the need for self-direction may preclude the use of these assessment methods. These technologies differ in terms of how similar the administration and response procedures are to traditional face-to-face test administration, and explored here are issues concerning the validity of these alternative modes of test administration.

Study of the normal aging process provides the contextual backdrop necessary for identifying and managing age-associated disease processes. In Chapter 5, we explore approaches to the development of normative comparison standards for measures of cognitive functions and issues relevant to the application of these standards.

SCD is an emerging clinical syndrome characterized by performance within normal expectations on measures of cognition and daily functioning in the context of significant concern about decline in cognitive abilities. In Chapter 6, we provide a thorough description of the state of current knowledge concerning this condition and provide guidance for clinicians in terms of assessment strategies and clinical decision making.

Concepts related to MCI have been studied as prodrome to dementia, and particularly AD, for over 20 years. Definitions and procedures for assessment of MCI have evolved over this period and are described in Chapter 7. In addition, we consider the utility of this construct, given that progression to dementia is not a forgone conclusion.

Finally, in Chapter 8, we focus on the differential diagnosis of prevalent age-related conditions. In so doing, key features in the clinical presentation will be identified for consideration when distinguishing among conditions. We have chosen to organize our discussion of these disorders according to their onset and progression (e.g., rapid onset, potentially reversible with intervention, variable, maximal neurological deficit at onset, insidious onset with progressive decline). We then review the impact of dementia on everyday functioning, including capacity assessment. Finally, we discuss the practice of assessment for the evolution of cognitive and behavioral symptoms as dementia progresses. Some measures lend themselves more toward care planning to enhance quality of life, while others have been shown to be useful for monitoring functional change over time.

KEY POINTS

✓ The assessment process is holistic and integrative.

✓ A lifetime of experiences, including early attachments, interpersonal relationships, educational and occupational attainment, and core cultural values and beliefs, affect later-life cognitive functioning.

✓ Information for the assessment is collected through multiple methods such as observation, interviews, objective testing from multiple sources such as the person being assessed, a knowledgeable informant, and existing records documenting educational, occupational, and medical functioning.

✓ Educational, linguistic, and cultural influences can affect the interpretation of cognitive assessments.

✓ Advances in technology have moved cognitive assessment beyond traditional face-to-face test administration.

✓ The unique characteristics of the aging process and age-related vulnerabilities give rise to specific ethical considerations for clinicians and researchers.

Key Interview Information to Be Obtained

This information can be obtained from the client or from a collateral informant about the client.

1. *Reason for referral.* Describe why you are here today.
   - What types of problems are you experiencing?
   - What are your goals for taking part in this assessment (i.e., what would you like to find out about yourself)?
   - Do these problems concern you?

2. *Onset.* When was each of these problems first noticed?
   - Was there something specific going on when you first noticed the problem?

3. *Course of progression.* Do you think these changes are getting worse, staying the same, or getting better?
   - If getting worse, has there been a rapid or slow change?
   - Do you experience fluctuations in your functioning (e.g., better and worse times)?

4. *Social situation.* What is your current living situation?
   - Are you married?
   - Who lives in the home?
   - Who else are you close to (e.g., children, friends)?
   - In what types of activities or hobbies do you take part (e.g., social activities including religious or cultural activities)?
   - Are there particular groups with whom you identify (e.g., cultural, ethnic)?

5. *Medical history.* Describe medical/physical conditions prior to the onset of the current condition (e.g., past injuries, surgeries, psychiatric or neurological conditions, chronic conditions such as diabetes, heart disease, cancer).
   - Did you receive treatment for this condition? When? By whom?
   - Are you taking any medications? What are these for?

6. *Prior functioning.* Describe your educational and occupational background.
   - How many grades did you complete in school?
   - Where did you obtain your education?
   - Were there any special problems during your schooling?
   - In what types of jobs have you been employed?

(continued)

7. *Current functioning.*

   - Sensory/motor: Do you have any difficulty seeing or hearing? Do you wear corrective lens or hearing aids? Do you have any difficulty with motor movements like walking or writing?

   - Have you noticed any changes in your memory (e.g., new learning, remembering where objects have been placed, recalling names or faces of friends or family members, finding way around familiar places, recalling past life events, recalling personal dates such as birthdays and anniversaries)?

   - Have you noticed any changes in your language skills (e.g., finding words, recalling names, understanding what others are saying, pronouncing words, initiating speech, stuttering)?

   - Have you noticed any changes in your mood? (e.g., irritable, sad or depressed, anxious, aggressive, suspicious of others, upsetting thoughts)?

   - Have you noticed any changes in your ability to perform everyday tasks (e.g., performing household chores, handling money, reading, driving, using the telephone, dressing, bathing, grooming)?

Cognitive Domains for Administration and Interpretation

Cognitive domain	2 *SD* below mean	1 *SD* below mean	Mean	1 *SD* above mean	2 *SD* above mean
Memory (acquisition and retention of new information)					
Memory measure 1		←			
Memory measure 2	←				
Reasoning/judgment (decision making, planning, risk taking)					
Reasoning measure 1				→	
Reasoning measure 2			→		
Visuospatial (recognizing faces, objects, operating simple implements, orienting clothing)					
Visuospatial measure 1			→		
Visuospatial measure 2			→		
Language (expressive and receptive language; speaking, reading, writing, comprehension)					
Language measure 1			→		
Language measure 2			→		
Behavior (personality, mood, motivation, interest, acceptable)					
Depression measure		←			
Anxiety measure		←			
Complex attention (sustained divided or selective attention; processing speed)					
Attention measure 1			→		
Attention measure 2			→		

(continued)

Cognitive domain	2 *SD* below mean	1 *SD* below mean	Mean	1 *SD* above mean	2 *SD* above mean
Executive function (planning, decision making, working memory, inhibition, mental flexibility)					
Executive measure 1		←			
Executive measure 2			→		
Perceptual–motor (visual perception, visual construction, praxis, gnosis)					
Perceptual–motor measure 1			—————→		
Perceptual–motor measure 2			————→		
Social cognition (recognition of emotions, perspective taking)					
Social cognition measure 1			→		
Social cognition measure 2			→		

Ethical Principles and the Assessment Process
(Russo et al., 2013a, 2013b)

Check the core ethical principles (in parentheses) addressed at each stage in the assessment process.

Prior to Assessment

_____ Boundaries of competence and maintaining competence (beneficence, nonmaleficence)

_____ Assessment by qualified person (beneficence, nonmaleficence)

_____ Client has right to know (respect for autonomy, beneficence, nonmaleficence):

    _____ the nature and purpose of the service

    _____ who will receive a report

    _____ who will have access to the information obtained

    _____ how the information may be used

    _____ the impact the service may have on her/his life

    _____ the limits of confidentiality

    _____ the involvement of third parties

    _____ the fee

_____ Client has the right to refuse service

_____ Client has the right to privacy and decides how much information may be shared with others (for exceptions, see Russo et al., 2013a)

Preparing for the Assessment

_____ Obtain multiple sources of information (beneficence, nonmaleficence):

    _____ Interview with older adult and carers

    _____ Biographical and medical information

    _____ Behavioral observations

    _____ Measures of cognition

(continued)

_____ Measures of emotion

_____ Measures of behavior

_____ Selection of age-appropriate, psychometrically sound measures, supported by research (beneficence, nonmaleficence)

During the Assessment Session

_____ Conduct the assessment in a manner to support autonomy, and dignity and to avoid harm (Respect for autonomy, beneficence, nonmaleficence)

Feedback

_____ Provide detailed information about the condition in a manner to support autonomy and dignity and avoid harm (respect for autonomy, beneficence, nonmaleficence)

_____ Emphasize strengths, ways to support capabilities, find ways for continued meaning and engagement (respect for autonomy, beneficence, nonmaleficence)

_____ Introduce resources and support/care options (respect for autonomy, beneficence, nonmaleficence)

CHAPTER 5

Normal Age-Related Cognitive Decline

Researchers have been studying cognition, or how the mind works, for approximately 150 years. As this work has evolved, domains of cognitive functions (e.g., memory, intelligence, attention, executive functions) have been defined and redefined to describe proposed underlying processes, the impact that aging may have on these processes, and the implications of these age-related changes. As noted already, some cognitive functions appear to decline with advancing age (e.g., tasks requiring motor speed, working memory, fluid intelligence, visuospatial tasks), whereas others remain relatively spared (e.g., semantic memory, crystallized intelligence). Here, we will focus on describing how this information can be applied in a clinical context.

Studies of normal cognitive aging may involve comparing people in different age groups at one point in time (i.e., cross-sectional age differences), following the same group of people over time as they age (i.e., longitudinal), following individuals over time (i.e., intraindividual longitudinal), or some combination of these approaches to take into consideration the shortcomings of each approach. These studies may focus on one domain or task within that domain of cognition (e.g., memory recall) or cognitive measures may be embedded in a broader context (e.g., with biological and social) to allow for a more holistic approach to understanding how cognitive functions interact with other factors across the aging process.

Findings from early studies of normal cognitive aging prompted the generation of theories to explain the developmental trajectories observed. From these studies, various approaches to the development of theories of cognitive aging have been, and are continuing to be, refined (Rodríguez-Aranda & Sundet, 2006). In Chapter 1, some of these approaches were described: information processing, intraindividual differences, contextual, biological, and integrative. Over time, these theories have moved from a singular focus on normal cognitive aging to incorporate observations and elements emerging from the study of disorders of cognition.

As these studies of normal cognitive aging make apparent, some cognitive functions decline while others remain relatively stable or may even improve. For example, it is generally accepted that fluid intelligence, or abilities requisite to flexible and adaptive thinking such as drawing inferences and understanding the relations among concepts, decline with age, whereas crystallized intelligence, or knowledge acquired through life experience and education in a particular culture, is maintained or may even improve (e.g., knowledge continues to be acquired) (Horn, 1982). Similarly, some forms of memory decline with age (e.g., working memory, explicit or declarative memory; Light, 2012; McCabe & Loaiza, 2012), whereas other forms are relatively spared (e.g., semantic memory; Grady, 2012). These changes are considered normal in that they represent typical changes associated with advancing age. However, it must be acknowledged that not all people will show the "typical" cognitive declines. Some people may show little to no discernible change in cognitive functioning as they age. It must also be acknowledged that, from a clinical perspective, a person's performance on measures of cognitive functioning may fall within the age-associated normal range but that person may be cognitively challenged in his or her everyday living for reasons other than neurodegenerative disorders. For example, some very old individuals may perform within the expected range on individual measures of cognition but be challenged in complex decision making as a consequence of difficulty integrating multiple sources of information, rapidly changing sociocultural circumstances, or physical frailty.

The study of normal aging, then, can provide the foundational information required to understand expected changes in cognitive functions associated with primary aging and provide comparison standards for the identification of impairment within and across cognitive domains. In this chapter, we will address the ways in which knowledge emerging from the study of normal cognitive aging provides the information necessary for the detection and management of conditions reflective of underlying pathological processes. In so doing, approaches to the development of normative comparison standards for measures of cognitive functions are described and issues relevant to the application of these standards are addressed.

Normative Comparison Standards

The strategies used in the assessment of older adults include observations, interviews, self-report of behaviors and concerns, and use of instruments or tests to assess how a person objectively performs a particular task within a cognitive domain. This last-named approach is dependent on understanding the strengths and limitations of these test instruments and their appropriateness for use with adults at various points in the lifespan. Through application of these tools with normal older adults, the characteristics of measures of cognitive functioning can be determined and comparison standards or norms developed for use in clinical contexts.

Approaches to Norms

Most measures for use in clinical practice have been developed by commercial companies and have information available on large samples of individuals, who are often representative of the population of interest (e.g., U.S. residents). Measures that have been published or updated recently have information on test performance available for older adults. However, this may not extend to the oldest-old (i.e., those over 80 years of age), where the greatest increase in the population of older adults is expected. The normative information available through these sources, then, is not always relevant for the clinician. Moreover, measures developed in the past or those developed by researchers may not have such extensive information available concerning older adults.

Regardless of the source of normative information, the nature of the *standardization sample* used to develop norms is critically important for identifying impairments in function. The purpose of standardization, in terms of test administration or in relation to the development and application of norms, is to reduce the amount of measurement error and provide a stable estimate of what is considered to be indicative of typical functioning for a specific segment of the population. That said, studies differ in terms of the samples that have been used to identify age-related changes in cognitive functioning and to develop comparison standards. Sometimes the norms are developed from a random sampling of individuals from a particular source (e.g., census lists). For example, measures of cognitive functioning may be collected as part of population-based epidemiological studies and used to create norms (Ganguli et al., 2010). In other instances, samples of convenience may be recruited through a variety of means (e.g., through media advertisements or via local recreation centers). Norms developed in different samples may therefore not be comparable and may not be equally applicable in all clinical contexts. That is, an appropriate standardization sample needs to be as similar as possible in terms of important demographic characteristics (e.g., age, gender, education, occupational background) to the people for whom it is being applied (i.e., the specific clinical context). Given the differences that exist between standardization samples and the observation that appropriate norms may not be available for all people seen in a clinical context, it is important to seek out the 'best' samples for comparison and, when necessary, apply several sets of norms. This allows the clinician to situate the person's performance in relation to other groups when determining the course of action to be taken.

Standardization samples may be further divided into segments to capture specific categories of interest. Certainly, performance on measures of cognitive functioning has been observed to differ across age groups, so comparison standards may take this into consideration and provide normative data stratified by age. Normative data have frequently been stratified by gender, and educational attainment as performance on cognitive measures has often been shown to be affected by (i.e., correlated with) these characteristics. However, as illustrated in earlier chapters, many other sociodemographic factors have been linked to healthy cognitive aging as protective or risk factors (e.g., facility with languages, cognitive leisure activities, social interactions, physical activity, nutrition) and may need to be taken into consideration when developing comparison standards. It is important to note, though, that these individual factors may not be independent but instead occur together in the same individuals (Poortinga, 2007). Moreover, distinguishing between risk factors for decline and causes of the decline is becoming increasingly blurred as we learn more about the interrelations among them (Geldmacher, Levin, & Wright, 2012).

Defining the standardization sample, then, is becoming more complex as we learn more about factors influencing healthy cognitive aging. By defining the sample characteristics in different ways, the comparison standard is necessarily altered. A randomly selected representative sample of the population of older adults may include individuals with disorders that affect cognitive functioning. This is true even when screening is done for obvious medical complications such as specific neurological or psychiatric conditions. It has become clear over the past two decades in particular that neurodegenerative conditions that underlie NCDs often have lengthy subclinical or presymptomatic stages (Albert et al., 2011) that may be undetected by the individual or those around him or her. Cross-sectional samples may be susceptible to including such individuals. However, it may be that this sample is indicative of the typical older adults in this population and provides a useful comparison. Restricting sample selection to those who are highly active and in extremely good health may be particularly useful for studying the nature of cognitive processes but may yield an elite comparison standard rather than a typical or normal comparison group.

Some of these concerns can be addressed in the context of longitudinal data collection where incident rates for cognitive impairment can be determined and factored into the process of developing modified comparison standards. One such approach, typically referred to as robust norming, has been to remove incipient cases of dementia from normative samples, as their inclusion tends to decrease the mean and increase the variability of test scores (De Santi et al., 2008; Holtzer et al., 2008; Pedraza et al., 2010; Ritchie, Frerichs, & Tuokko, 2007).

Once the standardization sample has been determined, the *test scores* can be represented for comparison purposes in a number of ways. Most often the distribution of raw scores will be examined, and some form of metric will be selected that characterizes the distribution against which comparisons can be made. This may be as simple as generating means and standard deviations of the raw scores from the normative sample and using these for comparisons. More commonly, the scores are converted to a common metric that helps determine where a person falls within the normative distribution (i.e., in relation to other people) and permits direct comparison of performance on different tests. When raw test scores are normally distributed, they can be converted to standard scores (Z-scores) or converted to have a mean of 100 and a standard deviation of 15 (e.g., as in IQ scores) or T-scores having a mean of 50 and an SD of 10. Some non-normally distributed scores (i.e., skewed) can be normalized to create a normal distribution (Crawford, 2004). In other instances (e.g., acute skewness), scores can be expressed in other ways for comparison purposes such as percentiles (Crawford, Garthwaite, & Slick, 2009).

While demographic characteristics known to influence cognitive test performance (e.g., age, gender, educational attainment) are commonly taken into consideration when developing normative standards, this practice is not without some controversy (O'Connell & Tuokko, 2010; Sliwinski, Buschke, Stewart, Masur, & Lipton, 1997; Sliwinski, Lipton, Buschke, & Wasylyshyn, 2003). This controversy has arisen in the context of screening for, or diagnosing, dementia. Advancing age is associated with the prevalence of dementia, and so applying age corrections to instruments that are used to detect dementia may remove important predictive variance. A distinction has been proposed between demographically corrected norms used to determine clinical strengths and weaknesses (i.e., "comparative norms") and "diagnostic norms" that combine uncorrected raw scores with age-corrected base rate information on dementia prevalence (Sliwinski et al., 1997, 2003). To examine the utility of this distinction, O'Connell and Tuokko (2010) used Monte Carlo simulation techniques in which the associations between demographic characteristics (i.e., age and education) and diagnosis (i.e., dementia) were manipulated while maintaining the association between test scores and demographic characteristics. They found that correcting for age in the context of dementia diagnosis does reduce classification accuracy when age is moderately associated with dementia risk. This is particularly problematic if a single test (e.g., screening tool) is being used to diagnose dementia, in which case it may be most appropriate to use raw scores. The use of multiple tests within a neuropsychological assessment approach offsets the reduction in classification accuracy associated with the use of demographically corrected scores.

Demographic corrections can be incorporated into the development of comparison standards in a number of ways. Simple raw score means and standard deviations can be presented for specific strata within the normative sample (Kang et al., 2013). Strata are typically included for demographic characteristics that correlate with the test scores (e.g., age, educational attainment, gender) but typically are not included when no correlations exist. Other approaches to demographic correction that have been proposed include overlapping cell tables or regression equations. Overlapping cell tables (Pauker, 1988; Saxton et al., 2000) are particularly useful when the number of stratification cells is large and sample sizes within each cell may be relatively small. By constructing the norm tables where the stratified variables are broken into relatively small increments (e.g., 5-year age intervals; 3-year education intervals) and comparison data are presented at the midpoint of each age range, the information in the cells will overlap and an individual participant's score may be represented in several cells (see Table 5.1). For example, from Table 5.1, a test score (not shown) for a person 70 years of age can be compared with scores for a normative sample across multiple cells. This allows for more direct comparisons of people falling at upper and lower ends of traditional groupings and maximizes normative data available for comparison purposes. The use of regression equations to develop demographically corrected comparison standards takes into consideration possible interaction effects between the demographic variables. This approach converts raw scores to scaled scores, and the demographic variables are regressed onto the scaled scores in a single step. The variable weightings derived from this regression analysis are then used to create predicted scores based on the demographic characteristics. This allows for a more precise prediction of expected normal performance than is available when providing normative data in stratified tables. The predicted scaled scores based on demographic characteristics are then subtracted from the participant's actual score, and the resulting difference (i.e., residual score) indicates whether they are performing better or worse than predicted by their demographic characteristics. These residual scores can then be converted to *T*-scores for use in clinical interpretation. Clinicians can then determine what cutoff *T*-score to use for their purposes (Heaton, Grant, & Matthews, 1991; Tuokko & Woodward, 1996).

TABLE 5.1. Example of Overlapping Cell Format

Cell test score	Cell age range and midpoint of age range					
Range	65–72	67–74	69–76	71–78	73–80	75–82
Midpoint	68	70	72	74	76	78

Note. Ages are in years.

It is not uncommon for some poor cognitive test performances to be observed for people with no cognitive impairment. For example, in the context of an entire battery of neuropsychological tests (eighteen measures), 88% of participants clinically determined to have no cognitive impairment in a Canadian epidemiological study had at least one test score falling in the impaired range, with a median of three abnormal scores (Tuokko & Woodward, 1996). Similarly, Mistridis et al. (2015) observed one or more scores at or below the 10th percentile for 60.6% of a healthy older adult sample (*n* = 1,081) administered the German version of the Consortium to Establish a Registry for Alzheimer's Disease–Neuropsychological Assessment Battery. This familywise error issue can result in overdiagnosis, increased burden for clients, and unnecessary costs to the health system. Procedures to address this issue are being developed and are being applied in the context of large cognitive test batteries (Huizenga, van Rentergem, Grasman, Muslimovic, & Schmand, 2016).

Each of the approaches to demographic correction noted thus far requires a standardization sample of substantial size. There are occasions when comparisons need to be made to small normative or control samples. Crawford and his associates have developed approaches and computerized programs for conducting such comparisons (Crawford, 2004; Crawford & Garthwaite, 2004; Crawford, Garthwaite, Azzalini, Howell, & Laws, 2006; Crawford, Garthwaite, & Howell, 2009; Crawford & Howell, 1998).

Finally, it should be noted that the availability of appropriate norms sometimes interacts with the choice of actual assessment instrument to be used. Although psychologists are ethically obligated to use the most up-to-date versions of tests available, at times it may be more ethical to use an older version of a test until sufficient clinical evidence exists to support the reliability, validity, and diagnostic accuracy of a newer form of a test within a given population (Loring & Bauer, 2010). For example, several issues were identified with the use of various subtests of the Wechsler Memory Scale—Third Edition (WMS-III; Wechsler, 1997) in older adults. Lezak, Howieson, Bigler, and Tranel (2012) note that impairment on Logical Memory is underestimated in persons with higher education, and Word Lists were generally insensitive to impairment in older adults. In such cases, it may be more ethical to use an older version of the test with more sensitive norms. The widely used Mayo Older Adult Normative Studies (MOANS; Ivnik, Malec, Smith, Tangalos, & Petersen, 1996; Lucas et al., 1998) have co-normed many frequently used neuropsychological tests for older adults at different ages and levels of education. The MOANS norms reference to the Wechsler Memory Scale–Revised (WMS-R; Wechsler, 1987); although this is an older test, the WMS-R may be preferable to WMS-III due to greater sensitivity in norms. To address these concerns, the latest revision of the WMS (WMS-IV; Wechsler, 2009) was designed with particular attention to older adults, with particular subtests designed for this population (e.g., the Brief Cognitive Status Exam). In this case, using WMS-IV as the most up-to-date test may be the most appropriate option. However, the advantage of using normative studies such as MOANS is that many frequently used tests are co-normed, which reduces variation in true score estimate due to the use of multiple different normative studies. As always, the most important consideration is that any normative studies used have a population that closely matches the demographics of a particular client. Where such matching is limited, diversions based on race/ethnicity, culture, and socioeconomic status should be acknowledged in the interpretation of test results. This further underscores the utility of repeat assessment, where intraindividual change over time is more relevant than comparison to normative standards.

Assessing Change over Time

In a clinical context, comparison of neuropsychological test performance to normative standards may be used to identify apparent changes in cognitive functioning or cognitive decline. However, identifying change in functioning from a single assessment can be challenging. While comparison with appropriate (e.g., similar demographic profile) normative standards may yield areas of relative strength and weakness, determining whether or not a decline in performance is evident requires additional scrutiny before such a conclusion can be drawn. It is typically recommended that clinicians obtain additional information about an individual's prior functioning by conducting interviews with collateral informants or by estimating a premorbid level of functioning. These estimates may be determined from demographic characteristics by examining performance on measures relatively insensitive to change or by noting 'best performance' whether reflected on test performance, from historical information or any current aspect of behavior (Lezak et al., 2004).

For individuals for whom English is the first or primary language, reading-based tests such as the Test of Premorbid Function from the Wechsler Adult Intelligence Scale–Fourth Edition (WAIS-IV; Wechsler, 2008) can provide a useful estimate. However, reading-based tests can be limited in persons who have limited English proficiency and in those who had limited formal schooling opportunities in Western countries. This refers not only to individuals with different ethnic or cultural backgrounds, but also to persons from the oldest-old cohorts, particularly women, where formal educational opportunities may have been quite limited. Years of education in and of itself can be used as a proxy for premorbid function; however, the work of Manly and others (e.g., Manly, 2006) suggests that it is not simply years of education but the actual quality of that education that matters. Occupational attainment is another important variable used to estimate premorbid function; for example, certain individuals may have failed to excel in school but through their own resilience and creativity have gone on to successful careers. In summary, to be able to speak to the question of decline, particularly at the initial assessment visit, accurate assessment of premorbid function is essential.

Although these approaches can be useful in practice, direct, objective measurement of change over time is generally preferable. Serial assessments are particularly important for monitoring changes in cognitive functioning. This may be useful to monitor disease progression and is particularly important in the context of interpreting mild indications of cognitive decline. However, several factors need to be considered when interpreting the results of serial cognitive assessments. First, not all measures that are of use for detecting cognitive deficits may be sensitive to change. Measures with floor or ceiling effects are examples; some of these measures may be particularly useful for screening purposes or as pathognomonic (i.e., highly suggestive) signs of a disorder of cognition but may be insensitive to subtle changes. Most neuropsychological measures, even those with full dispersions of scores, were initially adopted to detect cognitive deficits and so their sensitivity to change cannot be assumed. Although many of these measures have been demonstrated to be sensitive to change at the group level (e.g., differences in pretest–posttest comparisons), the clinician is most interested in the individual level of analysis.

One of the biggest challenges in the interpretation of serial assessments is distinguishing true changes in cognitive functioning (presumably due to an underlying pathological process) from changes that are due to other factors such as random errors and biases (Heilbronner et al., 2010). Random errors may occur as a result of the unreliability of a measure or in relation to statistical effects such as regression to the mean; common biases include practice effects. Classical test theory posits that any observed test score reflects both the individual's true performance score and an unspecified amount of measurement error. This measurement error is a function of the reliability of the measure, and some degree of unreliability is to be expected of all measures. Various approaches have been taken to estimate the amount of error inherent in test scores, and the types of error estimation selected will affect procedures for determining change in neuropsychological test performance. Similarly, regression to the mean, or the tendency for baseline scores to move toward the mean upon retesting (Nesselroade, Stigler, & Baltes, 1980), is a potential complicating factor in the assessment of change over time, though its actual impact on the interpretation of clinical data has not, as yet, been clearly delineated (McGlinchey & Jacobson, 1999). Practice effects, or improvements in test performance seen on readministration of the same measure to the same person, are thought to be an indication of learning (i.e., exposure to the task); some research suggests that these effects will disappear after the second exposure to the task (Ivnik et al., 1999; Theisen, Rapport, Axelrod, & Brines, 1998).

Practice effects, or retest effects, are of particular concern when the overall level of performance may be expected to decline across a number of cognitive domains (Duff, Beglinger, Moser, & Paulsen, 2010; Maassen, 2000; Maassen, Bossema, & Brand, 2008). These competing forces may work to cancel each other out, as practice effects decrease with advancing age, especially in persons over age 75 (Mitrushina & Satz, 1991; Ryan, Paolo, & Brungardt, 1992). However, it has also been noted that retest effects on neuropsychological tests can be substantial and persistent (Wilson, Watson, Baddeley, Emslie, & Evans, 2000). Practice, or retest, effects and their interaction with other variables may vary across measures (Heilbronner et al., 2010). It is critically important for clinicians to take these effects into consideration when interpreting change over time. An understanding of the normal individual variability that may occur with repeated assessments is important for the clinician when interpreting the meaning of observed cognitive change for a given person.

Unfortunately, data concerning the distribution of cognitive change scores for normative samples are limited (Heilbronner et al., 2010; Stein, Luppa, Brähler, König, & Riedel-Heller, 2010) and are rarely available in test manuals. Even when available, test–retest intervals can vary greatly from a few weeks to years, and the information available may not be ideal for use in clinical settings.

Many methods for assessing change at the individual level have emerged over the past 50 years (Chelune, Naugle, Lüders, Sedlak, & Awad, 1993; Crawford & Howell, 1998; Payne & Jones, 1957). These include indices of reliable change (RCIs) and more sophisticated standardized regression-based methods (SRBs). RCIs have been refined, and many variants are available (see Table 5.2) that differ in terms of the manner in which error terms are included (Chelune et al., 1993; Hageman & Arrindell, 1993; Hageman & Arrindell, 1999a, 1999b; Hsu, 1999; Jacobson & Truax, 1991; Temkin, Heaton, Grant, & Dikmen, 1999). For example, some RCI formulas correct for practice effects (Chelune et al., 1993) or for regression to the mean (Hsu, 1999). Also, SRBs can be used to assess cognitive change at the individual level and can control for confounding factors such as practice effects and regression to the mean for a particular measure (McSweeney, Naugle, Chelune, & Luders, 1993). In addition, SRBs can be expressed in a common metric (e.g., Z- or T-scores), facilitating comparisons of scores across different measures.

There remains considerable debate in the literature concerning the "right" way to address error and biases in the measurement of change. Several of these procedures have been applied to neuropsychological measures administered to older adults over time (Frerichs & Tuokko, 2005; Ivnik et al., 1999). Different cognitive domains have been shown to have varying degrees of stability in normal adults; consequently, different magnitudes of change are required to be considered reliable. Assessment of change is particularly challenging in memory testing, for the reliability of memory

TABLE 5.2. A Nonexhaustive List of Examples of Reliable Change Formulas (Frerichs, 2004)

Description	Formula	Source
Difference in observed test scores that exceeds the amount of variation that could be reasonably attributed to measurement error; standard error of measurement (*SEM*) in the denominator.	$RCI = (X_2 - X_1) / SEM$	Jacobson, Follette, & Revenstorf (1984)
Correction with a regression adjustment to the numerator by replacing the observed pretest score with an estimate of the individual's true initial score (which is always closer to the mean).	$RCI_{SPEER} = [X_2 - (r_{xx} (X_1 - M) + M)] / SEM$	Speer (1992)
Correction to replace the *SEM* in the denominator with the standard error of difference (*SED*) between two observed test scores.	$RCI_{JT} = (X_2 - X_1) / SED$	Jacobson & Truax (1991)
Correction that accounts for practice effects by subtracting a constant value (typically, the mean amount of group improvement or decrement over a specified interval in a control sample) from the observed difference score.	$RCI_{CHEL} = [(X_2 - X_1) - (M_2 - M_1)] / SED$	Chelune et al. (1993)
Correction for the effects of regression to the mean by replacing the observed difference score with a "residualized gain" score to take into account an individual's level of performance relative to the group mean; standard error term relevant to a residual change score is the standard error of prediction (*SEP*).	$RCI_{HSU} = [(X_2 - M_2) - r_{xx} (X_1 - M_1)] / SEP$	Hsu (1989, 1999)
Correction to account for regression to the mean due to measurement unreliability using the reliability of the difference score (r_{DD}); the *SED* term is retained but is calculated based on separate *SEM*s for the pretest and posttest.	$RC_{ID} = [r_{DD} (X_2 - X_1) + (1 - r_{DD}) (M_2 - M_1)) / (SEM_1^2 + SEM_2^2)^{1/2}$	Hageman & Arrindell (1993, 1999a, 1999b)

measures can be quite poor (Heilbronner et al., 2010). Given the importance of memory assessment and the requirement for evidence of cognitive decline (American Psychiatric Association, 2013) for dementia diagnoses, clinicians must be cognizant of these issues when interpreting change in diagnostic contexts. Some studies have shown the application of RCI and SRB procedures to be significantly associated with diagnostic change in older adults (Frerichs & Tuokko, 2006). Which approach a clinician chooses to employ may be dependent on the clinical condition of interest, the interval between assessments, and the ease of application within the clinical context.

With repeat administrations of tests, intraindividual change becomes more salient than norm-referenced performance per se. For example, for older adults with limited formal schooling, the very process of "taking a test" may be unfamiliar and result in an underestimate of performance at the first testing (Meyer & Logan, 2013). This may partially explain the observation that people seem to show the biggest practice gains between the first and second administration (Goldberg, Harvey, Wesnes, Snyder, & Schneider, 2015). Various data-driven and theoretical papers have recently been written on the consideration of practice effects in serial assessment: we refer the reader to Duff (2012), Goldberg et al. (2015), and Heilbronner et al. (2010) as a starting point. These papers consider the influence of demographic variables, different testing contexts, and different types of tests, and describe how each of these may influence intraindividual change through repeat assessment.

Normal Cognitive Aging in Context

The availability and application of normative comparisons standards are of critical importance for identifying impairment within and across cognitive domains. Often, however, this information does not consider all important demographic characteristics of the individuals seen in a clinical context. As noted, while normative standards often allow for age, gender, and educational attainment, many other factors can influence test performance. Clinicians need to be aware of these factors and, whenever possible, seek out additional information to help interpret test scores.

Physical Health

One potential factor contributing to cognitive deterioration among persons without neurological conditions such as dementia is decline in physical health stemming from a wide range of medical conditions, including cardiovascular disease or disorders affecting the endocrine and metabolic systems (Armstrong & Morrow, 2010). As is well known, the prevalence of many medical conditions rises with age, and by 80 years of age, the majority of older adults will exhibit at least one medical condition. As noted earlier, to restrict the normative sample to only those older adults with no medical conditions would be highly selective and not typical. When a standardization sample is derived from an unselected population that includes people with a range of medical conditions except those with specific conditions known to directly affect cognitive functions (i.e., NCDs such as AD), some degree of cognitive impairment related to these medical conditions may be present. While this type of sample may represent what is typical or normal in the context of daily life, comparison standards based on this group may underestimate the cognitive expectations for those individuals without these medical conditions. As yet, there is no consensus on the magnitude of these effects; some authors assert that these effects are small (Aarts et al., 2011), while others have shown that they can be substantial (Bergman & Almkvist, 2015). In Bergman and Almkvist's (2015) study of 118 healthy volunteers ages 26–91, controlling for physical health clearly mattered for older adults with normative scores on a variety of cognitive measures, rising by up to .8 of the test-specific *SD* at age 80. For example, performance on the Controlled Oral Word Association Test (COWAT) showed a plateau at age 70, when health factors were not controlled, but showed a continuous rise with age, when health factors were controlled. Using unadjusted scores increases the risk of making false-positive errors for healthy people who have no common medical concerns. That is, norms uncontrolled for health factors overestimate the negative influence of advancing age. This appeared to be related to the greater degree of interindividual variability that occurs with increasing age (Christensen et al., 1994).

Linguistic and Cultural Diversity

Other factors that can affect performance on cognitive measures include linguistic and cultural diversity. Yet, the availability of normative standards for comparison purposes in a broad range of language and cultural context is only beginning to emerge. Particularly in the context of diagnostic assessment of older adults, linguistic and cultural biases can lead to false-positive identification of neurocognitive disorders (McCurry et al., 2001). Typically, cognitive measures developed in English have been translated for use across populations differing in preferred language (Tuokko et al., 2009), and people fluent in that language would administer, score, and interpret the findings. Certainly, normative comparison standards can be developed for these translated measures (i.e., with speakers of that language), but this does not ensure that the same constructs are being measured or that the content and difficulty level is comparable to the original version of the test (American Educational Research Association, American Psychological Association, & National Council on Measurement in Education, 2014).

Evidence on the reliability, validity, and comparability of scores would need to be reported. For example, Fortin and Caza (2014) have demonstrated the utility of measures of memory and executive functions in older French-speaking Canadians and have provided normative data for a composite score for use in assessing older adults. When information about translated tests is lacking, the clinician must be cautious in drawing conclusions based on test performance alone. When translated measures are not available, an interpreter who has a basic understanding of the process of psychological assessment, who speaks the language of the test taker, and who is familiar with the cultural background may be involved in the assessment but cannot provide assistance to the test taker that may compromise the validity of the assessment. For people who are multilingual, the language of administration and response may need to be carefully considered because switching languages may, in fact, change the nature of the task at hand and the norms available (in either language) may no longer be valid comparison standards.

In addition to issues related to language administration and response, cultural context may affect cognitive test performance in that the strategies and elements contained within the assessment process may not be common to all cultures (Ardila, 2007). At least five different aspects of culture have been identified that potentially can affect cognitive test performance. These include patterns of abilities, cultural values, familiarity, language and educational attainment. It may not be feasible to have normative information available for all languages and cultures; it is critically important that clinicians understand the variables that can potentially affect cognitive test performance and take them into consideration when making clinical judgements under less than ideal conditions.

Lifelong Disadvantage

In cases of those who have experienced lifelong disadvantages, it may be that performance on measures of cognitive functioning has always been poor relative to age-associated normative standards. The challenge is to determine whether any changes in functioning experienced as the person ages reflect the consequence of biological, psychological, and social factors associated with normal aging or are indicative of underlying pathological change. While it has been shown that people with low educational attainment are at increased risk of an AD diagnosis, it cannot be assumed that any decline in cognitive or everyday functioning is necessarily indicative of underlying brain pathology.

Intellectual Disabilities

Individuals with intellectual disabilities (ID) present as a particularly vulnerable group for whom the impact of aging is of rising concern and is only beginning to be understood. This is in part because the life expectancy of people with ID has increased markedly in recent decades owing to advances in medical and public health care and changes in societal attitudes (Krinsky–McHale & Silverman, 2013). Life expectancy for those with mild ID is near parity with the general population, and those with moderate or severe ID are living into their late 60s and 50s, respectively (Bittles et al., 2002; Patja, Iivanainen, Vesala, Oksanen, & Ruoppila, 2000). Individuals with ID experience physical aging changes (including brain changes) and age-related chronic diseases, but, as yet, their changing needs often go unrecognized or are poorly managed (Hassiotis, Strydom, Allen, & Walker, 2003; Perkins & Moran, 2010). A number of factors contribute to this situation, including, in some cases, the diminished abilities of individuals with ID to communicate their needs and diagnostic overshadowing, or the tendency of clinicians to dismiss changes in functioning as part of the ID profile rather than acknowledging the co-occurrence of other conditions with ID (Holland, Hon, Huppert, & Stevens, 2000).

One of the greatest areas of concern when assessing people with ID is the lack of a comparison standard for determining change. There is large interindividual variability in cognitive and functional abilities within the population of people with ID, making use of a normative group approach difficult, if not completely inapplicable (Krinsky–McHale & Silverman, 2013; Zeilinger, Stiehl, & Weber, 2013). Instead, each individual will present with a lifelong profile of strengths and weaknesses that will provide the basis for identification of change (Krinsky–McHale & Silverman, 2013). The Working Group for the Establishment of Criteria for the Diagnosis of Dementia in Individuals with Intellectual Disability (Burt & Aylward, 2000) recommends that an objective baseline level of performance be obtained when individuals with ID are cognitively "healthy" before the age at which risk increases. This allows for ipsative comparisons (i.e., within the person) over time to assist in a more accurate detection of decline than can be achieved without such a baseline for comparison.

In recent years, a growing number of assessment tools have been evaluated for use in detecting cognitive decline in people with ID (see Table 5.3) (Elliott-King et al., 2016; Pyo, Kripakaran, Curtis, Curtis, & Markwell, 2007; Zeilinger et al., 2013). The use of instruments not designed for people with ID may not take important characteristics of people with ID into consideration, and their use is not typically recommended (Zeilinger et al., 2013). Measures useful for assessing the cognitive functioning of people with ID can be grouped into three categories: (1) test batteries that include various subtests for direct assessment of the person with ID and an informant report; (2) cognitive tests for direct assessment of the person with ID; and (3) informant reports (Elliott-King et al., 2016; Zeilinger et al., 2013). Many measures appear suitable for use with people with ID, and test batteries provide the most information concerning the assessment of cognition (Elliott-King et al., 2016; Zeilinger et al., 2013). However, each measure should be reviewed with respect to length, level of ID for whom it is most suitable, and setting where the measure will be used. In addition, physical and sensory impairments, language skills, and capacity for reflection and introspection of the person with ID being assessed need to be taken into consideration (Kuske, Wolff, Govert, & Muller, 2017; Pyo et al., 2007). Shorter cognitive measures and a reliance on informant reports may be most suitable for people with severe disability (Elliott-King et al., 2016). Direct assessment of cognition with test batteries or other measures of cognition can be used effectively for people with mild ID (Zeilinger et al., 2013), typically in association with informant reports. As yet, there is no agreed upon procedure for assessing cognition in people with ID as a baseline or for detecting changes in functioning. Further research is clearly needed. From both clinical and research perspectives, facilitating communication about, and comparability of, measures will prove beneficial.

Observed changes in behavior and functioning may occur as a consequence of many precipitants. With the aging process for people with ID comes changes in physical, psychological, and social domains similar to those changes seen in the general population (Kalsy-Lillico, Adams, & Oliver, 2012). Social networks and opportunities may diminish. Environmental changes may occur more frequently than in the past (e.g., loss of a loved one, change in residence), as may changes in physical functioning, some of which may be syndrome-specific. For example, older adults with cerebral palsy (who often have ID) show accelerated musculoskeletal system aging that may lead to loss of mobility, chronic fatigue, and chronic pain (Perkins & Moran, 2010). Older adults with Down syndrome (DS) show accelerated aging characterized by increased rates of hearing loss, osteoporosis, hypothyroidism, sleep apnea, and a genetically elevated risk of developing AD (Lott & Dierssen, 2010; Lott et al., 2012; Perkins & Moran, 2010). While not all people with DS will show clinical signs of dementia, when present, disturbance in cognition (e.g., memory, praxis) and changes in personality with behavioral disorders can markedly compromise everyday functioning (Anderson-Mooney, Schmitt, Head, Lott, & Heilman, 2016). Individuals with some other forms of ID are also at increased risk of dementia, and the onset of age-related declines in people with ID occurs at younger ages than in the general population (Lin, Wu, Lin, Lin, & Chu, 2011). The clinical presentation of incipient dementia in people with ID can differ from that seen in non-ID populations. Early behavioral and personality changes have been reported, especially in persons with DS (Zeilinger et al., 2013). Much of the work related to cognitive assessment in people with ID has been within the context of diagnosing dementia in adults with ID, including those with DS.

TABLE 5.3. Cognitive Assessment Tools for Intellectually Disabled People

Measure and authors	Comments
Examples of test batteries	
Test Battery for Dementia in Intellectual Disability (Burt & Aylward, 1998)	Developed for the American Association on Mental Retardation (now the American Association on Intellectual and Developmental Disabilities); includes an informant report
Neuropsychological Assessment of Dementia in Adults with Intellectual Disability (Crayton, Oliver, Holland, Bradbury, & Hall, 1998)	Developed for people with ID
Neuropsychological Test Battery for Dementia in Down Syndrome (Jozsvai, Kartakis, & Collings, 2002)	Developed for people with ID; includes an informant report, the Dementia Scale for Down Syndrome
Battery for Early Detection of Dementia in Down Syndrome (Johansson & Terenius, 2002)	Developed for people with ID; includes an informant report; all measures are newly developed (i.e., no previously existing measures included)
Examples of cognitive tests for direct assessment	
Dementia Rating Scale (Mattis, 1988)	Suitable for use with people with ID
Down's Syndrome Mental Status Exam (Haxby, 1989)	Developed for use with people with ID
Modified Selective Reminding Test (Buschke, 1973)	Measure of memory; suitable for use with people with ID
Shultz MMSE (Shultz et al., 2004)	Developed for use with people with ID
Examples of informant reports	
Dementia Screening Questionnaire for Individuals with Intellectual Disabilities (Deb, Hare, Prior, & Bhaumik, 2007)	
National Task Group on Intellectual Disabilities and Dementia Practices— Early Detection Screen for Dementia (NTG-EDSD) (*https://aadmd.org/index.php?q=ntg/screening*)	Designed to be a baseline assessment for longitudinal follow-up; available in many languages

Other Special Circumstances

The situation for high-functioning people is somewhat different in that significant cognitive changes may go undetected as they continue to perform within the age-associated average or high-average range on neuropsychological tests (Rentz et al., 2000). This has significant implications for prognosis and treatment. High-functioning people have greater cognitive reserve and may be able to compensate both behaviorally and neurologically for ongoing neural damage (Stern, 2002). As a consequence, when cognitive impairments are detected, subsequent decline may be far more rapid than seen in the general population (Stern, 2002), with no opportunity for intervention. For these reasons it is extremely important to ensure that appropriate comparison standards (e.g., education-adjusted; ipsative comparisons over time) are employed for detecting cognitive changes in this segment of the population.

Other highly vulnerable groups are very old individuals who may be of low educational attainment, physically frail, or confronted with rapidly changing sociocultural circumstances. While a person's cognitive functioning may fall within the expected age-associated range on individual measures of cognition, they may face challenges in complex problem solving as a consequence of difficulty effectively integrating multiple sources of information (Willis, 1996). Basic cognitive functions are necessary components of complex decision making but may be insufficient for generating alternative solutions, evaluating the options for feasibility given the circumstances, prioritizing the viable options, and formulating an action plan (Willis, 1996). Some assistance in everyday decision making may be required, even though their cognitive functioning is typical of their age cohort.

Selection and Use of Normative Standards

The selection of appropriate normative datasets for interpretation of raw test data rests on the assumption that the characteristics of the standardization sample are similar to the characteristics of the person being assessed. However, given the number and types of cognitive measures administered, it may be necessary to use a number of normative data sets derived from different standardization samples. If these norms differ with respect to the application of adjustments for demographic characteristics known to influence cognitive test performance (e.g., age, gender, educational attainment), the interpretation of the data may be dramatically affected (Kalechstein, van Gorp, & Rapport, 1998). In their comparison across different normative datasets, it was observed that the same test score could yield as many as four different clinical classifications (e.g., Average, Low Average, Borderline, and Impaired) (Kalechstein et al., 1998). The magnitude of variability observed across datasets varied as a function of test-specific (e.g., reliability of the measure) and population-specific (e.g., corrections for age and gender) factors. In the absence of a single, comprehensive set of normative data that is large, demographically broad, and representative of the specific population to which it is to be applied, most clinicians are likely to turn to multiple sets of comparison standards developed on standardization samples with differing characteristics (e.g., norms controlled and uncontrolled for common medical conditions). For example, the clinician may select: (1) norms that consider the moderating variable that is most likely to affect the individual's performance (e.g., age is most likely to affect speeded tasks, whereas education may be expected to influence scores on measures of verbal achievement); (2) norms that take into account the moderating effect of extreme deviations in demographic characteristics (e.g., no or very low educational attainment); (3) norms where samples sizes within cells are large enough to provide precise estimates of population parameters; (4) norms developed relatively recently as increases on measures of cognitive functions have been observed over time (e.g., the Flynn effect) and older norms may underestimate expected levels of performance; (5) norms matched in terms of geographical and socioeconomic distribution; or (6) norms relevant to the level of functioning being addressed in the referral question (e.g., identification of deficits versus competence level in rehabilitation or decision-making contexts) (Kalechstein et al., 1998).

Summary and Conclusions

Knowledge concerning the expected, universally experienced trajectories of age-associated change in cognitive functioning forms the necessary foundation for the identification of atypical deterioration. In developing and selecting appropriate comparison standards for detecting impaired functioning within and across cognitive domains, numerous factors need to be considered. Characterization of the standardization sample used to develop normative information is critically important. However, many factors have been identified that influence cognitive aging, and defining the "best" comparison standard is becoming increasingly complex. While it is well known that age, gender, and educational attainment are often associated with cognitive performance, health status and linguistic and cultural diversity also play a role in determining what may be considered a "typical" performance on a measure of cognition. The availability of longitudinal data from large epidemiological studies that contain suitable measures of cognitive functioning (e.g., do not have floor or ceiling effects) is providing the opportunity to examine the equivalency of normative data generated for medically heterogeneous groups, adults with specific medical conditions known to impact cognition, and medically healthy groups.

Other factors found to influence cognitive function such as fluency in the language of test administration can also be examined in many of these large datasets. Being able to adjust normative expectations based on these empirical investigations may improve diagnostic accuracy and reduce the possibility of misdiagnosis. Access to longitudinal data on large epidemiological samples is providing the opportunity to confront some of the drawbacks arising from dependence on cross-sectional data (e.g., inability to identify cases with underlying disorders of cognition at a single assessment). However, when using longitudinal data, the challenge becomes how best to distinguish between true change in cognitive functions and measurement error. Knowing what type and how much cognitive change is associated with primary or normal aging is crucial for determining how much change, and in what cognitive domains, is diagnostically significant. Given the increasing complexity inherent in interpreting change, multiple sets of comparison standards will likely need to be addressed from samples with differing characteristics and carefully considered when assessing for impairment.

KEY POINTS

✓ Expected age-associated changes in cognition are reflected in normative comparison standards.

✓ Multiple sets of comparison standards may be required to address the particular characteristics of a client.

✓ Several methods for assessing change in cognitive function over time have been proposed, and the "best" approach for clinicians to adopt will depend on the clinical condition of interest, interval between assessments, and ease of application.

✓ Many factors can influence test performance (e.g., health status, linguistic and cultural diversity).

✓ Individuals for whom premorbid functioning falls at the extreme ends of the normal distribution of cognitive functioning require special consideration to ensure appropriate interpretation of change.

CHAPTER 6

⚕ Subjective Cognitive Decline

In the field of cognitive aging and dementia, the phenomenon of SCD is rapidly gaining interest and traction in the literature, including a relatively recent special issue of the *Journal of Alzheimer's Disease* devoted entirely to this topic (Tales et al., 2015). SCD refers to a syndrome whereby older adults complain or are concerned about perceived declines in cognitive abilities, yet they perform within normal limits on standardized neuropsychometric and other clinical measures and retain normal function in instrumental activities of daily living (Jessen et al., 2014). While this might sound characteristic of the average healthy older adult, accumulating evidence suggests that persons with SCD are distinct from those with normal aging and that SCD is a valid clinical entity with diverse etiologies and phenomenologies. A major driving force behind interest in SCD is its relationship to preclinical AD. Longitudinal research suggests that SCD confers an increased risk of developing AD (Jessen et al., 2010; Reisberg et al., 2008; Reisberg, Shulman, Torossian, Leng, & Zhu, 2010), particularly in persons who present with relevant biomarkers such as amyloid pathology or who are *APOE* ε4 positive (e.g., Dik et al., 2001; van Harten et al., 2013). Conversely, cross-sectional studies show that persons with SCD are more likely to manifest biomarkers of AD as compared to healthy controls (Amariglio et al., 2012; Perrotin, Mormio, Madison, Hayenga, & Jagust, 2012; Visser et al., 2009). This suggests that, at least for some individuals, SCD may be the first prodromal sign of AD, particularly those with positive biomarkers of the disease (Jessen et al., 2014). However, even for individuals without preclinical AD, SCD may be associated with important cognitive and emotional outcomes that warrant clinical attention. In this chapter, we discuss the current state of the science on SCD, factors that can influence the report of cognitive complaints in older adults, and assessment methods and preliminary recommendations for the care of these older adults.

Evolution and Operationalization of the Construct of SCD

In routine clinical practice, older adults with significant concerns about cognitive decline, in the presence of normal clinical assessment, may previously have been regarded as "worried well" and provided with reassurance about the normalcy of their cognitive status. However, over the past decade, retrospective analyses of longitudinal data from large epidemiological studies have begun to reveal that persons who developed MCI and dementia, particularly AD, often complained of perceived decline in cognitive abilities for many years before objective symptoms emerged—as long as 15 years prior to a diagnosis (Amieva et al., 2008; Reisberg et al., 2008). Subsequently, researchers and clinicians believe that SCD presents a unique window of opportunity not only to detect people who may be at risk for AD, but also to implement interventions that could slow the progress of decline (Jessen et al., 2014; Smart et al., 2017).

The Subjective Cognitive Decline Initiative Working Group

SCD is a complex construct with heterogeneous etiologies and phenomenologies. A significant proportion of individuals with SCD are estimated to decline to AD, and this has largely been the group of most interest to date. However, SCD may also occur as a prodrome to other dementias (e.g., vascular dementia; Slot et al., 2016), or it may be associated with chronic, nondegenerative psychological and physical health conditions that nevertheless impair quality of life. As such, regardless of etiology, older adults with SCD are an important population for assessment and treatment, whether to improve current function or to bolster existing reserves to buffer against anticipated cognitive decline. In 2012, the Subjective Cognitive Decline Initiative (SCD-I) Working Group was formed in response to the challenge of understanding the complex and evolving construct of SCD. The SCD-I is an international group of clinician–scientists with expertise in AD/dementia research that has conducted research on SCD.

Proposed Diagnostic Criteria for SCD

The first task of the SCD-I was to create consensus criteria for the empirical study of SCD in aging studies, and the so-called Jessen criteria for SCD were published in 2014 (Jessen et al., 2014). In brief, to be classified as having SCD, the individual must report self-experienced persistent decline in cognitive ability relative to prior levels of function and unrelated to an acute event, occurring in the context of normal neuropsychological test performance and normal functional abilities. The decline cannot be better accounted for by either a psychiatric or neurologic condition, medication, or substance use. This paper also presented "SCD *plus*" guidelines for persons at particular risk for preclinical AD, requiring that the individual have subjective decline in memory (versus other cognitive domains), have an age of onset of SCD greater than 60 years, have specific concerns or worries about SCD, particularly relative to same-age peers, and show positive biomarkers of preclinical AD.

Rabin et al. (2015) found that, across international sites, a great diversity of participants and methods are currently being used to study SCD, and it is therefore unlikely that one could impose one set of strict, homogeneous criteria that all researchers should follow. Follow-up work by Molinuevo et al. (2017) provides guidelines on how the Jessen criteria can be operationalized and implemented within research studies, promoting harmonization across studies while acknowledging that individual studies may differ in aims and scope.

The SCD-I is rapidly growing in membership and continues to focus on projects related to promoting harmonization across international groups in order to facilitate the most nuanced understanding of this complex construct. Emerging areas of focus include establishing rates of decline associated with other dementias (Slot et al., 2016), using biomarkers in conjunction with SCD to determine risk for AD (Buckley et al., 2016b), identifying self-report items that differentiate those with SCD from healthy older adults (Sikkes et al., 2017), and ascertaining the quality of evidence for nonpharmacological interventions in SCD (Smart et al., 2017).

Rates of Cognitive Decline in SCD

As noted earlier, an accumulating evidence base indicates that SCD—particularly SCD with AD biomarkers—confers increased prospective risk of decline to AD. Knowledge of the base rates of SCD associated with future decline is critical in being able to appropriately inform clients regarding the magnitude of risk and realistic likelihood of pathologic cognitive decline. For example, giving someone a diagnosis of SCD will mean significantly different things if the estimated rate of non-normal cognitive decline from SCD is 5% versus 50%. Unfortunately, with the relatively recent emergence of SCD as a distinct concept of study, the exact rates of decline remain unclear and can differ substantially across studies. For example, Reisberg and colleagues (2010) found that, over a 7-year period, more than half of the sample with SCD (54.2%) declined to either MCI or dementia diagnoses, as compared to only 14.9% of persons without SCD. Furthermore, persons with SCD declined more rapidly, at about 60% greater than the rate of healthy controls. In contrast, a recent meta-analysis found that 10.9% of older adults with SCD were at risk of developing dementia over four years, twice the number of those with no such complaints (Mitchell, Beaumont, Ferguson, Yadegarfer, & Stubbs, 2014). Other research has focused on longitudinal prediction of decline using SCD in concert with relevant biomarkers. Here again, the evidence is mixed, often showing dissociations between cognitive decline and clinical conversion. Scheef et al. (2012) found that persons with SCD demonstrated memory declines that were associated with glucose metabolism in brain regions associated with AD. In a sample of persons with SCD and evidence of preclinical AD based on cerebrospinal fluid markers, van Harten et al. (2013) also found evidence of declines on tests of memory, executive functions, and global cognition, but not progression to clinical diagnosis over a 2-year period. Finally, Buckley and colleagues (2016a) assessed a sample of clinically normal persons who were beta-amyloid positive based on PET imaging. Classifying individuals as having "high" or "low" SCD, they found that having high SCD was associated with an approximately fivefold greater rate of progression to MCI or dementia, but this was not associated with decline on episodic memory over 3 years.

There are at least four major difficulties in ascertaining the rate and frequency of decline of persons with SCD to AD and other dementias. The first is the *sampling window within which the estimates are taken.* For example, if SCD is a preclinical phase that lasts approximately 15 years (Amieva et al., 2008; Reisberg et al., 2008), then those in the 4-year period at the beginning of that phase may show significantly less decline than those in the 4 years closer to the end of the window, where people are very close in time to emergence of a clinical diagnosis because of objective cognitive impairment. Thus, a sampling window of participants older in age and closer to time of diagnosis is likely to reveal higher estimates as compared to a sampling window with younger participants more distal from time to diagnosis.

The second issue is the *demography of the sample in question.* For example, one source of data on SCD may be from participants in community-based studies of older adults where assessment of complaints is cursory and is part of a much larger battery of self-report measures. Some degree of complaint is typical and to be expected in a healthy older adult population (Cooper et al., 2011; Slavin et al., 2010). However, complaints in this context are likely to mean something different than complaints that come from individuals who present to a memory disorders clinic, which likely denotes a much higher level of concern and also higher probability of actually having preclinical AD (Coley et al., 2008).

A third issue is the *terminology used to describe SCD.* An evolving entity in the literature, SCD was variously referred to in the past as subjective cognitive impairment (Reisberg & Gauthier, 2008; Reisberg et al., 2008), subjective memory impairment (Jessen et al., 2010), and cognitive complaints (Saykin et al., 2006). Obviously, different operational definitions of SCD could result in significantly different estimates of prevalence of the phenomenon itself, as well as anticipated rates of decline to MCI and dementia. Further compounding this issue is the use of SCD as a diagnosis versus a descriptive term, something that the study of MCI has struggled with for the last decade. The lack of a consistent definition for SCD was noted by Abdulrab and Heun (2008), who called for the creation of consensus criteria to define this phenomenon. The SCD-I Working Group was formed in 2012 for this express purpose and to harmonize international research on this topic.

The fourth and final issue is the focus on *memory as the primary criterion of complaint*. SCD has garnered significant interest because of the proportion of such persons who are at risk of declining to AD. Persons with AD show prominent episodic memory impairment, and individuals with the amnestic variant of mild cognitive impairment (aMCI) show the greatest risk of conversion to AD as compared to other dementias (Albert et al., 2011), which likely explains an almost-exclusive focus on the measurement of memory complaints in prior studies (Rabin et al., 2015). However, SCD itself is emerging as an etiologically heterogeneous syndrome and may be predictive of other conditions beyond AD, including other dementias (Slot et al., 2016). Moreover, even in the case of AD, memory complaints per se are somewhat common in the healthy older adult population (Cooper et al., 2011; Slavin et al., 2010) and may have limited specificity and predictive value when it comes to ascertaining SCD with preclinical AD (St. John & Montgomery, 2002; Wang et al., 2000). As such, researchers have acknowledged that, rather than focusing on memory exclusively, the term *cognitive* may better capture the phenomenon of SCD (Jessen et al., 2014; Reisberg et al., 2008), acknowledging the fact that other cognitive domains may be differentially pathognomonic of different trajectories of cognitive decline. Further longitudinal studies using the new "Jessen criteria" (Jessen et al., 2014) may promote harmonization of approaches to researching SCD and subsequent answers to outstanding questions such as the rate and frequency of decline in persons with SCD.

What does all of this mean for the individual clinician working with the individual client? Clinicians would be advised to consider the following: (1) the age of the individual in question relative to the duration of perceived decline, (2) who initiated the referral (e.g., the individual based on his or her own concern, general practitioner check-up), (3) complaints in cognitive domains beyond memory, particularly those beyond complaints of normal aging such as word-finding and episodic memory retrieval difficulties, and (4) the severity of complaints and/or their perceived impact on functioning.

Many, or even all, of these challenges in predicting rates of decline have plagued the field of MCI for at least a decade and have no easy answers. In turn, perhaps the study of SCD can learn from shortcomings in the MCI literature to move expeditiously forward in understanding those for whom SCD truly represents a dementia prodrome.

Objective Markers of Decline in Persons with SCD

A core feature of neuropsychological assessment is standardized neuro-psychometric testing, whereby an individual's performance is compared to that of persons with similar age, education, and other demographic backgrounds. According to the Jessen criteria (Jessen et al., 2014), normal performance on neuropsychometric tests is a core criterion for diagnosis of SCD. Given the significant numbers of individuals predicted to decline to AD and other dementias, this suggests that neuropsychometric tests, as typically administered, lack the requisite sensitivity to detect the subtle levels of decline experienced by older adults with SCD. As such, one of the biggest challenges that remains is being able to prospectively discriminate persons with SCD from healthy older adults before clinically significant decline is manifest. As SCD is largely based on self-report of cognitive decline, significant work has already been conducted to isolate specific types of cognitive complaints that may be unique to persons with SCD and hold concurrent and predictive validity in terms of decline. In parallel, the field has continued to look for objective indicators to corroborate these self-reports of decline, given the relative insensitivity of standardized neuropsychometric tests as typically administered. Three areas of research foci have emerged: (1) use of biomarkers that suggest preclinical AD or other disorders that could influence cognitive status, (2) experimental–cognitive paradigms sensitive to group differences between healthy older adults and those with SCD, and (3) novel application of existing neuropsychological tests and constructs.

Biomarker Evidence

A variety of studies have shown that self-report of SCD is associated with higher frequency of biomarkers, particularly AD biomarkers of amyloidosis and neurodegeneration. Several studies have shown cross-sectional association between occurrence of SCD and AD-like neurodegeneration, including reduced hippocampal volume (Perrotin et al., 2015; van der Flier et al., 2004), bilateral entorhinal cortex (Jessen et al., 2006), gray matter atrophy (Peter et al., 2014), and cortical thinning and atrophy in medial temporal and frontotemporal regions (Meiberth et al., 2015; Saykin et al., 2006). PET with novel tracers such as Pittsburgh Compound B (PiB) has revealed cross-sectional associations between amyloid burden and SCD, although the evidence is more mixed as compared to that found in studies on neurodegeneration. For example, some studies have found that amyloid burden is positively associated with higher numbers of endorsed memory complaints (Amariglio, Townsend, Gradstein, Sperling, & Rentz, 2011) and perceptions of worse memory compared to peers (Perrotin et al., 2012). However, other studies have found no such association (e.g., Buckley et al., 2013; Chételat et al., 2010; Rodda et al., 2010). Still other work has examined cerebrospinal fluid (CSF), looking for associations between AD profiles and presentation of SCD. For example, Visser and colleagues (2009) found that a CSF profile similar to AD was more common in persons with SCD compared to healthy controls. In terms of *APOE* ε4, a known genetic risk for AD, there have again been mixed findings. Mosconi et al. (2008) found that in persons with SCD who were carriers, they were more likely to show a CSF profile similar to AD, although not in the entire group. Likewise, Antonell and coworkers (2011) failed to find group differences between SCD and healthy controls in terms of their CSF profiles.

Work establishing relationships between biomarkers and self-report of SCD is important, providing an objective means by which to corroborate an individual's complaints before clinical symptoms are manifest. Although the evidence is somewhat mixed, several studies show associations between AD biomarkers and SCD. Perhaps the reason for the mixed evidence has to do with the different operational definitions of SCD that have been used, as well as the fact that not all persons with SCD decline to AD. Future studies that can elucidate subtypes of SCD may reveal associations with biomarkers related to other neurodegenerative disease processes (e.g., vascular disease).

Experimental–Cognitive Paradigms

Obtaining information on biomarkers is an important source of information in establishing whether changes in brain structure and function underlie an older adult's report of concern. However, a limitation of relying on biomarkers alone is that there is not always a 1:1 relationship between underlying biomarkers, including those of preclinical AD, and observable cognitive function (Stern, 2009, 2012). Moreover, biomarkers beyond simple structural MRI are expensive and sometimes invasive, and access to these outside of specialty academic medical centers may be limited. Given the insensitivity of standard neuropsychometric tests, some researchers have focused on the application of experimental–cognitive paradigms that could detect group differences between healthy older adults and those with SCD. This has at least two benefits. First, experimental paradigms may be more sensitive to detect the kinds of subtle declines experienced by persons with SCD. For example, evidence suggests that reaction time intraindividual variability, or inconsistency in moment-to-moment responding, declines with normal aging and is also a harbinger of later decline and death (Bielak, Hultsch, Strauss, MacDonald, & Hunter, 2010). However, standardized tests, even those using reaction times, do not typically yield a sufficient number of trials to conduct this type of analysis. Second, there already exists a robust literature on cognitive aging and cognitive/affective neuroscience in typical older adults (Kensinger & Gutchess, 2016; Mather, 2016; Peters, Hess, Västfjäll, & Auman, 2007; Verhaeghen, 2013), which provides a comparison point for the performance of persons with suspected SCD.

Memory is a popular focus within studies on cognitive aging and dementia, possibly because AD is the most common form of dementia, and persons with amnestic MCI seem to have the greatest risk of conversion to AD (Albert et al., 2011; Blacker et al., 2007). For example, Koppara et al. (2015) drew on previous work suggesting that memory feature binding—an aspect of visual short-term memory—is a sensitive and specific marker of AD. They found that persons with SCD showed evidence of subtle cognitive deficits on a short-term memory-binding task, even when their standardized memory performance did not differ from controls.

Emerging literature has also examined the role of attention and executive functions in SCD, consistent with prior literature indicating that these constructs may be more sensitive markers at the very earliest stages of nonnormal decline, including both MCI and AD (Saunders & Summers, 2011; Silveri, Reali, Jenner, & Puopolo, 2007; Wylie, Ridderinkhof, Eckerle, & Manning, 2007). Smart and colleagues (Smart, Segalowitz, Mulligan, & MacDonald, 2014a) examined attention capacity as an objective marker of SCD. They administered a computerized go/nogo task and simultaneously recorded the P3 event-related potential (ERP), a biomarker of attention capacity. As compared to demographically matched controls, persons with SCD showed a clearly attenuated P3 ERP, even after controlling for any differences in mood, anxiety, and neuroticism. This is consistent with existing literature showing that the P3 is attenuated in persons with AD (Jeong, 2004; Olichney & Hillert, 2004; Polich, 2004). Interestingly, despite the P3 attenuation, persons with SCD did not perform worse behaviorally on the task. This could suggest that, despite objective changes in brain function, individuals are early enough in the decline process that they can actively compensate for such changes. However, in the same sample of older adults, Mulligan, Smart, and Ali (2016) found evidence of behavioral differences on the Multi-Source Interference Test, a task with low and high cognitive control conditions. While there were no differences in mean reaction time (RT), persons with SCD showed reduced accuracy across all trial types and greater RT variability as compared to healthy controls.

Decision making, considered a higher-order aspect of executive functions, has also been examined in SCD. Delay discounting is the phenomenon whereby most people tend to weight future outcomes less heavily than immediate ones when making decisions. Hu, Weber, Kleinshmidt, and Jessen (2014) administered a computer-based delay-discounting task to persons with SCD and healthy controls (both older and younger) and found that the SCD group had a higher rate of discounting than the older controls and a trend toward higher discounting as compared to the younger control group. Moreover, for persons with SCD, the discounting rate significantly negatively correlated with the MMSE and immediate recall on the Consortium to Establish a Registry for Alzheimer's Disease (CERAD), and positively correlated with self-report of present fatalism as measured on the Zimbardo Time Perspective Scale. Smart and Krawitz (2015) examined performance on the Iowa gambling task (Bechara, Damasio, Damasio, & Anderson, 1994), developed as an experimental measure of decision making but now available as a standardized clinical neuropsychological test (Bechara, 2007). Commensurate with the Jessen criteria, groups did not differ on performance on the test based on standardized clinical scoring. However, Bayesian parameter estimation of trial-to-trial performance demonstrated that, compared to healthy controls, individuals with SCD showed evidence of discounting of prior outcomes in favor of temporally contiguous outcomes when making decisions. These studies taken in concert provide interesting insights into the potential decision-making capacity of persons with SCD. Specifically, they present evidence of discounting of both prior and future outcomes, resulting in a more present-moment focus, which could be reflective of difficulties with attention and aspects of executive control such as updating/working memory.

One of the greatest challenges in studying SCD is to separate those individuals from healthy older adults, given normal neuropsychological test scores in both groups. Experimental–cognitive paradigms hold promise to detect cognitive differences in SCD that provide corroboration for their concerns. This work is in the early stages, however, and the predictive validity of these measures requires further study.

Novel Application of Neuropsychological Tests and Constructs

Studies on MCI have suggested that adding specific neuropsychometric criteria to diagnostic decision making, above and beyond clinical consensus, improves the reliability and validity of resultant diagnoses (Bondi et al., 2014). Applying this approach to SCD becomes challenging, given that affected persons are, by definition, a population that scores within normal limits on standardized tests. This has led researchers to examine neuropsychological tests in novel ways in order to seek reliable and valid metrics of objective decline in persons with SCD. The aforementioned study by Smart and Krawitz (2015) is one such example, where a standardized test, the Iowa gambling task, was subjected to more advanced statistical analysis using Bayesian parameter estimation to uncover group differences compared to healthy controls. Rabin and colleagues (2014) sought to determine whether prospective memory could reveal cognitive difficulties in persons with SCD. Prospective memory, defined as memory for future intentions (Einstein & McDaniel, 1990; van den Berg, Kant, & Postma, 2012), is more complex than other forms of memory. It involves not only episodic encoding and consolidation of a cue (e.g., hear an alarm) and its associated activity (e.g., go to the dentist), but executive control in terms of being vigilant to the future occurrence of the cue and following through on the desired action. They administered a novel clinical test, the Royal Prince Alfred Prospective Memory (RPA-ProMem) test, to persons with SCD and MCI, as well as healthy controls. Despite intact performance on typical episodic memory tests, persons with SCD scored significantly lower than healthy controls on long-term, naturalistic subtasks (i.e., those that more closely mimic real-world events) of the RPA-ProMem. Given the additional executive demands of this task, this finding is consistent with the aforementioned studies indicating that difficulties in attention and executive control in persons with SCD may be more sensitive to objective cognitive impairment than traditional episodic memory tasks. Research on prospective memory is also important, given its ecological relevance to the daily lives of older adults.

Recently, Edmonds and colleagues (2015b) discussed the concept of "subtle" cognitive decline, defined in actuarial terms based on neuropsychometric test performance. They defined subtle cognitive decline as impaired scores (>1 *SD* below age-corrected norms) on two measures in different cognitive domains, as well as a score of 6–8 on the Functional Assessment Questionnaire. They found that this criterion had predictive value in determining who would decline to MCI and AD using data from the Alzheimer's Neuroimaging Disease Initiative and that it provides an operational definition of the subtle cognitive decline referenced in the National Institute on Aging–Alzheimer's Association (NIA-AA) criteria on preclinical AD (Sperling et al., 2011).

Emerging literature suggests that highly educated persons with SCD show greater likelihood of showing concurrent (Mulligan et al., 2016; Smart et al., 2014a; Smart & Krawitz, 2015) and future non-normal cognitive decline (Jonker, Geerlings, & Schmand, 2000; van Oijen, de Jong, Hofman, Koudstaal, & Breteler, 2007). Such persons may score normally on standardized tests due to greater cognitive reserve and compensatory capacity (Stern, 2009, 2012), yet have greater awareness of premorbid abilities and associated sensitivity to subtle performance declines. Rentz et al. (2004) discussed the use of IQ-adjusted norms to predict progressive decline in older adults with above-average intelligence. While this work was published before the proliferation of research on SCD, reanalysis of existing datasets with highly educated older adults may reveal the same types of subtle cognitive declines discussed by Edmonds and colleagues (2015b).

In sum, clinical-neuropsychological tests remain the gold standard for ascertainment of current clinical impairment in cognitive abilities, yet as typically applied and scored, these seem insensitive to impairment in persons with SCD. The studies discussed show promise for novel ways of employing these tests or analyzing the associated data in order to provide objective corroboration of the cognitive concerns of persons with SCD.

Operationalizing the Diagnosis of SCD in Clinical Practice

While a great many tools exist to capture brain and behavioral functioning in older adults, standardized neuropsychometric testing remains the gold standard for assessing current cognition and for ascertaining clinically significant deviations from normative functioning. Moreover, even at stages where objective impairment is more evident (i.e., MCI), the addition of neuropsychometric data is known to increase diagnostic sensitivity and precision (Bondi et al., 2014). However, given that SCD by definition denotes normal performance on neuropsychological testing, understanding the meaning of complaints and concerns in this context becomes a clinical conundrum for neuropsychologists and other professionals conducting assessments of older adults. Reisberg et al. (2008) referred to SCD as the stage "where the patient knows, but the doctor doesn't know" (p. S105). However, this does not mean that the clinician cannot use the wealth of other information at his or her disposal to characterize a person's current functioning.

Neuropsychological assessment is a holistic and integrative assessment process whereby test results are interpreted within a biopsychosocial framework, including in-depth clinical interview with the client and a relevant informant (e.g., partner, family member), detailed information on medical and psychiatric history, as well as review of available neuroimaging studies. As with any diagnostic presentation, the clinician understands that a client's current cognitive function is multiply determined and likewise amenable to improvement through multiple avenues. This is perhaps no more evident than in the case of SCD, given the fact that self-reported complaints are in and of themselves nuanced, complex, and multiply determined (Buckley, Saling, Fromann, Wolfsgruber, & Wagner, 2015). Practically speaking, neuropsychological assessment of persons with suspected SCD should include, at a minimum, a comprehensive clinical interview documenting premorbid and comorbid mood/anxiety disorders and physical health conditions, personality, and complaints pertaining to a broad sampling of cognitive domains, not solely memory (Rabin et al., 2015). Ideally, the client would at some point obtain a comprehensive work-up through his or her primary care provider or neurologist in order to rule out reversible causes of cognitive impairment such as metabolic disturbances (McConnell, 2014).

SCD versus MCI or Dementia

This differential diagnosis is a relatively straightforward proposition. Assuming that the test administration is valid, the presence of impairment on formal neuropsychological testing scored according to appropriate normative comparisons, in conjunction with self/informant reports of decline, effectively rules out SCD and rules in diagnoses associated with objective cognitive impairment. Comprehensive medical examination, including neuroimaging and reversible dementia work-up, will provide supporting information with regard to specific etiology. The extent of impairment, particularly relative to instrumental activities of daily living, will indicate whether MCI or dementia is the more appropriate diagnosis.

SCD versus Normal Aging

This is likely to be the more common—and more challenging—differential diagnosis a clinician will have to make. Although some studies have shown subtle cognitive differences between those with SCD and healthy older adults (e.g., Hu et al., 2014; Smart et al., 2014a; Smart & Krawitz, 2015), these tend to be group-level differences using experimental measures. At the individual client level, there are still no reliable objective measures to corroborate the diagnosis of SCD and differentiate it from normal aging. This necessarily places the emphasis on self-report of decline (Rabin et al., 2015). That said, even in the absence of objective test findings, the clinician can take steps to increase the likelihood of identifying someone who has SCD, particularly individuals who may be at risk for decline to AD or other dementias; these we discuss in the next sections.

Self-Report of Cognitive Complaints

The clinical interview should include a thorough survey of complaints of impairment across all cognitive domains, not just memory. Although memory items are among those most commonly administered (Rabin et al., 2015), several studies suggest that memory, particularly episodic memory, may not have the requisite specificity to differentiate SCD from healthy older adults. For example, Amariglio and coworkers (2011) found that, in the Nurses Health Study, items such as way-finding (i.e., spatial navigation) better predicted incipient cognitive decline. In addition, Smart and colleagues found that objective tests of attention and executive function discriminated those with SCD from healthy controls (Smart et al., 2014a; Smart & Krawitz, 2015; Mulligan et al., 2016) as well as self-report of conscientiousness, items that overlap with self-report of executive function (Smart, Koudys, & Mulligan, 2015). Many of the questionnaires currently available to assess cognitive complaints are individual difference measures (i.e., do not have cut scores to separate clinical from nonclinical groups). Other measures in use have been designed for MCI and dementia samples, assuming that SCD differs from these conditions by degrees of severity only, which has yet to be established (Rabin et al., 2015). Thus, such measures should be used as supporting evidence in the context of a comprehensive assessment, but they will likely not be sufficient to provide definitive answers as to whether someone does or does not meet criteria for SCD.

In terms of recommendations for specific measures, there is no current gold-standard "complaints" measure that can reliably categorize persons with and without SCD. Rabin and colleagues (2015) conducted a comprehensive review and analysis of the various means by which self-report of complaints was being assessed across nineteen international research studies affiliated with the SCD-I. Thirty-four self-report measures were currently in use, comprising 640 self-report items of cognition. There was little overlap across studies, with 75% of measures being used by only one single study. Unsurprisingly, assessment of memory predominated (accounting for 60% of items), with other domains such as executive function (16%) and attention (11%) being represented at a much lower frequency. Many of these measures were being used within the context of large-scale longitudinal studies that had been underway for several years before SCD gained significant attention. Therefore, assessment of SCD was often not the primary driving factor in selection of measures. Rather, the measures being used were often chosen based on practical decisions such as brevity of administration or availability. Research is currently underway within the SCD-I to harmonize self-report items across these international research studies in order to derive items with the greatest sensitivity and specificity for SCD and predictive validity in terms of objective cognitive function and biomarkers (Sikkes et al., 2017).

Based on this review, it was not possible to make specific recommendations for the use of individual measures. Moreover, it may not be possible to identify gold-standard self-report measures, given that complaints are likely to differ as a function of the demographic and cultural context of the assessment. A thorough and detailed clinical-neuropsychological interview will always provide a rich body of information within which to understand the individual's current biopsychosocial function. That said, if individual cognitive complaints measures are to be chosen to supplement the interview, Rabin and colleagues (2015) have offered some preliminary recommendations, including the following:

1. Use measures where item stems are simple and readily understandable (e.g., avoid double-barreled items where the referent of a positive item endorsement is unclear).
2. Use measures that assess individual constructs (e.g., cognition) as opposed to combining multiple constructs within a measure (e.g., cognition associated with mood, health).
3. Assess complaints using cognitive issues that are most pertinent to a given individual's daily life (e.g., it is less reliable to ask about financial ability when the person's spouse has always handled finances).
4. Assess domains beyond episodic memory, given that some episodic

memory changes are observed in normal aging and other aspects of memory—and cognition in general—may be more pathognomonic of non-normal decline at this early stage of SCD.

5. Where possible, assess complaints using a narrow and specific time-frame (e.g., days, weeks, months). Using temporal referents that are more distal (e.g., 5 or 10 years) could decrease the reliability of reporting and make it problematic for respondents to remember individual events.

Cross-Cultural Expression of Complaints

Many of the data on SCD come from Westernized, industrialized samples. As such, a question remains as to the cross-cultural meaning of complaints and how these are expressed. In other words, items that may have construct validity in European or Caucasian samples may not have the same validity in other populations. For example, Jackson and colleagues (2016) examined data from the Harvard Aging Brain Study to examine the relationship between objective and subjective memory performance, specifically comparing Caucasian and African American participants. While both groups complained at a similar rate, those cognitive complaints were associated with objective cognition in the Caucasian sample ($r = -.401$) but not in the African American sample ($r = -.052$). These findings are intriguing because they indicate that the lack of association is not simply a function of a lower endorsement of complaints in the African American sample; the results remained even after controlling for socioeconomic and educational factors.

The first-person, phenomenological experience of SCD is still largely unknown. One cannot assume that measures designed in Westernized (and primarily Caucasian) samples—much less those being used that were originally designed for non-SCD samples—can effectively capture experience across a diversity of populations. Given the emphasis that is placed on self-report of cognitive complaints, this underscores the need to augment item-based, psychometric approaches to assessment of complaints with qualitative approaches that provide rich descriptions of a person's first-person experience of cognitive decline (Buckley et al., 2015; Rabin et al., 2015). In practical terms for the individual clinician, this underscores the importance of asking detailed questions in the clinical interview, and not relying solely on self-report measures for ascertaining cognitive complaints.

Concern as Distinct from Complaints

Emerging studies suggest that, while complaints about cognitive change may be relatively frequent in the older adult population (Cooper et al., 2011; Jonker et al., 2000; Slavin et al., 2010), specific concern or worry about those changes may be a more sensitive indicator of SCD. For example, Jessen and coworkers (2010) analyzed data from the AgeCoDe study, a large-scale, general practice, registry-based study in Germany. Participants were asked, "Do you feel like your memory is becoming worse?" Response options were "no"; "yes, but this does not worry me"; and "yes, this worries me." The researchers assessed participants at baseline and at 1.5- and 3-year follow-up intervals, finding that subjective memory impairment with worry was associated with greatest risk for conversion to any dementia (hazard ratio [HR] = 3.53) or AD (HR = 6.54), with 69% sensitivity and 74.3% specificity. Researchers drawing on data from the same AgeCoDe study investigated whether the temporal stability of SCD report influenced AD dementia risk in healthy older adults. They found that SCD with worry that was consistently reported over time was associated with greatly increased risk of AD (Wolfsgruber et al., 2016). Such findings indicate that concern or worry about decline has incremental predictive validity over report of complaints per se. In separate research conducted in a community sample of volunteers, persons were classified as having SCD based on level of concern or worry using the question, "Are you concerned or worried about changes in your thinking abilities, more than just normal aging?" This classification based on concern was associated with several objective markers of change in both brain (Smart et al., 2014a; Smart, Spulber, & Garcia-Barrera, 2014b) and cognitive function (Mulligan et al., 2016; Smart & Krawitz, 2015).

As cognitive decline progresses to more pathological levels as observed in MCI and dementia, concerns may dwindle as individuals develop anosognosia, or loss of awareness of deficits (Wilson et al., 2016). However, the findings of the aforementioned studies suggest that concern may have specific value at this very early stage of decline in SCD, when individuals retain awareness of their current function. Moreover, because individuals at this stage are likely compensating for subtle changes, they may be more aware of changes that are not obvious to family and health care providers. As such, clinicians are advised to inquire about concern as distinct from report of cognitive complaints, and concern specific to cognitive function rather than generalized worry such as that seen in conditions such as generalized anxiety disorder (although mood/anxiety should still be assessed, as detailed below).

Self-Report of Other Constructs That Could Influence Report of Cognitive Complaints

Just as cognitive function is multiply determined, so is self-report of cognitive function (Buckley et al., 2015). More specifically, self-report of complaints is likely to be influenced by factors such as mood, anxiety, personality (particularly neuroticism and conscientiousness), and current physical health status (Rabin, Smart, & Amariglio, 2017). Clinician-based and self-report assessments of depression, anxiety, personality, and physical health symptoms are a standard component of clinical-neuropsychological assessment, and these take on particular importance in the context of SCD. Understanding the unique sources of variance in self-reported complaints is useful insofar as it may elucidate different subtypes of SCD associated with different etiologies, particularly given that not all persons with SCD will decline to AD (Jessen et al., 2014). Of course, individual measure selection should be appropriate to the particular demographics of the individual under evaluation and may be subject to variation across countries and cultures. That said, some widely used self-report measures that are applicable and relevant in older adult samples include the Geriatric Depression Scale (Yesavage et al., 1983), the Adult Manifest Anxiety Scale–Elderly Version (Lowe & Reynolds, 2006), and the Minnesota Multiphasic Personality Inventory—Second Edition, Restructured Format (Ben-Porath & Tellegen, 2008). Again, a thorough clinical interview can always be used to augment any information obtained through self-administered measures.

Informant Report of Individual's Cognitive Function

The informant report provides an important supplementary piece to augment an individual's self-report of SCD. A reliable informant may provide information to corroborate the manifestation of subtle signs of cognitive decline, even in older adults who lack objective evidence of impairment (Mulligan et al., 2016). Moreover, some studies have shown that informant reports have incremental validity in predicting who will decline to MCI and dementia, as well as the rate of associated cognitive decline (Gifford et al., 2014; Rabin et al., 2012; Slavin et al., 2015). It should be borne in mind, however, that any informant report is liable to be influenced by the respondent's own cognitive function and current mood state (including depression and anxiety), as well as the respondent's level of familiarity with the individual in question. This includes the frequency of contact in any given week, as well as the longevity of the relationship. These are all factors that should be taken into consideration when weighing the impact of the informant report.

The informant report is important at every stage of assessment along the trajectory of cognitive decline, and it is an issue we discuss in each assessment chapter. With respect to specific measures that have been examined in research on SCD, the Informant Questionnaire of Cognitive Decline in the Elderly (IQCODE; Jorm & Jacomb, 1989) has been investigated in several studies. The IQCODE is one of the most widely used informant measure to screen for dementia in older adults, with good reliability and validity to assess a general factor of cognitive decline. The informant is asked to rate the individual across a variety of domains, relative to the individual's performance 10 years ago. Included are items such as recognizing the faces of family and friends, remembering details about family and friends such as names, birthdays, addresses, and autobiographical information (e.g., one's own address and phone number), as well as a variety of items that tap domains such as new learning, episodic memory, semantic knowledge, attention control, and executive function. The original IQCODE included twenty-six items, although a comprehensive review of the available literature by Jorm (2004) suggests that the sixteen-item version performs just as well and is actually preferred.

Another measure that has been specifically examined in the SCD population is the Everyday Cognition Scale (ECog; Farias et al., 2008), a more contemporary measure of cognitive complaints. Like the IQCODE, it asks about the individual's present performance relative to his or her performance 10 years ago on items of memory, language, and attention/executive function. While both of these measures have strengths, a significant limitation is that both use a 10-year time referent which, as discussed above in the context of self-reports, can significantly decrease the reliability and validity of reporting, in this case being influenced by the longevity of the client–informant relationship and the informant's own memory status. As usual, these measures should be considered only one piece of data and supplemented with informant interview, where possible.

Possible Subtypes of SCD Relative to Potential Etiologies

SCD associated with preclinical AD has probably garnered the most attention in the research, likely because AD is the most prevalent dementia, and certain studies report that more than half of participants with SCD eventually decline to MCI and AD (Reisberg & Gauthier, 2008; Reisberg et al., 2010). However, this leaves a large proportion of affected individuals who present with SCD associated with a different etiology. It remains to be seen whether these SCD subtypes have different cognitive and behavioral phenotypes, much as the variants of MCI can differ according to neurodegenerative causes such as AD, PD, and cerebrovascular disease. Although research and clinical guidance on this topic are in their infancy, it behooves clinicians to attempt to ascertain the major contributors to a given client's SCD presentation. As current cognitive function is multiply determined, there is unlikely to be a single explanatory factor. That said, obtaining some understanding of the underlying causes this early in the process could allow for significant early intervention to slow or delay the onset of further decline (Smart et al., 2017).

Obtaining Information on Relevant Biomarkers

Persons with SCD show normal neuropsychometric test performance, which is the usual gold standard of objective evidence of cognitive decline.

However, biomarkers can provide a useful source of objective brain dysfunction and facilitate consideration of different etiological contributions to a given presentation of SCD. The first consideration would be SCD associated with preclinical AD, given the prevalence of AD as the most commonly diagnosed form of dementia. According to the "Jessen criteria" for SCD (Jessen et al., 2014), "SCD *plus*" denotes persons with SCD who also have positive biomarkers of preclinical AD. In 2011, the NIA-AA Workgroup provided recommendations for using biomarkers to define the preclinical stages of AD (Sperling et al., 2011). They proposed a hypothetical model of dynamic biomarkers of AD based on a previously proposed AD pathophysiological cascade model. In their model, the first stage of pathology is cerebral beta-amyloid accumulation, as evidenced via CSF and PET scanning. The next emergent sign is synaptic dysfunction, as evidenced on fluorodeoxyglucose positron emission tomography (FDG-PET) and/or functional magnetic resonance imaging (fMRI). Following on from this, signs of tau-mediated neuronal injury (CSF) and neurodegeneration (volumetric MRI) become evident, as do declines in cognitive and clinical status. Access to these biomarkers is most common at major research centers. However, clinicians at other facilities may only have access to volumetric MRI data. According to Sperling et al.'s (2011) model, negative MRI findings would not preclude an SCD *plus* diagnosis, but would simply denote that the underlying pathophysiology has not yet progressed to a level that is manifest on structural MRI. In this case, then, clinicians should also consider other markers suggestive of SCD *plus* as outlined in Jessen et al. (2014).

Interestingly, this pathophysiological cascade model proposed by Sperling and colleagues (2011) has recently been challenged in the literature. Analyzing data from the Alzheimer's Disease Neuroimaging Initiative (ADNI), Edmonds et al. (2015b) classified 570 cognitively normal participants based on NIA-AA criteria and separately based on each individual's number of abnormal biomarkers or cognitive markers associated with preclinical AD. They found that neurodegeneration alone was 2.5 times more common than amyloidosis alone at baseline. Moreover, for those who demonstrated only one abnormal biomarker at baseline and later progressed to MCI or AD, neurodegeneration was the most common, followed by amyloidosis alone or subtle cognitive decline (defined in a previous section), both of which were equally common. Perhaps this is not surprising, given that persons can show evidence of amyloidosis and neurofibrillary tangles without necessarily developing AD dementia. Rather, the work of Edmonds et al. (2015b) suggests that structural MRI has value in ascertaining early signs of preclinical AD, which is important given that this biomarker is relatively accessible for most clinicians in routine practice.

In the case of preclinical AD, neurodegeneration would likely be evidenced by a characteristic pattern of atrophy involving the medial temporal lobes, as well as paralimbic and temporoparietal cortices (Sperling et al., 2011). However, structural MRI can also be used to evidence patterns of neurodegeneration and disease associated with other etiologies. Thus, structural MRI remains useful in ascertaining other etiologies of SCD beyond preclinical AD. For example, neurodegeneration in the frontal and temporal lobes might indicate signs of FTLD, particularly in younger clients in their 40s or 50s. Conversely, small-vessel ischemic disease or white matter lesions could suggest an underlying process of cerebrovascular etiology.

Non-neurological Etiologies of SCD

If major neurodegenerative diseases have been considered less likely, then the clinician might consider the relative contribution of psychological factors to self-report of SCD. As noted in Chapter 3, depression elevates the risk of all-cause dementia, including AD, and can be associated with cognitive difficulties as well as structural brain changes including gray matter abnormalities within frontal-subcortical and limbic networks (Sexton, McKay, & Ebmeier, 2013) as well as white matter integrity (Allan et al., 2016). Thus, the seriousness of depression as an etiology for SCD should not be minimized; rather, if depression is a significant current concern, it should be rigorously managed not only to improve current mood and quality of life, but also to possibly decrease risk for future cognitive decline. Anxiety disorders might also heighten report of cognitive complaints. In this case, anxiety may stem from a lack of knowledge about expected changes with normal aging; in this instance, provision of psychoeducation around normative age-related cognitive change may serve to decrease anxiety and concomitant report of cognitive complaints. However, as noted previously, worry specifically about cognitive decline (i.e., *concern*) should be considered a potential indicator of SCD and not be dismissed as evidence of being "worried well," particularly if psychoeducation does not abate the client's concerns. Certain personality traits are also worth considering in a diagnostic formulation of SCD. There is an accumulating body of research that focuses on the role of neuroticism and conscientiousness in particular, with both higher neuroticism and lower conscientiousness being associated with risk for MCI and dementia (Duberstein et al., 2011; Low et al., 2013).

Finally, current physical health status should be considered as a contributing etiology, as discussed at length in Chapter 3. This can manifest in the form of both acute and more chronic medical conditions, as well as side effects of medications used to treat those conditions. Aside from acute medical etiologies, self-report of cognitive complaints is known to be influenced with the experience of chronic health difficulties (Boone, 2009).

Summary of Differential Diagnosis of SCD

Following a biopsychosocial framework is essential to understanding and characterizing a person's current cognitive status and the various factors contributing to their presentation. Aside from standardized neuropsychometric testing and clinical interview, a comprehensive assessment should always include a comprehensive medical work-up (provided by an appropriate physician) as well as recent neuroimaging studies, with structural MRI being a minimum. Moreover, the first assessment should be considered primarily to establish baseline functioning, with repeat assessment being recommended to objectively establish the presence of clinically significant decline in cognitive and functional status (Heilbronner et al., 2010). Use of appropriate RCIs, discussed in Chapter 5 (Duff, 2012; Frerichs & Tuokko, 2005), will allow ascertainment of whether statistical changes in test scores bear clinical relevance while considering the influence of practice effects due to repeat exposure to testing.

Ethical Issues in Providing a Diagnosis of SCD

As has already been clearly elaborated, SCD is an evolving and complex topic. As such, researchers and clinicians must consider the ethical implications of classifying persons with SCD and disclosing SCD status to older adults in clinical and research contexts. Individual countries and jurisdictions within those countries have governing bodies that regulate the profession of psychology, and include their own individual ethics codes. By way of example, we consider here the codes of the American Psychological Association (2010) and the Canadian Psychological Association (2017), and discuss how these codes provide clear guidelines about how to consider ethical issues associated with providing a diagnosis of SCD. One can consider broadly the principles and standards of these codes, and how these become relevant in the context of issues that are specific to the evaluation of persons with suspected SCD.

Beneficence versus Nonmaleficence

The most pressing ethical concern the clinician must consider is the need to weigh the risks and benefits in providing a diagnosis of SCD or disclosing SCD status, given the current state of knowledge regarding the condition (APA Principle A: Beneficence & Nonmalfeasance; CPA Principle II: Responsible Caring). Although SCD as a field of research and clinical investigation is relatively new, work has already been done to consider the ethical issues associated with disclosing *APOE* ε4 genotype status to persons who are currently asymptomatic. Schicktanz and colleagues (2014) have provided a comprehensive overview of this topic, with relevant issues highlighted here.

Benefits of Diagnosis

Being informed about having a condition that may confer risk for future decline could encourage individuals to take better care of their health and engage in preventive measures to mitigate risk for further decline. This might include, but not be limited to, improving cardiovascular health, known to be associated not only with VaD but also AD (Attems & Jellinger, 2014), as well as enhancing cognitive reserve through mental, social, and physical activity (Stern, 2009, 2012). Providing a diagnosis also respects individuals' autonomy by not withholding information that could influence their decision making (e.g., future planning).

Risks of Diagnosis

The risks are largely psychological, and there is a need to consider the implications of providing a diagnosis when the rates of decline are unknown, the state to which someone will decline is unknown (e.g., AD vs. other dementias), and when there is no known cure for dementia and limited empirical evidence for treatments to alter its course. Minimally, clinicians should consider how they wish to present the information, as well as factors that could increase psychological risk for adverse outcomes, including current or prior history of depression or suicidality (Draper, Peisah, Snowdon, & Brodaty, 2010). Both the American Psychological Association and the Canadian Psychological Association make provisions for circumstances under which it may be determined that it is in the client's best interests to withhold diagnostic information to avert adverse outcomes (American Psychological Association Principle C: Integrity; Canadian Psychological Association Principle III: Integrity in Relationships).

Responsibility to Society

Beyond the care of individual clients, psychologists have a responsibility to society at large. They are therefore urged to consider the broader societal impact of knowledge obtained and used in a clinical or research context and to decide whether it promotes good or could do harm, such as promote stigmatization (American Psychological Association Principle B: Fidelity & Responsibility; American Psychological Association Principle D: Justice; Canadian Psychological Association Principle IV: Responsibility to Society). The prevalence rates for SCD in clinic versus community samples remain to be established, along with the meaning of the diagnosis being given in such differing contexts. Certain individuals in the field have raised concern that overly inclusive assessment of older adults in the community could create a health crisis among typical healthy older adults who are not currently experiencing SCD (Fox, Lafortune, Boustani, & Brayne, 2013). Aside from the obvious psychological harm, this could also unnecessarily burden an already taxed health care system, as growing numbers of individuals would seek unnecessary assessment. Although a prevention agenda may save money and resources in the long run, this approach should only be undertaken if it does not unduly deprive access to care in persons already diagnosed with MCI and dementia who have documented needs for support. In other words, one must consider the ethical context of distributive justice (Schicktanz et al., 2014).

In sum, a systematic, ethically guided approach should be taken with regards to giving an individual older adult a diagnosis of SCD, considering the following factors:

- One must base the diagnosis on the most comprehensive assessment possible, bearing in mind that SCD is a diagnosis of exclusion (i.e., one has already ruled out reversible causes of cognitive impairment, mood/anxiety disorders, etc.).
- The potential for self-harm (e.g., suicidality, impulsive decision making) must be established, and the associated risks and benefits of diagnostic disclosure weighed accordingly.
- When diagnostic information is provided, it should be given in a balanced and transparent way, being forthright about the available evidence and its limitations, as well as the practical implications of the diagnosis.
- Any distress associated with an early diagnosis may be tempered by providing the individual with tractable recommendations to promote cognitive, physical, and emotional health. While limited evidence exists for empirically supported treatments specifically for SCD (Smart et al., 2017), recommendations can be given to empower the individual to take care of their overall health and well-being (e.g., building cognitive reserve, cardiovascular health) (see Part III of this book for recommendations).

Summary and Conclusions

The current world population is rapidly aging, and people are becoming better educated about and more proactive in advocating for their own health care. Neuropsychologists will begin to see larger numbers of older adults in their practice in general and will likewise be faced with increasing frequency of requests to determine whether an apparently cognitively normal older adult may nevertheless be at risk for future decline. Although SCD by definition denotes within normal limits performance on standardized neuropsychometric testing, clinical neuropsychologists still remain uniquely positioned to integrate and make meaning from the vast variety of sources that could contribute to perceived cognitive decline. Moreover, they also have at their disposal a varied skill set for how to support implementation of skills and strategies that can enhance current cognitive function and could delay the onset or rate of future cognitive decline.

In terms of future directions, further research is needed to understand the features that elevate risk of SCD portending future cognitive decline. This includes more multimethod assessments, as well as novel and more sensitive subjective and objective markers beyond those currently in use. Collaboration should be fostered across international lines, such as that espoused by the SCD-I. This will promote understanding of cross-cultural differences in the expression of SCD, as well as allow for more rapid accumulation of large-scale, harmonized datasets that can expedite our understanding of the condition. As our understanding is rapidly growing, it is also incumbent on researchers to enter into dialogue with those providing direct care to clients, both psychologists and medical professionals. Researchers must seek to understand how well educated providers are about SCD and how they are approaching the issue of diagnosis. Such knowledge can inform future research questions, the findings of which must, in turn, be made meaningful and accessible to individual practitioners. This last step is essential if we are to realize the potential of SCD in detecting people who may be at risk for decline, years before such decline is clinically manifest.

KEY POINTS

✓ Persons with SCD represent a distinct group of older adults who may be at risk for future non-normal cognitive decline. Standardized neuropsychological assessment may lack the requisite sensitivity to distinguish persons with SCD from healthy older adults, and the clinician should be aware of false-negative diagnoses in this regard.

✓ There is no gold-standard method of predicting which persons with SCD will decline to MCI and dementia. However, certain factors may elevate this risk, including (but not limited to) increased age, higher education, depressed and/or anxious mood, and positive biomarker status.

✓ Given that cognitive complaints are relatively typical in the older adult population, clinicians should be sensitive to complaints that seem to be beyond the scope of normal aging (e.g., spatial navigation difficulties). Moreover, *concern* about one's cognitive abilities—as distinct from complaints—may increase the predictive value of SCD for future decline.

✓ SCD is likely associated with multiple factors. To the degree that any of these factors are treatable (e.g., mood and anxiety), secondary prevention–intervention should be pursued, to avert or slow the rate of future decline, as well as improve current cognitive and emotional function.

✓ Providing a diagnosis of SCD has ethical implications and should be undertaken with care and transparency, mindful of factors that might increase the risk of a deleterious effect of providing such a diagnosis (e.g., suicidality).

CHAPTER 7

Mild Cognitive Impairment

Significant research and clinical attention has been focused broadly on the concept of MCI over the past two decades (Petersen et al., 2014). Identifying individuals with cognitive impairment who do not yet meet clinical criteria for dementia held promise for implementing interventions that might slow or alter the trajectory toward dementia. However, the concept of MCI has been controversial, with disparities ranging from the creation and implementation of diagnostic criteria to the diagnostic and prognostic utility of the construct itself. In this chapter, we present current diagnostic approaches to MCI, situated within the historical context of the evolution of the MCI as a clinical construct. We then discuss practical assessment strategies for operationalizing the diagnosis of MCI in clinical practice, and we conclude with ethical considerations in providing such a diagnosis.

Evolution of the Construct of MCI

Researchers and clinicians have known for some time that there is a transitional period between healthy aging and cognitive decline associated with dementia. In the previous chapter, we discussed the construct of SCD as a condition of interest that is being widely recognized as a potential preclinical prodrome to dementia. Prior to awareness of the condition of SCD, MCI was the primary area of focus with regard to identifying the condition intermediate between healthy aging and dementia. In brief, MCI refers to a syndrome whereby an individual presents with self-reported cognitive decline, often corroborated by informant report. However, unlike SCD, persons with MCI show objective evidence of cognitive impairment in at least one cognitive domain that is clearly beyond the scope of normal aging, albeit with limited to no appreciable impact on everyday function (Albert et al., 2011).

While researchers and clinicians have agreed about the existence of MCI, over the years they have disagreed about the best way to characterize this stage. As early as 1962, Kral (1962) proposed a distinction between benign and malignant forgetfulness, distinguishable on the basis of cognitive symptoms and the course of progression. Twenty years later, everyday functioning was added as a consideration, and the term *limited cognitive disturbance* was proposed to describe people who reported and demonstrated mild memory impairment but who were able to perform everyday tasks adequately (Gurland, Dean, Copeland, Gurland, & Golden, 1982). Subsequently, numerous distinctions have been made to specify the types, magnitude, and duration of cognitive impairment considered adequate to be clinically useful. Many of the classification systems emerging in the late 1980s and 1990s seemed purely descriptive and did not specify expectations regarding an underlying pathology or prognosis (e.g., Blackford & La Rue, 1989; Levy, 1994).

In 1996, Rediess and Caine (1996) proposed a spectrum of cognitive functions and identified five clusters or levels of cognitive functioning: (1) successful or optimal cognitive aging; (2) age-related cognitive decline; (3) mild cognitive impairment; (4) mild neurocognitive disorder or questionable dementia; and (5) dementia (ranging from mild to severe). Clusters 1 and 2 included people for whom decline in function was not anticipated, whereas clusters 3 and 4 captured a heterogeneous group of people with objective evidence of cognitive impairment, many of whom were considered likely to exhibit a progressive course and be diagnosed with dementia over time. In addition to identifying these distinctly different levels of cognitive functioning, Rediess and Caine (1996) also provided specifications as to the characteristic profiles for these groups in terms of types and magnitude of cognitive impairment, everyday functional status, and potential protective and risk factors. Operational definitions for the term *mild cognitive impairment* were proposed by Zaudig (1992), based on the DSM-III-R and ICD-10 criteria for dementia, and by Petersen and colleagues (1999).

An international working group revised prior criteria to acknowledge the fact that MCI progressing to AD only applies to one subtype of MCI (i.e., amnestic variants) and that other subtypes may not progress in the same manner or at all (Winblad et al., 2004). Similarly, Petersen and Morris (2005) have proposed how the clinical features of MCI may map onto different underlying pathologies beyond AD. Presumably, if one can identify subtypes of MCI that are more likely to be associated with AD, one could better estimate rates of decline; however, this assumption is controversial. Moreover, the issue of MCI as diagnosis versus descriptor should be borne in mind, as we discuss the various classification systems currently in use for MCI. Despite the various controversies, of all the terms used to describe this intermediary condition, MCI seems to have been the most enduring (Petersen et al., 2014), and this is the primary term that we use in the remainder of this chapter.

Current Diagnostic Approaches to MCI

In this section, we discuss the most frequently used diagnostic approaches to MCI, along with significant issues and limitations associated with those classification systems.

Current Classification Systems for MCI

Neuropsychologists and other professionals can make a diagnosis of MCI in several different ways. The most recent MCI criteria, compiled by the NIA-AA working group (Albert et al., 2011), include specific guidelines for the diagnosis of MCI, both in research contexts ("Clinical Research Criteria") and in clinical practice ("Core Clinical Criteria"). Broadly speaking, the core clinical criteria include (1) concern regarding a change in cognition, (2) impairment in one or more cognitive domains, (3) preservation of independence in functional abilities, and (4) not demented. In terms of criterion (2) specifically, this is operationalized as objective cognitive impairment that is typically 1–1.5 *SD* below age and education-corrected normative scores, although it is emphasized that these are guidelines and not absolute cut scores. For example, for a person who had high premorbid function, scores in the average range relative to peers may represent a relative decline, yet fail to meet the MCI criterion if interpreted strictly. Persons with episodic memory impairment (i.e., amnestic MCI) are anticipated to have greater risk of declining to AD as opposed to individuals who have preserved memory but impairment in other cognitive domains. Additionally, regarding criterion 3, it is acknowledged that individuals may show minor difficulties in activities of daily living, but they are able to compensate to a degree that significant functional impairment is not observed. The diagnosis is further substantiated by the presence of AD biomarkers such as autosomal genetic mutations for AD and one or two ε4 alleles in the *APOE* gene.

As noted, the NIA-AA criteria treat MCI as a diagnosis, presumed to be associated with underlying AD pathology. This is commensurate with early conceptualizations of MCI—a prodrome to AD eventually leading to AD dementia (e.g., Petersen et al., 1999). However, researchers and clinicians have acknowledged that not all individuals with MCI decline to AD. For example, Petersen and Morris (2005) provided four subclassifications of MCI: (1) amnestic MCI, single domain; (2) amnestic MCI, multiple domain; (3) nonamnestic MCI, single domain, and (4) nonamnestic MCI, multiple domain. These different subclassifications were anticipated to represent different underlying pathologies, such as frontotemporal dementia, DLB, VaD, and depression. The Albert et al. (2011) criteria note that persons with episodic memory impairment (i.e., amnestic MCI) are more likely to decline to AD. This finding implies that persons with the nonamnestic variants may be more likely to decline to non-AD dementias. Despite the popular application of these subclassifications of MCI, recent neuropsychometric studies have called their utility into question.

Beyond the NIA-AA criteria, other classification systems allow for the specification of alternative etiologies to explain the presence of MCI as a descriptive condition denoting an intermediary stage between healthy aging and dementia. The particular classification system a clinician chooses may be dictated, in large part, by the setting and prevailing guidelines about reimbursement of care. Two of the most commonly used of such classification systems are the DSM-5 (American Psychiatric Association, 2013) and the ICD-10 (World Health Organization, 1993). The ICD-10 provides different codes based on the presumed underlying etiology of the observed cognitive impairment, such as cerebral degeneration (G31.9) and mild memory disturbance (F06.8). DSM-5 provides a greater operationalization of the diagnostic criteria pertinent to MCI, referred to as mild NCD. Unlike the NIA-AA criteria, the DSM-5 criteria are not exclusively focused on MCI associated with AD. In fact, earlier editions of the DSM were criticized for having criteria that were "Alzheimerized," as the requirement of memory impairment did not equally apply to other types of dementias (Brown, Lazar, & Delano-Wood, 2009). Rather, the criteria for mild neurocognitive disorder allow the clinician to choose from a variety of potential etiologies (e.g., AD, as well as DLB, FTLD, among others). A majority of neuropsychologists in routine clinical practice will likely use the DSM-5 criteria to make a diagnosis of MCI. In addition, several expert working groups have convened to codify criteria similar to those of Albert et al. (2011) but for non-AD etiologies, with the criteria for vascular cognitive impairment (VCI; Gorelick et al., 2011; Skrobot et al., 2017) and Parkinson's-related cognitive impairment (Litvan et al., 2012; Szeto et al., 2015) as two such examples.

Classifying the Presumed Etiology of MCI

As we discuss subsequently, controversy has arisen over whether MCI represents a diagnosis associated with a specific neurodegenerative disease process, or whether it simply represents a descriptor of current function. Regardless of how the term is used, the clinician must work to establish (or generate reasonable clinical hypotheses about) the presumed etiology. In the NIA-AA criteria, MCI due to AD is corroborated by the presence of certain AD biomarkers. Although AD cannot be definitively diagnosed until autopsy, a separate NIA-AA workgroup recently proposed *in vivo* markers of preclinical AD that can be used to corroborate a diagnosis of MCI associated with AD (Sperling et al., 2011). The Albert et al. (2011) criteria additionally treat MCI due to AD as a diagnosis of exclusion, meaning that all other systemic or brain-related etiologies must be ruled out in order to have the strongest likelihood that underlying AD neuropathology is the cause of MCI. This can prove challenging because AD itself may be comorbid with other pathologies, particularly vascular pathology (Albert et al., 2011). Mixed AD-vascular dementia is one of the most common dementias in late life, increasing in frequency with advancing age (Schneider, Arvanitakis, Bang, & Bennett, 2007; James, Bennett, Boyle, Leurgans, & Schneider, 2012). Moreover, accumulating research suggests that vascular mechanisms may be an intrinsic aspect of AD itself, which may account for the apparent high comorbidity of these two conditions (Snyder et al., 2015).

Petersen et al. (2014) note that while both NIA-AA and DSM-5 criteria suggest an increasing role for biomarkers in differential diagnosis, most markers are not validated—or practical—for use in routine clinical practice and remain a focus of current research investigation. Although biomarkers can provide compelling evidence of neuropathology, positive biomarker status does not have a 1:1 relationship with objective cognitive impairment or future decline to dementia. Rather, only neuropsychometric assessment can provide objective evidence of current cognitive impairment. Moreover, where objective medical evidence of presumed etiology is harder to obtain, a neuropsychologist might use the particular pattern of test results, in conjunction with clinical interview data, to make an informed clinical opinion about the underlying etiology, neurodegenerative or otherwise. If we assume that MCI is a step intermediate between healthy aging and dementia, then we can likewise assume that, if a person has a particular neurodegenerative condition, his or her test profile will differ in degrees of magnitude from the actual dementia diagnosis. For example, a person with vascular-related cognitive impairment might show a less severe form of the common profile observed in VaD, consisting of cognitive slowing, executive dysfunction, and a memory retrieval deficit as hallmark findings. Conversely, in the cases where there is no objective biomarker evidence of underlying neuropathology, and neuropsychometric test performance does not map to any known neurodegenerative etiology, a clinician may endeavor to use MCI as a descriptive rather than diagnostic term. In DSM-5 nomenclature, this would be codified as mild NCD of unspecified etiology. One example might be an older adult who presents with various medical comorbidities, multiple medication use, and perhaps some issues with mood, all of which could contribute to current cognitive function. Table 8.3 in Chapter 8 includes information on some of the more common dementia profiles that can be used as a point of reference to inform hypotheses about MCI etiology.

MCI as a Prodrome to Dementia

Much of the confusion surrounding MCI stems from use of the term as a diagnosis versus a description about a person's current functioning. Used as a diagnosis, MCI would, at least in theory, hold prognostic value for prediction of decline to subsequent dementia associated with an assumed underlying neurodegenerative process. Many studies have examined the incidence and prevalence of MCI and the rates of conversion from cognitive impairment to dementia, with virtually all studies noting wide variations across their findings (Ward, Arrighi, Michels, & Cedarbaum, 2012). Much of this variation is related to key differences between studies in terms of their operational definition of MCI, study recruitment and design, the samples studied, how cognition is measured, how findings are reported (e.g., relative odds of conversion versus percent conversion), and study duration (Clark et al., 2013; Tuokko & McDowell, 2006). Many of these studies observe stability or even improvement in cognitive functions over time, in addition to decline for some (i.e., rates of conversion to dementia ranging from 1–15% [Busse, Bischkopf, Riedel-Heller, & Angermeyer, 2003] or 2–31% [Bruscoli & Lovestone, 2004]). Even when using the Petersen criteria, the way those criteria are operationalized can result in drastically different rates of progression. For example, Loewenstein et al. (2009) compared rates of diagnosis and progression based on how many psychometric tests were used to give an MCI diagnosis. When one test was used to diagnose amnestic MCI, 56% of individuals improved, 25% remained stable, and 19% declined over an approximate 3-year period. Compare this with the rates observed when two impaired scores in a domain were used to make the diagnosis—in this case, no individuals improved, 50% remained stable, and 50% declined. Estimated rates of progression are typically derived from large-scale longitudinal studies, where researchers may be mindful of participant burden in the number of tests administered. However, the findings of Loewenstein et al. (2009), as well as other researchers since then, indicate that using fewer tests may come at a significant cost in terms of obtaining accurate assessments of the rate of expected decline, and even conferral of the diagnosis itself. In subsequent sections, we discuss some of the ways researchers have investigated to improve the predictive validity of MCI with regard to decline.

Early versus Late MCI

One approach used to better gauge progression is to classify individuals as having "early" MCI (EMCI) versus "late" MCI (LMCI). The Alzheimer's Disease Neuroimaging Initiative (ADNI) is a longitudinal, multicenter study designed to ascertain clinical, imaging, genetic, and biochemical biomarkers for early detection and tracking of AD (ADNI, n.d.). In 2009, EMCI was introduced as a way to gather biomarker data earlier in the clinical progression toward AD. In ADNI2, the second wave of data collection, the study protocol differentiated persons with EMCI and LMCI based on a single score, delayed recall of paragraph A from Logical Memory on the WMS-R (ADNI, 2011). The clinical utility of EMCI and LMCI is still being investigated. Jessen and colleagues (2013) examined data from the Age-CoDe study, a general practice registry-based longitudinal study in older adults designed to identify predictors of cognitive decline and dementia. A baseline sample of 2,892 participants was classified as having subjective memory impairment (SMI, a previous term for SCD), EMCI, and LMCI. The groups were classified according to performance on the delayed recall task of the CERAD: SMI was associated with <1.0 *SD* below demographically adjusted norms, EMCI with 1–1.5 *SD* below norms, and LMCI with greater than 1.5 *SD*s below norms. Further, participants were subdivided as to the presence of concern associated with experienced memory impairment. Over the 6-year follow-up period, risk of AD dementia was greatest in LMCI, which is unsurprising. However, among the individuals with SMI and EMCI, risk was similarly elevated in the subgroups of participants who reported concern. This suggests that, early in the trajectory of decline, perceived concern has additional prognostic value over and above self-reported cognitive complains, the presence of which may elevate the risk for subsequent decline to AD or other dementias. Emerging research on SCD likewise points to the importance of distinguishing *concern* from *complaints* as an additional marker to identify risk for decline.

Biomarkers

Another approach to tracking progression is through the use of biomarkers. An important question is whether positive biomarker evidence elevates a person's risk to decline to dementia as compared to individuals with no such biomarkers. According to the NIA-AA criteria, suggested markers for pursuit in research studies are those that show evidence of amyloid deposition and/or neuronal injury. As Petersen et al. (2014) note, however, a large number of neuropathological studies indicate that not all persons who are positive for such biomarkers at autopsy express the clinical syndrome of cognitive impairment or dementia during their lifetime. In other words, being biomarker-positive does not definitively predict that someone will develop pathological cognitive impairment and/or decline to dementia in the future. Stephan et al. (2012) conducted a systematic review of investigating the neuropathology of MCI, which included 162 studies from a variety of settings, including epidemiological, population-based studies to clinic samples. With respect to neuropathology, MCI was broadly construed to contain both AD and non-AD pathology. Considering this broad definition of MCI, it is perhaps not surprising that the authors found a large number of neuropathological mechanisms observed in MCI, ultimately concluding that this syndrome cannot be understood within a single framework. Moreover—and perhaps most pertinent to the question of progression—they found that there was no clear relationship between typical neuropathological markers of AD and progression from healthy aging to MCI. Taken together, the findings leave unresolved the question of whether neuropathological findings in MCI represent risk factors that may lead to decline (i.e., in a diathesis–stress relationship), or whether they represent intrinsic factors of an impending disease process associated with dementia.

Necessity of Neuropsychometric Testing as Part of Diagnosis

Neuropsychologists have strongly advocated for the necessity of using neuropsychometric test data to improve the reliability of MCI diagnoses, regardless of presumed etiology. Research on persons with MCI frequently occurs within the context of large-scale epidemiological and longitudinal studies with very large sample sizes. These large sample sizes facilitate reliable detection of the phenomenon of interest and how it may change over time. However, Bondi and Smith (2014) note serious concerns with this approach. Given the time and cost resources to conduct such studies and the associated participant burden, participant characterization may be limited to brief screening measures or clinician rating scales that do not adequately provide an objective quantification of current cognitive function. Less in-depth characterization may mean that people are misclassified as MCI, which in turn *decreases* the reliability of detecting the phenomenon of interest. In this same vein, Morris (2012) has raised concern that the revised NIA-AA criteria may mean that individuals with mild or very mild AD could be reclassified as MCI based on CDR scores and activities of daily living performance, undermining the reliability of the diagnosis. A similar concern could be raised regarding the differentiation of mild and major NCD based on subjective clinical opinion alone.

Even though objective cognitive impairment is one of the main criteria for MCI, there is currently no gold standard for operationalizing this criterion. Jak and colleagues (2009) analyzed data from a community-based longitudinal study on aging in order to demonstrate how applying different neuropsychometric criteria would lead to different rates of diagnosis and subsequent decline, stability, or reversal. They used five different sets of criteria: the original Petersen et al. (1999) criteria (a score of <1.5 *SD* below normal on WMS-R Logical Memory recall), the historical Petersen and Morris (2005) typical criteria (any measure in any domain <1.5 *SD* below normal), liberal criteria (any single test being 1 standard deviation below normal), conservative criteria (two measures within a domain being 1.5 SD below normal), and comprehensive criteria (two measures within the same domain at 1 SD below normal). Each of these approaches had different estimates of MCI diagnosis as well as predicting status at follow-up (average = 17 months). The liberal criteria were the most unstable over time; this is not unexpected, given the work of Heaton and others, where studies of cognitively normal individuals have shown that having at least one impaired test score in a comprehensive assessment battery is relatively common and reflects normal variation (Heaton et al., 1991; Heaton, Miller, Taylor, & Grant, 2004; Palmer, Boone, Lesser, & Wohl, 1998). The historical criteria had most stability over time (98%); however, the authors estimated that these criteria missed a significant proportion of people with both amnestic and nonamnestic MCI, given the reliance on a single test of paragraph recall. This suggests that the historical criteria have high specificity for amnestic MCI but low sensitivity to discriminate healthy individuals from those with other forms of MCI. The authors determined that the comprehensive criteria struck the greatest balance between sensitivity and specificity, as well as showing greater stability than either typical or liberal criteria.

Subsequent authors have built on the work of Jak et al. (2009) in applying the comprehensive versus conventional Petersen and Morris (2005) criteria to estimate rates of diagnosis and decline in MCI. Clark et al. (2013) used data from a longitudinal study on aging run in conjunction with University of California, San Diego and the San Diego Veterans Affairs Healthcare System. In applying the conventional MCI criteria (Petersen & Morris, 2005; Winblad et al., 2004), 134 individuals met the criteria for MCI, with most being single-domain nonamnestic (n = 74), followed by multidomain amnestic (n = 29), single-domain amnestic (n = 16), and multidomain nonamnestic (n = 15). To meet MCI criteria, individuals only needed to have one test score more than 1.5 SDs below normal in any cognitive domain. By comparison, when using Jak et al.'s (2009) comprehensive criteria, only eighty individuals met the criteria for MCI. The rate of single-domain nonamnestic dropped dramatically to only twenty-nine participants, while the other rates remained relatively similar (multidomain amnestic = 27, single-domain amnestic = 14, and multidomain nonamnestic = 10). These findings suggest that using too few measures—as little as one measure—can result in false-positive diagnoses of MCI, and may further explain the conflicting rates of progression to dementia. The other striking finding of the Clark et al. (2013) study is the comparatively fewer individuals diagnosed with amnestic MCI using conventional criteria. If AD is the most commonly diagnosed dementia, and persons with amnestic MCI are those anticipated to have highest rates of decline to AD, then one would predict a majority of persons in the sample to have amnestic MCI. The participants in this study were from a community-based longitudinal study, as opposed to a clinic sample, which draws attention to the fact that differing rates of diagnosis and subsequent decline may vary as to whether the sample comes from a clinic-based sample versus a community-based sample.

Aside from the issue of having insufficient data to reliably make a diagnosis, recent neuropsychological research has called into question the conventional classifications of amnestic versus nonamnestic and single-domain versus multidomain MCI. Clark and colleagues (2013) applied cluster-based analyses to persons diagnosed with MCI using either the conventional criteria (Peterson & Morris, 2005) or more stringent criteria requiring at least two impaired test scores in a domain (Jak et al., 2009). Using the conventional criteria, three subtypes emerged, representative of an amnestic/language subgroup, a mixed/multidomain subgroup, and a normal subgroup. Using the Jak et al. (2009) criteria, four clusters emerged, representing dysexecutive problems, amnestic MCI, mixed MCI, and a group that had a single impaired test score on a measure of visuospatial function. Edmonds et al. (2015a) applied this cluster-based approach to 825 individuals enrolled in ADNI and classified as MCI. In this dataset, four clusters emerged, representing amnestic ($n = 288$), dysnomic ($n = 153$), dysexecutive ($n = 102$), and cluster-derived normal ($n = 282$). The normal group had fewer *APOE* ε4 carriers than the other groups, fewer individuals who progressed to dementia, and cerebrospinal fluid AD biomarker profiles that were not significantly different from the healthy normative reference group. These findings suggest that taking an empirical or actuarial approach to classification results in more reliable diagnoses and more reliable associations to biomarker outcomes and rates of decline.

Given these issues, Bondi and Smith (2014) have little difficulty advocating strongly for the input of clinical neuropsychologists in the codifying of MCI, specifically including objective neuropsychometric evidence to improve the reliability of MCI diagnoses. Although research studies are often limited in the scope of their neuropsychometric test administration due to cost and participant burden, clinicians in routine practice are not bound by these same considerations. They can use results from a comprehensive test battery to make the most informed clinical judgment about the scope of impairment and the appropriateness of an MCI diagnosis. Jak et al. (2009) note that their comprehensive approach is more akin to what is used in routine clinical practice, where consistency of findings and patterns of impaired test scores are used to make clinical judgments. In working with individual clients, conveying the meaning of an MCI diagnosis—and what this means for subsequent decline—raises ethical issues, which we discuss in a separate section later in this chapter. At a minimum, this underscores the importance of routine monitoring and repeat neuropsychometric assessment over time, in order to corroborate the presence of any objective decline.

Operationalizing the Diagnosis of MCI in Clinical Practice

We next discuss the practical implementation of the current state of knowledge on MCI to working with individual clients. In Chapter 4, we introduced some foundational principles that apply to assessing individuals at any stage along the trajectory of decline. We refer the reader back to this chapter to contextualize the additional information we provide here with specific regard to MCI. In particular, we draw attention to the introduction to Chapter 4, which outlines the APA's recent guidelines for the evaluation of age-related cognitive change.

Medical Work-Up

If MCI is taken as a descriptor of current function (rather than a harbinger of neurodegenerative disease), then any number of factors may give rise to significant cognitive impairment, not least of which are reversible medical causes. Likewise, adequate treatment of these underlying medical causes could stabilize or reverse manifest cognitive impairment, or at the very least provide further information as to the likely etiology. As with any older adult assessment, it is imperative to ensure that the client has had a thorough medical work-up, at a minimum including a comprehensive medical work-up to rule out contributory medical factors such as vitamin deficiencies, infectious processes, and metabolic disorders. Note that certain medications may have iatrogenic effects on cognition, particularly when used in older adults; psychologists should be apprised of some of the more commonly used medications in geriatric populations, and their potential side effects.

Clinical Interview

The clinical interview provides a wealth of information that can be used in making an MCI diagnosis. We refer the reader back to Appendix 4.1 (in Chapter 4), which provides a foundational set of questions that should be asked in every older adult assessment. In terms of questions specific to MCI, these should additionally include (1) perception of decline and (2) course of decline.

Perception of Cognitive Decline

MCI implies the perception of a significant decline from prior levels of functioning, one that is observed by the individual or an informant, or one that is extracted by a trained clinician. The interview can be used to ascertain information about perceived decline, as well as significant discrepancies between self and informant report, which in and of itself can be a valuable data-point. The further a client progresses toward dementia, the more likely it is that he or she will experience *anosognosia,* that is, decreased awareness of their deficits. Research has suggested that, in later stages of MCI and dementia, clients tend to underestimate their deficits relative to their informants, whereas in SCD and earlier stages of MCI the opposite is true, where clients overestimate (or at least more readily report) their deficits relative to informants (Edmonds et al., 2014; Mulligan, et al., 2016; Rueda et al., 2015).

Course of Decline

Inquiring about the scope and course of decline provides valuable information in terms of differential diagnosis. Following are three questions regarding decline that can be posed to individual clients:

1. "Can you pinpoint an exact time in your life when your thinking seemed to get worse? Was there some specific life event or stressful situation going on when you noticed your thinking getting worse?"
2. "Is your thinking consistently bad, or are there times when you seem to be thinking more clearly?"
3. "Since you noticed a change in your thinking abilities, do you feel that these abilities are getting worse over time, or are your thinking abilities fairly stable, even if worse than before?"

Most neurodegenerative disease processes have a slow, insidious course, until the impairment reaches some critical point that finally precipitates the evaluation. In these types of cases, it may be difficult for the client or informant to pinpoint when cognitive decline started. Moreover, such impairment tends to be relatively stable across time and context, although there are unique exceptions where waxing and waning of cognition can occur with neurodegeneration, specifically DLB. Finally, neurodegeneration implies deterioration over time, so it is expected that the client or informant will report some type of continued decline over time, even if subtle. The exception to this typical insidious course is certain presentations of vascular cognitive impairment, which can have either an abrupt or an insidious onset and course.

Conversely, there are other times when a client or an informant is able to identify a salient life event that is temporally contiguous to the onset of cognitive decline. Medical procedures and seemingly routine surgeries that do not involve the central nervous system can nevertheless negatively impact cognitive function. For example, while not necessarily a common occurrence, coronary artery bypass graft surgery can, in some cases, be associated with hypoxic-ischemic events that cause abrupt onset of cognitive impairment (Fink et al., 2015). With this in mind, it is important to ask the client about specific events that may occur close in time to the perceived onset of decline, despite how unrelated they appear to be.

In other cases, a clearly identifiable event temporally contiguous to cognitive decline signals the role of mood in cognitive impairment. For example, a significant life stressor such as medical illness or bereavement can trigger the onset of depression, which if severe enough can cause cognitive impairment. One way to ascertain the role of mood is to ask the client, "Do your symptoms seem to wax and wane with how you are feeling? Think about the times your mood is improved; do you tend to be thinking more clearly at those times?" Affirmative answers to these questions typically corroborate the role of a mood disorder in current cognitive impairment. Moreover, persons with late-life depression would not be expected to show further decline over time, and if the depression is adequately treated, cognitive function may improve. One complicating factor is the well-known comorbidity of depression and VCI, so well established that some have argued that depression may in fact be a prodrome to VaD (Diniz et al., 2013). This is further complicated by the fact that both conditions have similar neuropsychometric test profiles (i.e., the "subcortical" profile of slowed processing speed, memory retrieval difficulties, and executive dysfunction). In this case, it may be prudent to aggressively treat the depression and, with improvement in symptoms, reassess in order to ascertain whether cognitive function has at least stabilized or even improved. This is especially important, given the evidence demonstrating that late-life depression is a risk factor for the subsequent development of dementia (DaSilva et al., 2013; Diniz et al., 2013).

Psychometric Test Performance

Given the issues discussed previously regarding reliability of diagnosis, most or all of the contemporary classification systems for MCI explicitly discuss the necessity to include formal neuropsychometric testing. In distinguishing mild from major NCDs in DSM-5, neuropsychometric test data, along with functional status, seem essential to differentiating these two conditions. Next we discuss some specific considerations in compiling an appropriate neuropsychometric test battery to assess for the presence of MCI.

Use of Appropriate Norms

As is true for any older adult assessment, instruments should be carefully chosen and appropriate norms available with demographic characteristics most relevant to the client. We refer the reader back to Chapter 5 for a detailed discussion of norms.

Estimating Decline

At the initial visit, decline is usually inferred based on current test performance that is lower than predicted based on norms and/or estimated premorbid function, as well as self and/or informant complaints of decline. This speaks to the need to use an appropriate measure of premorbid function, which is a complex and multifaceted construct to assess. By definition, two time-points of test data are required to definitively demonstrate objective evidence of decline, and ideally a more robust diagnosis of MCI will be arrived at with multiple assessments.

Psychometric Test Selection

In terms of actual test selection, there is no gold-standard test battery for assessing individuals with MCI. Rather, the clinician is likely to use a battery of tests similar to those used with healthy older adults and persons with subjective cognitive decline, focusing on degrees of impairment in order to corroborate the diagnosis of MCI. As noted previously, research on MCI has been hampered with inconsistent estimates about rates of decline to dementia versus stability or reversal to cognitive normality; part of the issue may be due to inadequate or inconsistent neuropsychometric characterization. We believe the Jak et al. (2009) criteria to be the most tractable for routine clinical-neuropsychological practice, where at least two tests within a domain at 1 *SD* below normal corroborates the presence of impairment within that domain (and therefore evidence toward MCI). We recommend a broad screening of all cognitive functions to arrive at the most comprehensive diagnosis. To avoid false negatives in persons with high premorbid function, tests should be sufficiently challenging to show a range of performance and avoid ceiling effects, for example, using the California Verbal Learning Test-II Standard Form as opposed to the Short Form (Delis, Kramer, Kaplan, & Ober, 2000). Aside from cognitive functions, mood and anxiety should be assessed at a minimum, and if time permits, personality as well. Psychological assessment is discussed in more detail in Chapter 12

The Use of Profiles to Determine Etiology

To the extent that MCI is a transitional stage toward dementia, one would expect that individuals with MCI would exhibit profiles of cognitive decline that differ in orders of magnitude from those observed in dementia diagnoses. Again, the criterion of 1.5 *SD* below normal can be applied to these profiles, and where such impairment is observed, this can be used in support of a particular etiological factor.

Self- and Informant Report of Decline

As noted previously, comparison of self and informant report is valuable for assessment at any stage along the trajectory of cognitive decline, and a variety of measures are available for this purpose. Similar to SCD, two frequently used and investigated measures in the MCI population are the IQCODE (Cherbuin & Jorm, 2013) and the E-Cog (Farias et al., 2008). The E-Cog in particular has recently been gaining traction in the literature, appealing because it has both a self- and an informant report, as well as surveying a broad swath of cognitive domains beyond memory (which tends to be the focus of many cognitive complaint questionnaires). However, both of these measures are limited by their temporal referent, which asks individuals to rate themselves/their loved one compared to 10 years ago. Having such a protracted temporal referent could affect the reliability of information provided, as a function of the length of time the client and informant have known each other as well as the informant's own memory function. Given this limitation, these measures provide important supplemental information about specific symptoms, but they should not be used as a substitute for asking such questions in the interview itself. The Frontal Systems Behavior Scales (FrSBe; Grace & Malloy, 2001) have parallel forms for self and informant. Although the FrSBe was designed for ratings of self and others before and after acute events such as head injury, the benefit of this measure is that the client and informant can establish the temporal referent of the estimated onset of decline. The FrSBe targets symptoms associated with frontal lobe functioning, specifically, apathy, disinhibition, and executive dysfunction, and has been shown to discriminate persons with frontotemporal dementia (which tends to have a younger onset) from those with AD (Malloy, Tremont, Grace, & Frakey, 2007).

Functional Impairment in MCI

One of the most important criteria that differentiates the diagnosis of MCI from dementia is the absence of functional impairment. That is, individuals with MCI are expected to present with significant cognitive impairment, yet retain relatively preserved function in instrumental activities of daily living. However, it stands to reason that if persons with MCI are on a trajectory of cognitive decline toward dementia, the erosion of functional abilities is likely to occur in a gradual, insidious fashion rather than in an abrupt deterioration. This implies that subtle changes in functional abilities may be observed in persons with MCI but are less manifest because the affected individual retains the awareness and ability to actively compensate for said changes.

Recent work by Lindbergh, Dishman, and Miller (2016) supports this contention. The authors conducted a systematic review and meta-analysis of functional disability in persons with MCI. A total of 151 effect sizes from 106 studies was included in the final analysis. Random effects models indicated a large overall effect size of functional disability that was significantly more pronounced in persons with MCI versus healthy controls. Persons with multidomain MCI had significantly worse instrumental activities of daily living performance compared to single-domain MCI. This finding is perhaps unsurprising given that increasing cognitive burden may supersede the individual's attempts to successfully compensate for erosion of functional abilities. This is consistent with findings from Gold's (2012) previous review of the literature on instrumental activities of daily living in MCI. The authors also found that nonamnestic MCI was associated with greater impairment in instrumental activities of daily living than amnestic MCI, despite the fact that the latter predisposes most strongly to later AD. This makes sense given that a preponderance of prior research indicates that, of the various cognitive domains typically assessed, general intellectual function and executive functions contribute most strongly to everyday functional abilities (Tuokko & Smart, 2014). Given that AD is the most frequently occurring dementia and that memory impairment is a hallmark of this disorder, many large-scale aging studies focus heavily on memory, with relatively less attention paid to other cognitive domains. These findings on performance of instrumental activities of daily living further underscore the importance of comprehensive screening of cognitive domains beyond memory, not only for detecting other neurodegenerative processes beyond AD but also for predicting likely decline to dementia. Overall, the findings corroborated the notion that, similar to cognitive decline itself, functional decline exists on a continuum and may gradually erode as individuals progress from healthy aging to MCI, and further on to dementia.

In terms of how to assess instrumental activities of daily living, Lindbergh and colleagues (2016) noted that the highest effect sizes were observed for performance-based measures and informant reports, which again makes sense considering that decreasing awareness may impact self-report of functional abilities. They also noted that a combination of self and informant reports provided a medium effect size that was intermediate to the use of either self-report or informant report measures used alone. Thus, where performance-based measures are not practically applicable, self and informant reports used together may provide a reasonable approximation of actual instrumental activities of daily living abilities. One of the most widely used measures is the Lawton–Brody Instrumental Activities of Daily Living scale (Lawton & Brody, 1969). It contains eight items that pertain to a broad array of daily activities and is relatively brief to complete. It can be administered in interview form to the client and/or informant together. The Functional Activities Questionnaire (FAQ; Pfeffer, Kurosaki, Harrah, Chance, & Filos, 1982) would be another alternative, as there is some evidence to suggest that it can discriminate persons with MCI from mild AD (Teng et al., 2010). The Test of Practical Judgment (TOP-J; Rabin et al., 2007) can provide valuable information on the client's judgment in a variety of everyday, practical situations, although the limitation of this test is that it assesses practical knowledge but not necessarily the real-world application of such knowledge. This limitation is particularly important given that, with MCI comes the possibility of diminishing awareness, such that a client retains semantic knowledge but fails to effectively implement said knowledge.

In assessing instrumental activities of daily living, it is also important not to assess simply the occurrence of a certain behavior but also the opportunity to engage in this behavior. For example, a client may present with reports that she is not managing her finances; however, this may be because her partner always managed the finances, and now that he is deceased, her children have opted to take over this task on her behalf. In addition, for decline in performance of instrumental activities of daily living to be used in the differential diagnosis of MCI versus dementia, such decline must be due to cognitive and not physical reasons (e.g., the client has difficulty driving because of poor attention versus cataracts impairing vision).

Repeat Assessment

Typically, the criterion of decline is met using subjective evidence from the client and any available informant. However, in order to objectively corroborate the presence of decline, we recommend regular follow-up and repeat assessment. Not only does this permit monitoring for the presence of decline, but repeat assessment can also be used to track response to intervention. In Chapter 5, we discussed in detail the considerations associated with repeat assessment and ascertainment of clinically meaningful change.

Psychological and Ethical Considerations in the Diagnosis of MCI

Following a diagnosis of MCI, a client will understandably have questions and concerns about prognosis (meaning progression to dementia). One of the most challenging aspects of MCI is the lack of precision with which this diagnosis does, in fact, predict future decline. As noted before, while MCI does seem to confer a greater risk for decline to dementia in certain individuals, significant numbers of those diagnosed remain stable or even revert to cognitive normality. The meaning of an MCI diagnosis may be more descriptive than anything else, as it may be difficult to predict the future course for these individuals.

Psychological Reactions to MCI

Considering the ambiguity surrounding progression, it stands to reason that providing an MCI diagnosis, whether in descriptive or etiological terms, has psychosocial and psychological implications for the client. Persons with MCI are expected to retain some awareness of cognitive function—and ergo cognitive difficulties—that may cause adjustment difficulties as individuals adjust to their new level of functioning. Many individuals may reasonably assume that a diagnosis of MCI foreshadows subsequent decline to dementia, which can create its own fears (Corner & Bond, 2004). However, this issue is further complicated by the very fact that there are few reliable predictors of progression from MCI to dementia. As a result, affected individuals are left in a limbo state where it may be hard to move forward into such an uncertain future. Several qualitative studies have illuminated the psychological experiences of individuals diagnosed with MCI. For example, Frank and colleagues (2006) reported that individuals with MCI identified salient themes as including uncertainty of diagnosis, skill loss, change in social and family roles, embarrassment and shame, emotionality, and (fear of being a) burden. The theme of ambiguity was echoed in the work of Beard and Neary (2013), who found that participants struggled to define MCI and determine whether or not it was a disease, as well as reporting difficulty grappling with the social implications of an MCI diagnosis. Ali and Smart (2016), in a pilot qualitative study of the experience of grief in persons with MCI, found that the MCI experience tended to be characterized as one of ambiguous loss that is disenfranchised and associated with loss of important roles and aspects of one's identity. This study parallels work conducted in persons with stroke and brain injury, suggesting that neurological diagnoses are often associated with the experience of loss (Alaszewski, Alaszewski, & Potter, 2004; Carroll & Coetzer, 2011; Kuluski, Dow, Locock, Lyons, & Lasserson, 2014).

These concerns of older adults are not unfounded, given the uncertainty in the diagnosis faced by clinicians and researchers themselves. Thus, the diagnosis of MCI and formal neuropsychological feedback must be provided with the utmost care. Some of the same provisions that apply to making a diagnosis of SCD would be prudent to consider in the context of MCI. This requires balancing the need to provide honest information about the assessment results with any limitations of those findings (particularly with regard to predicting later decline). It is also crucial to assess for current or past history of depression, as well as risk for suicide or other imminent harms, given the research showing that disclosure of *APOE* status has higher risk in such individuals (Schicktanz et al., 2014). Any neuropsychological assessment should focus on strengths as well as signs of impairment. To that end it would be prudent to emphasize what people can do to maintain function and to live their lives to the fullest in spite of the diagnosis.

Issues Surrounding Advanced Care Planning and Other Legal Decisions

As we have already discussed, there is a gray zone within which persons with MCI—specifically those who are declining to dementia—begin to evidence functional impairment. It is worthwhile at this juncture to have a discussion with the client and his or her family about the practical implications of the client's cognitive impairment and how it may impinge on the client's ability to engage in important decision making regarding health care and finances. In some ways, it is optimal to have these conversations while a person with MCI presumably possesses enough awareness to participate in autonomous decision making. Part of this conversation will likely involve advising the family to consult with an eldercare attorney or an attorney with experience in advanced care planning. In addition, we refer clinicians to an excellent resource on working with older adults with diminished capacity, created by the American Psychiatric Association in conjunction with the American Bar Association (American Bar Association Commission on Law and Aging & American Psychological Association, 2008). This manual discusses the assessment of capacity in the context of various domains of decision making, including medical, legal, and driving capacity (see the next section for further discussion of issues related to driving). While cognitive impairment does not presume a lack of capacity, and persons with MCI are not necessarily expected to lack capacity, being familiar with this approach to assessment provides a further set of tools that clinicians can use in repeat assessments as they track diminishing capacity and intervene accordingly.

Determining Limits to Confidentiality

As a person evidences diminishment in capacity or everyday function, issues of safety may arise. Psychologists are ethically mandated to break confidentiality when there is concern that clients may be at risk of harm to themselves or to others. As noted earlier, persons with MCI can show subtle changes in various aspects of daily functioning, some of which may or may not bring risk of harm to self or others. A specific issue that raises concerns about safety in persons with MCI is driving—both the emergence of concern about impaired driving and a client's receptivity to feedback about the need to stop driving (Kowalski et al., 2011). In clinical practice, we have found that driving cessation can be a contentious issue between clients and concerned family members, thereby presenting a challenging dilemma. First and foremost, psychologists should be aware of the specific legal obligations in their jurisdiction with regard to mandated reporting on driving. In some jurisdictions, the psychologist is required to document impairment that is of concern and to notify the referring physician, but ultimate responsibility lies with the physician. Conversely, in other jurisdictions, a psychologist is required to document and report someone who is at serious risk of harm from driving and who has failed to comply with a request to stop driving.

In terms of the assessment itself, psychologists should consult the literature on how to use their findings to answer the question of whether a client is likely to pose a safety threat while driving. Love and Tuokko (2015) surveyed clinical psychologists across Canada ($n = 84$) who reported having some older drivers in their clinical practice. Respondents noted that while they were aware of issues related to older drivers, they did not necessarily see the assessment of driving-related abilities as a routine part of their practice. Similarly, most respondents (75%) reported being receptive to further education about the evaluation of fitness to drive. While there is no gold-standard neuropsychometric test that predicts driving ability, common sense can be employed in considering whether impairments in domains such as attention, visuospatial function, executive function, and motor control elevate the risk of harm through driving (Rizzo & Kellison, 2010). It is incumbent that all clinicians have a straightforward, though not punitive, conversation with the client and their family regarding curtailment of driving, acknowledging the practical impact of this decision. Stopping driving may be a gradually unfolding process (e.g., first limit driving at night or under poor visibility conditions) in which the individual can still exercise some agency and autonomy in making the decision. In other cases, discussing concerns about driving with the individual may be challenging because of the individual's difficulties in awareness, either neurological or psychological. Love and Tuokko (2015) provide a variety of resources for psychologists to follow up, including psychoeducational materials that can facilitate discussion between clinicians, family members, and the affected individual.

Summary and Conclusions

Several decades of work have attempted to understand the condition of MCI, define its boundaries, and explore its clinical utility as a means of identifying persons at risk for subsequent decline to dementia. For the affected individual, MCI is a challenging condition because the distress associated with possible decline to dementia may be as troubling as current cognitive impairment itself. In terms of future directions, greater attention needs to be paid to consistent use and operationalization of the term *MCI* in published research, particularly with regard to whether it is a descriptor or a diagnosis. This would include greater characterization of presumed etiology, including biomarker status, as well as in-depth neuropsychological characterization using criteria that are sensitive to impairment beyond normal variation. These efforts will help ascertain who is at elevated risk for decline to dementia, as well as promote more targeted application of intervention to improve cognitive and emotional functioning in persons with MCI.

KEY POINTS

✓ Persons with MCI show significant cognitive impairment that is beyond the scope of normal aging, evidenced in one or more domains of cognitive abilities.

✓ Much like SCD, while MCI is considered a risk factor for future development of dementia, there is no gold-standard marker to determine which individuals will definitively show future decline.

✓ There is debate—and inconsistency—in the field as to whether MCI represents a descriptor of current function or whether it is indicative of progression of an underlying neurodegenerative disease that foreshadows future decline. This important factor has made it problematic to estimate rates of future decline.

✓ Assessment of individuals with suspected MCI should include a comprehensive assessment of medical as well as psychological functioning. This, along with the relative onset of cognitive decline, will help to clarify the presumed etiology and, in turn, may enhance the predictive ability of future decline (e.g., someone with MCI in the context of AD biomarkers, plus a strong family history of AD, may be at elevated risk for declining to AD).

✓ Providing a diagnosis of MCI can have significant psychological consequences, particularly given the uncertainty of the meaning of the diagnosis with regard to future decline. In providing this diagnosis, it is important to ensure that the older adult has adequate supports in place to address any adverse psychological response.

✓ An MCI diagnosis also has ethical implications in terms of decision making in areas such as driving, finances, and medical preferences. Providers are encouraged to work with individuals and their families so that their wishes are expressed and documented before any future cognitive deterioration occurs that will prevent them from doing so. This type of conversation, though difficult, will promote the older adult's autonomy and dignity at a time when he or she may feel these qualities are being eroded along with cognitive decline.

CHAPTER 8

Dementia

Dementia has been defined in many different ways in research and clinical practice, but typically it refers to a decline in cognitive functioning of sufficient severity to interfere with everyday functioning. It is often this interference with everyday functions that brings the condition to clinical attention, even though some subtle cognitive decline may have been evident previously. While historically the term *dementia* implied a progressive course, more recent definitions carry no connotations concerning prognosis (e.g., DSM-IV; American Psychiatric Association, 1994). Similarly, McKhann and colleagues (2011), when providing core clinical criteria for all-cause dementia, note that a diagnosis of dementia encompasses many different underlying diagnostic etiologies and a spectrum of degrees of cognitive impairment from mild to very severe. Specifically, all-cause dementia, according to McKhann et al.'s (2011) criteria, is diagnosed when cognitive or behavioral symptoms are present that (1) interfere with the ability to function at work or in usual activities; (2) represent a decline from previous level of functioning; (3) are not explained by delirium or a major psychiatric disorder; (4) are detected through history taking and objective cognitive assessment; and (5) involve a minimum of two domains (i.e., memory, reasoning, visuospatial abilities, language functions, personality/behavior/comportment). Here we use the term *dementia* to signify cognitive impairment without connotation as to prognosis and include conditions that may be static or progressive. The onset of the cognitive impairment (e.g., rapid, fluctuating, insidious) may vary and may be suggestive of an underlying pathology. Moreover, some underlying etiologies can present in multiple ways. For example, a single, large cerebrovascular event may show maximal deficits at onset, while the accumulation of small vascular events may appear as an insidious onset with progression of deficits over time.

Much neuroscientific research has been conducted linking cognitive impairment to underlying pathology through neuroimaging and biomarkers. Some forms of dementia are linked to specific causes identifiable with neuroimaging (e.g., probable vascular neurocognitive disorder) or through temporal relations between onset of cognitive impairment and an event (e.g., traumatic brain injury). However, definitive biologically based procedures for detection of most forms of dementia are not yet available, and cognitive impairment remains critical for differential diagnostic decision making. For these idiopathic forms of dementia, only presumptive diagnoses of an underlying disease process (e.g., AD) are made with varying levels of certainty premortem (McKhann et al., 2011). Neuropsychological assessment in the context of dementia can delineate a profile of cognitive strengths and weaknesses for use in diagnostic decision making and intervention planning. When observed over time, a trajectory of cognitive decline may be evident, and adjustments can be made to the context of care, as needed. In this chapter, we address the manner in which neuropsychological assessments are conducted at various points in the trajectory of cognitive decline evident in dementia.

Conducting the Assessment

The nature and content of the dementia assessment are likely to vary depending on the primary purpose of the assessment and the degree of cognitive impairment present. However, in all instances, it is important that the assessment is conducted with high ethical standards (see Chapter 4 for details). A variety of specific ethical issues can arise when conducting assessment of cognitively impaired older adults, and care must be taken to ensure that these issues are adequately addressed. The presence of cognitive impairment may, but does not necessarily, preclude engaging in the informed consent process. In some cases, a surrogate decision maker or guardian will need to be enlisted as support for the person in providing joint decision making. The assessment must be conducted in a manner that avoids harm and supports the autonomy and dignity of the older adult. It is important that appropriate assessment approaches and measures are selected, a process that may be particularly challenging as the severity of dementia increases. Later in this chapter, we address the assessment of cognitive capacity and continued decline after a diagnosis of dementia has been made. As dementia severity and dependency on others increase, joint decision making and sharing of information with caring supporters will be paramount.

Initial Diagnosis of Dementia

A diagnosis of dementia is considered when concern about an older adult's cognitive functioning arises and coincident difficulties with everyday functioning are evident. The assessment process as described in Chapter 4 is followed, and it is important to assess for other indicators of conditions (e.g., personality, mood) that may compromise cognitive functions for reasons other than dementia. In addition, the collection of information concerning daily functioning is particularly important, as this is a required element of a dementia diagnosis (McKhann et al., 2011). Typically, when an initial assessment for dementia is conducted, basic activities of daily living (e.g., eating, toileting) will be unaffected. The focus for assessment will be the more complex levels of functioning required for independent living such as shopping, use of the telephone, food preparation, and management of finances and medications (also known as instrumental activities of daily living). While objective measures of daily functioning such as the Everyday Problems Test (Diehl, Willis, & Schaie, 1995) and the Texas Functional Living Scale (Cullum et al., 2001) are available, subjective rating scales are frequently used to collect information about daily functioning. These include the Older American Resources and Services (OARS; Fillenbaum, 1988), the measures of activities of daily living and instrumental activities of daily living from the Multilevel Assessment Instrument (Lawton, Moss, Fulcomer, & Kleban, 1982), and the Index of Independence in Activities of Daily Living (Katz, Moskowitz, Jackson, & Jaffe, 1963). The primary advantage of the subjective measures is that they can be administered in a relatively short period of time (Tuokko & Smart, 2014). However, as with any self-report measures, they are subject to recall errors and biases.

The temporal relations between cognitive impairments and impairments of everyday behaviors are complex and multifactorial. A clear co-occurrence of cognitive and functional losses is evident in relation to dementias (Tuokko & Smart, 2014). While less clearly articulated in the literature, the hierarchy of loss in everyday behaviors typically identifies complex instrumental activities of daily living as likely to be affected earlier than less complex instrumental activities of daily living or activities of daily living. It is particularly important to assess for areas of high potential risk for clients (e.g., financial management, driving). We will address these areas of concern later in this chapter.

The breadth of cognitive domains and the types of detailed assessments required to determine the presence of dementia have been articulated by the NIA-AA workgroups on diagnostic guidelines for AD (McKhann et al., 2011) and DSM-5. In Table 8.1, we indicate the domains relevant to each of these sets of diagnostic criteria. Of note, these sets of criteria differ with respect to the minimum necessary number of cognitive domains where impairment is evident (i.e., one for DSM-5; two for McKhann et

TABLE 8.1. Key Information for Differential Diagnosis of Dementia

Domain	Example of types of information
	History
Onset	Sudden, variable, gradual
Duration of symptoms	Hours, days, months, years?
Course of progression	Maximal neurological deficit at onset, rapid deterioration, progressive decline, variable
Social situation	Marital status, living situation, cultural context
Past medical/physical conditions	Surgeries, anesthetics, psychiatric/neurological events, medications
Current medical/physical conditions	Vision, hearing, motor limitations, medications, psychiatric/neurological conditions
Prior functioning	Educational and occupational background
Current functioning	Daily activities, hobbies, social participation
	Testing
Memory[a,b]	Acquisition and retention of new information
Reasoning/judgment[a]	Decision making, planning, risk taking
Visuospatial[a]	Recognizing faces, objects, operate simple implements, orient clothing
Language[a,b]	Expressive and receptive language; speaking, reading, writing, comprehension
Behavior[a]	Personality, mood, motivation, interest
Complex attention[b]	Sustained, divided or selective attention; processing speed
Executive function[b]	Planning, decision making, working memory, inhibition, mental flexibility
Perceptual–motor[b]	Visual perception, visuoconstruction, perceptual–motor, praxis, gnosis
Social cognition[b]	Recognition of emotions, perspective taking

[a]Identified by McKhann et al. (2011); [b]identified in DSM-5 (American Psychiatric Association, 2013).

al., 2011). However, neither source provides specific direction as to the meaning of impairment. DSM-5 refers to "modest" or "significant" cognitive decline from previous level of cognitive performance. McKhann et al. (2011) merely specify the presence of deficits in two or more areas of cognition, as established through a combination of history taking from the affected person and a knowledgeable informant, and an objective cognitive assessment (i.e., mental status examination or neuropsychological testing). Formulation of a diagnosis of dementia then involves the application of clinical judgment, taking into consideration all available information, and requires a broad understanding of brain–behavior relations.

A number of factors should be considered when selecting measures to assess the cognitive domains of importance for the diagnosis and differential diagnosis of dementia. As is evident in Table 8.1, the application of diagnostic criteria for dementia requires that a broad range of cognitive domains be included in the assessment. For both sets of diagnostic criteria, documentation of cognitive impairment with standardized measures of cognitive function is preferred. In addition to the traditional face-to-face administration of measures of cognitive functions, some measures are available to collect collateral information about the cognitive functioning of people with dementia from informants. Table 8.2 provides a brief description of some of these measures. While these measures may be used when the person with dementia is inaccessible for evaluation, it is always preferable to obtain information concerning cognitive functioning directly from the person with dementia and to combine the information obtained through these different sources.

In DSM-5, the term *dementia* is subsumed under the entity "major NCD," and various etiological subtypes are described. Cognitive impairment of insufficient severity to be classified as a major NCD (or dementia) is recognized as mild NCD in the DSM-5 and is addressed elsewhere in this book (Chapter 7). Major NCDs include degenerative dementias such as AD as well as static conditions such as traumatic brain injury and conditions where a single cognitive domain may be impaired. In addition, cognitive impairments secondary to one or multiple medical conditions are also included as NCDs.

Differential Diagnosis

As the focus of this book is on cognitive decline and this chapter addresses dementia, only the most prevalent age-related conditions considered in formulating a differential diagnosis are described here and distinguished from other disorders that may compete with, or confound, the diagnosis of dementia. In so doing, some key features for consideration when distinguishing between conditions are identified (see Table 8.3). These features,

TABLE 8.2. Informant-Based Measures of Cognitive Decline

Measure and Authors	Description
Alzheimer's Questionnaire (Sabbagh et al., 2010)	Brief, informant-based screening questionnaire for AD; assesses *current functioning* in Memory (5 items), Orientation (3 items), Functional Ability (7 items), Visuospatial (2 items), and Language (3 items); administration time = 2.6 ± 0.6 minutes; in primary care, sensitivity and specificity for detecting AD (98.55, 96.00, respectively)
AD8 (Shaik et al., 2015)	Eight-item informant-based dementia screening instrument; has been used in community settings; assesses memory, orientation, and complex function *over the "past several years"*; acceptable construct validity versus CDR domains and neuropsychological testing ($R \geq .4$)
ECog (Rueda et al., 2015; Park, Harvey, Johnson, & Farias, 2015; Farias et al., 2011)	Informant-based rating scale with 39 items that measure different domains of everyday functioning in relation to 10 years earlier: Everyday memory, Everyday Language, Everyday Visuospatial Functions, Everyday Planning, Everyday Organization, and Everyday Divided Attention (latter three = executive functions); rates patients *in relation to 10 years earlier*; more strongly related ($Rs = .2$-ish) to objective markers of AD than self-report; 12-item short form strongly correlated with functional measures and neuropsychological scores (Blessed $R = .41$; CDR $R = .45$, episodic memory $R = .33$, executive function $R = .19$)
Multidimensional Assessment of Neurodegenerative Symptoms Questionnaire (MANS) (Locke et al., 2009)	Brief measure of cognitive, personality, functional, and motor symptoms potentially related to neurodegenerative etiologies; 87 questions assessing changes *in the past year* in daily habits, personality, and motor functioning; 5–10 minutes to complete; skip pattern for no change; if change present, inquire re: frequency of behavior; four factors = cognitive symptoms, behavioral symptoms, functional symptoms, and language symptoms
IQCODE (Sikkes et al., 2011; Nygaard, Naik, & Geitung, 2009; Cherbuin & Jorm, 2013; Butt, 2008)	Developed and validated to collect information on health and memory of community-dwelling older adults; asks informants to rate 26 changes in everyday cognitive functions *over the past 10 years* (e.g., remembering, learning new things, understanding verbal material, following events, composing written material, handling everyday tasks) of older adults with whom they are familiar; sensitivity and specificity for detecting dementia approximately .75–.85; useful for discriminating between normal, MCI, and AD

TABLE 8.3. Key Features of Disorders Affecting Cognition

Onset of cognitive change	Disorder	Cognitive/behavioral features and course
Rapid (hours to days)	Delirium	• Impaired attention, including ability to focus, sustain, and shift • Disturbances of awareness and levels of consciousness • May fluctuate throughout the day • Likely to resolve with treatment of underlying medical condition
Potentially reversible	Major neurocognitive disorder due to another medical condition	Decline from previous level of functioning in one or more areas of cognitive functioning commensurate with the underlying medical condition (e.g., improvement for treatable disorder, deterioration with progressive, untreatable disorder)
	Major depressive disorder and other disorders of mood	• Low motivation • Limited spontaneous elaboration • Preoccupation with affective state • Memory and executive deficits may be secondary to attentional problems • Cognition better than complaints indicate
Variable	Major neurocognitive disorder with Lewy bodies (DLB)	• Fluctuations in cognitive functions • Impaired attention and disturbance of awareness • Impaired executive functions and visuospatial abilities; recurrent detailed, well-formed visual hallucinations • Memory deficits appear later • At least 1 year after cognitive impairments, slowed movement, rigid muscles, tremors, or shuffling gait may emerge
Maximal neurological deficit at onset	Major vascular neurocognitive disorder (VaD)	• Subsequent to cerebrovascular event, evident history, physical examination, and/or neuroimaging • Cognitive and physical deficits heterogeneous, commensurate with location and extent of vascular lesions

(continued)

TABLE 8.3. *(continued)*

Onset of cognitive change	Disorder	Cognitive/behavioral features and course

Insidious onset with progressive decline	Major FTLD	• *Behavioral variant:* Prominent decline in social conduct that may include disinhibition; apathy; loss of empathy/sympathy; perseveration; compulsive or ritualistic behavior (e.g., hoarding); hyperorality or other changes in eating behavior; early cognitive deficits may include deficient executive functions (e.g., poor planning, distractibility, poor judgment); memory and learning relatively spared; perceptual–motor abilities preserved
		• *Language variants:* Deterioration of language skills with either semantic changes or loss of the ability to generate words and speak easily
		  ○ *Semantic*—fluent speech, difficulty generating or recognizing familiar words; comparatively spared episodic memory
		  ○ *Agrammatic/nonfluent*—halting speech, short phrases, grammar errors; comprehension, reading and writing preserved longer than speech
		  ○ *Logopenic*—spontaneous but slow speech output, word retrieval problems, difficulty repeating phrases or sentences, reading and writing preserved longer than speech

	Major neurocognitive disorder due to AD	• Early impairment in memory and new learning, sometimes deficits in executive functions • Later emergence of impairments of attention, language, and perceptual–motor abilities • Social cognition tends to be preserved until late in the course • Atypical variants: Language, visuospatial, and executive
	VCI	• Mild degrees of cognitive impairment may be evident prior to a stroke or may be indicative of a more insidious accumulation of vascular pathology either cortically or subcortically • Executive dysfunction may be present

including onset/course of decline and cognitive profile, are particularly useful for distinguishing between underlying conditions early in the disease process. In Table 8.4, we note prototypical signs for some forms of dementia, not all of which are described in detail. Of note, disorders that present primarily as movement disorders (e.g., PD, Huntington's disease [HD], PSP, and CBDS) are shown on the right side of Table 8.4 but are not described in detail in this chapter. As an underlying neurodegenerative disease progresses, cognitive deficits become more pervasive and may no longer be useful as indicators of specific etiological dementia variants. However, assessment in moderate and later stages of dementia may serve a number of purposes. For example, the temporal sequencing of changes in cognitive functions may provide confirmation of initial differential diagnosis. Conversely, marked departures from expected trajectories may be indicative of initial misdiagnosis and the emergence of comorbid conditions warranting further evaluation (e.g., medical disorders). Moreover, continued evaluation throughout the course of a dementing process can yield valuable information of relevance to care planning.

We have elected to focus on prevalent processes that affect brain function resulting in measurable cognitive changes in the geriatric population. For more in-depth discussions of the myriad forms of dementia, including those associated with prominent movement disorders, we refer the reader to Attix and Welsh-Bohmer (2006); Noggle, Dean, Bush, and Anderson (2015); and Parks, Zec, and Wilson (1993). We have organized our discussion of these disorders according to their onset and progression (e.g., rapid onset, potentially reversible with intervention, variable, maximal neurologic deficit at onset, insidious onset with progressive decline; Tuokko & Hadjistavropoulos, 1998; Tuokko & Ritchie, 2016), inasmuch as the clinical presentation may help formulate diagnostic hypotheses. However, as will become evident, some conditions may present in multiple ways, and these conditions are located in only one location in our organizational structure (e.g., vascular events of differing presentations appearing within VaD section).

Rapid Onset of Cognitive Impairment

A sudden change in cognitive functioning such that a person's abilities to focus, sustain, and shift attention are impaired is characteristic of a delirium. This impairment of attention may fluctuate over the course of the day, together with other indications of cognitive impairment, disturbances of awareness, and levels of consciousness. These disturbances develop over a short period of time (e.g., hours to days) and are likely to be the direct physiological consequences of underlying medical conditions (e.g., urinary tract infection) or exposure to toxins (including alcohol, withdrawal from

TABLE 8.4. Early Key Diagnostic Signs for Selected Dementias

Cognitive impairment	AD	PCA	VaD	FTD-SD	FTD-A	FTD-B	DLB	PD	HD	PSP	CBDS
STM loss	✓										
Word-finding	✓		✓	✓	✓						
Retrieval deficit			✓								
Attention dysfunction			✓				✓				
Executive dysfunction			✓				✓		✓		
Apraxia		✓		✓	✓						
Agnosia		✓		✓							✓
Agraphia		✓									✓
Language		✓		✓	✓						
Visuospatial		✓					✓				
Other features											
Mood/behavior change				✓		✓					✓
Hallucinations (visual), delusions							✓	✓	✓		
Gait change							✓	✓	✓	✓	
Tremor							✓	✓	✓		
Unilateral motor signs								✓	✓		✓
Eye-movement abnormalities										✓	

Note. FTD-SD, frontotemporal semantic variant; FTD-A, frontotemporal agrammatic variant; FTD-B, frontotemporal behavioral variant; CBDS, corticobasal degeneration syndrome.

alcohol, reactions to medications) occurring alone or in combination. Some instruments that have been developed for use in identifying delirium (Carvalho, de Almeida, & Gusmao-Flores, 2013) include the Confusion Assessment Method (Dosa, Intrator, McNicoll, Cang, & Teno, 2007), the Delirium Rating Scale (Trzepacz et al., 2001), and the Intensive Care Delirium Screening Checklist (Nishimura et al., 2016).

Delirium serves as a marker for serious illness in an older adult and necessitates immediate medical attention. Not attending to the underlying condition may result in stupor, coma, seizures, and possibly death. While recovery from delirium is possible following treatment of the underlying condition, there is presently no agreed upon terminology for defining recovery. It has been suggested that distinctions be made between general versus symptomatic recovery and between short- and long-term outcomes, and that cognitive recovery be central for defining recovery in delirium (Adamis, Devaney, Shanahan, McCarthy, & Meagher, 2015). The prevalence of delirium rises with age to 14% in those over age 85 and has been observed in 10–30% of older adults presenting to emergency departments. Delirium is especially prevalent among older adults in hospital (6–56%), postoperatively (15–53%), and in nursing homes (up to 60%), as well as among the terminally ill (80%) (DSM-5).

While delirium is in and of itself distinct from dementia, a delirium can be superimposed on an existing dementia, exacerbating the rate of cognitive decline, or it may herald the emergence of an underlying dementia (Fong et al., 2009). Delirium is also associated with falls in hospitalized patients and with poor outcomes when experienced postoperatively (Australian and New Zealand Society for Geriatric Medicine, 2016). Subsyndromal delirium is characterized by the presence of some, but not all, of the symptoms associated with the diagnosis of delirium. While subsyndromal delirium has been defined in various ways, it appears to be associated with some poor outcomes and is gaining attention in medical settings (Meagher et al., 2014).

Potentially Reversible Forms of Cognitive Impairment

Many medical conditions can adversely affect cognitive functioning and be mistaken for an idiopathic NCD such as AD. These conditions may not present as a delirium but may affect cognition in a variety of other ways that meet the criteria for major NCD. It must be noted that conditions affecting many different systems in the body may give rise to cognitive impairment, including those affecting the endocrine system (e.g., hypoglycemia, hypothyroidism), immune disorders (e.g., systemic lupus erythematosus), nutritional conditions (e.g., thiamine deficiencies), conditions resulting in hypoxia such as heart failure, and renal failure (DSM-5). Suffice to say that a thorough understanding of the older adult's medical history and medical condition is imperative when formulating a differential diagnosis involving cognitive impairment.

Key features to consider when associating cognitive deficits with medical conditions is the temporal sequence between the onset of the condition and the emergence of the cognitive deficit, as well as the cognitive response to treatment for the medical condition (American Psychiatric Association, 2013). While the presence of one or more of these serious medical conditions does not preclude the existence of another underlying neurodegenerative condition, it is imperative that all medical conditions commonly associated with cognitive impairment be evaluated and addressed before ascribing the cognitive impairment to another etiology (e.g., AD).

Other potentially reversible conditions that may affect cognitive functioning include disorders that affect mood. Depressive disorders are quite common in older adults, although the prevalence is approximately one-third that of individuals between 18 and 20 years of age (DSM-5). Several depressive syndromes are described in the DSM-5 including major depressive disorder, persistent depressive disorder (i.e., dysthymia), substance/medication-induced depressive disorder, and depressive disorder due to another medical condition. Depression in older adults may be accompanied by cognitive impairments such as memory impairment, executive impairment, or attentional deficits (Lockwood et al., 2000). It has been observed that cognitive impairments may remit with treatment (Lockwood et al., 2000). However, it has also been observed that there are high rates of comorbidity between depression and dementia (Snowden et al., 2015). Depressive symptoms may precede, and possibly be a risk factor for, dementia (Ownby et al., 2006). Whether or not depression is accompanied by cognitive impairment sufficiently severe to warrant a diagnosis of dementia, treatment for depression may alleviate any excess disability created by the depression.

Variable Cognitive Impairment

One of the core distinguishing features for the DSM-5 diagnosis of major NCD with Lewy bodies (also known as DLB) is fluctuating cognition associated with pronounced variations in attention and alertness. DLB may be mistaken for PD, but there are several important distinguishing factors. The first, and perhaps the most important, is the onset of symptoms; in PD, motoric features always, by definition, precede cognitive impairments. By contrast, in DLB the features of parkinsonism (e.g., slowed movement, rigid muscles, tremors, or a shuffling walk) emerge at least a year subsequent to cognitive deficits. Persons with DLB can also present with recurrent visual hallucinations that are detailed and well formed. Second, while the DLB and PD cognitive profiles overlap in terms of attention, executive functions, and visuospatial abilities, individuals with DLB also show cortical impairments such as memory emerging over time (Petrova et al., 2016). Third, persons with DLB often show waxing and waning cognitive status, and the early presentation of fluctuations in cognition may resemble delirium but with no discernible underlying medical cause.

The parkinsonism seen in DLB must be distinguished from neuroleptic-induced extrapyramidal signs. Features further suggestive of DLB include rapid-eye-movement sleep behavioral disorder, and severe narcoleptic sensitivity. For a DSM-5 diagnosis of probable major NCD with Lewy bodies to be made, two of the core features and one of the suggestive features must be present. Individuals with only one feature (core or suggestive) may be identified with possible major NCD with Lewy bodies. Other features such as repeated falls, unexplained loss of consciousness, nonvisual hallucinations, and depression may be associated with the disorder. While the early trajectory of the disorder is characterized by fluctuations in cognition, ultimately the disorder progresses to profound impairment of cognitive functions.

Given that this disorder is characterized by hallucinations, the common coexistence of severe narcoleptic sensitivity is important to note. Traditional antipsychotic medications used in the treatment of hallucinations (e.g., haloperidol) must be avoided. People with narcoleptic sensitivity may respond to such medications with worsening cognition, increased and possibly irreversible parkinsonism, or neuroleptic malignant syndrome, which can be fatal (Baskys, 2004). The treatment for hallucinations must be approached cautiously, using very low doses of medications under constant observation for adverse effects.

Maximal Neurological Deficit at Onset

Vascular Dementia

Dementias that occur as a consequence of cerebrovascular incidents (Onyike, 2006) are classified in DSM-5 as major vascular NCDs and may also be referred to as VaD. However, DSM-5 also provides for a milder form of vascular NCD. Moreover, at least some forms of cerebrovascular disease can be effectively managed to prevent or delay progression of cognitive impairment. VCI, then, can be the result of various types of cerebrovascular disease that may differ in terms of identification, severity of cognitive impairment, and management (Skrobot et al., 2017). VaD, the condition associated with the most severe form of cognitive impairment, is the second most common cause of neurocognitive disorders (after AD), and the prevalence increases with age. According to Skrobot et al. (2017), mild degrees of cognitive impairment may be evident prior to a stroke or may be indicative of a more insidious accumulation of vascular pathology, either cortically or subcortically.

Cerebrovascular incidents of sudden onset (i.e., poststroke) often are associated with significant cognitive and physical deficits. The Vascular

Impairment of Cognition Classification Consensus Study (Skrobot et al., 2017) notes that poststroke dementia includes various causes and changes in the brain and that the severe cognitive impairment occurs within 6 months of the stroke, differentiating it from other forms of VaD (i.e., subcortical ischemic vascular dementia, multi-infarct dementia). The type and severity of cognitive impairment in VaD is dependent on the location and cause of the cerebral damage. VaD may be the result of an occlusion of blood vessels in the brain that may affect subcortical structures, or it may occur subsequent to hemorrhage (i.e., rupturing) of intra- or extracranial blood vessels that may affect cortical regions. Lesions affecting subcortical regions tend to result in physical features such as muscle spasticity, rigidity, and limb weakness. The cognitive profile associated with subcortical damage varies but may include apathy and loss of tact. Cortical damage may result in well-defined focal syndromes related to the location of the damage (e.g., aphasia following damage to the cortical areas involved in speech production). Often, a clear temporal relationship exists between a vascular event and the onset of cognitive deficits that is supported by neuroimaging evidence, and a diagnosis of probable vascular NCD can be made. In other instances, the evidence may be less clear, and a presumptive diagnosis of possible vascular NCD is made.

VaD and other types of NCDs (e.g., AD) can coexist, resulting in a mixed cognitive profile. The temporal sequencing of the emergence and progression of cognitive deficits and evidence from neuroimaging may provide information as to the primary diagnosis (e.g., AD vs. VaD). It has been suggested that both VaD and AD may be linked to a common underlying pathology (de la Torre, 2004; Onyike, 2006; Snyder et al., 2015), but they are diagnosed as distinct entities.

Traumatic Brain Injury

Cognitive impairments, including those significant enough to interfere with everyday functions, have been observed to occur subsequent to traumatic brain injury (TBI) sustained at any age. Within DSM-5, a major NCD due to a TBI is diagnosed when there is evidence of an impact to the head with loss of consciousness, posttraumatic difficulties with memory, disorientation, and/or confusion or neurological signs, including neuroimaging evidence of injury. Outcomes after TBI vary depending on many factors such as the mechanism of injury (e.g., motor vehicle crash, fall), age at onset, severity of the TBI (i.e., mild, moderate, severe), and comorbid conditions (e.g., posttraumatic stress disorder, substance use disorders). While TBIs are often associated with motor vehicle crashes and sports injuries in people between the ages of 15 and 24 years, another peak in the incidence of TBI occurs for people ages 70 years and older. Falls are the most common cause of TBI in older adults (Lecours, Sirois, Ouellet, Boivin, & Simard, 2012), and TBIs sustained by older adults are a major cause of death, disability, and increased dependency on others (Testa, Malec, Moessner, & Brown, 2005). Those older adults who sustain a mild TBI may show little to no cognitive or functional sequelae after a period of recovery (Albrecht, Masters, Ames, & Foster, 2016; Rapoport et al., 2008), but this is not always the case (Kinsella, 2010); recovery from TBI in older adults generally is not strongly predicted by the level of severity (Testa et al., 2005). Certainly, medical complications occurring in concert with even mild TBIs can affect the recovery process. For example, because of age-related changes to the pathophysiology of the brain, older adults may be at greater risk than younger adults of delayed subdural hematoma or intracranial hemorrhage subsequent to a TBI (Papa, Mendes, & Braga, 2012; Rathlev et al., 2006). In addition, the traumatic experience itself (Kinsella, Olver, Ong, Gruen, & Hammersley, 2014; Kinsella, Olver, Ong, Hammersley, & Plowright, 2014; Testa et al., 2005) and the consequences of other injuries (e.g., pain; Moriarty, McGuire, & Finn, 2011) sustained at the time of the TBI can contribute to slower rates of recovery and poorer long-term outcomes in mood, everyday functioning, and cognition for older adults (Papa, Mendes, & Braga, 2012).

Other factors related to the person's preinjury status (e.g., medical or neuropsychiatric conditions, genetic predispositions) and postinjury environmental supports (e.g., access to rehabilitation, social engagement and support; Lecours et al., 2012) can also affect the recovery process. The person's preinjury status is influenced by the protective and risk or vulnerability factors for cognitive aging described in Chapters 2 and 3, which, in turn, may contribute to (or limit) the reserve capacity of the individual (Goldstein & Levin, 2001). A person's preinjury medical status may also increase the risk for recurrent falls and subsequent TBIs.

After a period of recovery, the residual cognitive and functional impairments due to the TBI are considered nonprogressive or stable (Cato & Crosson, 2006). The most frequently observed deficits in cognitive functioning post-TBI are in the areas of attention, memory, and executive functioning (Starkstein & Jorge, 2005). In accordance with the theory of brain reserve capacity, it is conceivable that some further cognitive decline may occur in association with the expected age-related changes. A link has been made between a history of TBI and the development of AD, but the evidence for this link remains unclear (Starkstein & Jorge, 2005). Differences between studies in the manner in which types and severity of TBI are characterized and how dementia is diagnosed contribute to this lack of clarity. In particular, the cognitive status of people prior to TBI is often unknown or not investigated, and it is well known that many neurodegenerative conditions (e.g., AD) may have long preclinical phases. It may be that for people predisposed to develop AD (e.g., genetic vulnerability), TBI accelerates the process by reducing cognitive reserve. Another possible explanation is that biochemical changes subsequent to TBI initiate a cascade of molecular changes within the brain leading to AD-like pathology (Starkstein & Jorge, 2005). That said, much more research is needed to establish a convincing link between TBI and AD.

Another complicating factor is that repeated concussive and subconcussive injuries may result in an apparent neurodegenerative condition known as chronic traumatic encephalopathy (CTE) or traumatic encephalopathy syndrome (TES). Specific diagnostic criteria have been proposed for these conditions (CTE: Jordan, 2013; Victoroff, 2013; TES: Montenigro et al., 2014), though none have been agreed upon at a national or international level (Iverson, Gardner, McCrory, Zafonte, & Castellani, 2015). These conditions have been identified most often in athletes and soldiers, with an average age of onset of 54 years (Turner, Lucke-Wold, Robson, Lee, & Bailes, 2016). The onset of symptoms can range from a few months posttrauma to several decades and include disturbance of mood (e.g., depression, paranoia, suicidality), behavior (e.g., deterioration in interpersonal relationships, criminal and violent tendencies), cognition (e.g., memory impairment, executive dysfunction, attention and concentration difficulties, language impairment, and visual spatial difficulties), and motor functions (e.g., dysarthria, tremor, gait disturbance, features of parkinsonism). Younger people with CTE are most likely to exhibit changes in mood, including explosive rage and substance abuse, whereas cognitive decline may be the primary presentation for those with an older age at onset (Stern et al., 2013). This is a relatively rare condition, and much more research is needed for a clear understanding of the diagnostic implications of the cognitive change observed following repeated head injury.

Insidious Onset with Progressive Decline

As indicated earlier, mild degrees of cognitive impairment may be indicative of the insidious accumulation of vascular pathology either cortically or subcortically; this condition in relation to MCI is described elsewhere (see Chapter 7). An insidious onset of vascular changes may appear prior to a stroke or in relation to other forms of VaD such as subcortical ischemic VaD, multi-infarct dementia, or dementia associated with mixed etiology (Skrobot et al., 2017). There are other neurodegenerative disorders such as Huntington's disease (HD) or PD, or rarer conditions such as CBDS and PSP that may also have cognitive and behavioral consequences, though these typically are not manifest in the early stages of the underlying disease process and are not addressed here. The major NCDs where cognitive impairment plays a central role emerges slowly and insidiously, shows gradual progressive deterioration, and interferes with everyday functioning include variants of FTLD and AD.

Frontotemporal Lobar Degeneration

FTLD can be characterized as a spectrum of disorders that affect changes in behavior and language functions. Two primary variants of FTLD are described in DSM-5: the behavioral variant and the language variant. The behavioral variant is characterized by a prominent decline in social conduct as well as three or more of the following behavioral symptoms: disinhibition; apathy; loss of empathy or sympathy; perseverative, compulsive, or ritualistic behavior; and hyperorality or other changes in eating behavior. The marked changes in behavior often occur early in the course of the disorder, with little evidence of cognitive impairment except for apparent deficits in executive or self-regulatory functions. Memory and perceptual–motor functions remain relatively spared early in the disease progression.

In the language variant, marked impairment of language is evident, and these deficits have been classified as semantic, agrammatic/nonfluent, and logopenic (The FTD Disorders, 2016). The semantic form of the language variant (or semantic dementia [SD]) is characterized by difficulty generating or recognizing familiar words with fluent speech being retained, allowing the person to talk around situations where a word cannot be recalled. In the agrammatic/nonfluent form of the language variant, there is great difficulty producing speech. It may be effortful and hesitant and appear uncoordinated. Mutism may occur. Comprehension, reading, and writing are preserved longer than speech but will eventually be affected. In the logopenic variant, there are problems with word-finding, speech may be slow, difficulty repeating phrases and sentences may be apparent, but repetition of words is typically retained. As with the agrammatic form, reading and writing will be maintained longer than speech but will decline over time and mutism may occur. Difficulty with comprehension of complex materials may become evident, and difficulty swallowing may occur late in the course of the disease.

A diagnosis of probable frontotemporal neurocognitive disorder can be made if there is evidence of a genetic component (e.g., family history, genetic testing) or neuroimaging evidence of disproportionate frontal and/or temporal lobe involvement. If these sources of information are not available, a diagnosis of possible frontotemporal neurocognitive disorder is made. It has been proposed that certain disorders primarily affecting movement such as ALS, CBDS, and PSP may also fall within the spectrum of FTLD disorders.

Alzheimer's Disease

The most prevalent form of major NCD is AD, accounting for approximately 60% or more of all cases of dementias (Terry, 2006, 2007). The prevalence of AD is age-associated, with a mean survival after diagnosis of approximately 10 years (DSM-5). While the diagnostic criteria for AD have been refined (McKhann et al., 2011), it continues to be a diagnosis of exclusion in that the diagnosis cannot be made if there is evidence of any other coexisting condition that could contribute to the observed cognitive impairment (DSM-5; McKhann et al., 2011). According to DSM-5 diagnostic criteria, there continues to be an emphasis on a decline in memory and learning, whereas the diagnostic criteria for probable or possible AD of McKhann and his colleagues (2011) can be fulfilled by either amnestic or nonamnestic (i.e., language, visuospatial, executive dysfunction) presentations. That said, it is acknowledged in the diagnostic features section of the DSM-5 that nonamnestic forms of AD exist. One such atypical variant of AD is posterior cortical atrophy (PCA) that presents with impairment of complex visual processing. The DSM-5 and McKhann et al. (2011) sets of diagnostic criteria also differ as to the meanings of the terms *probable* and *possible AD*. In DSM-5, a diagnosis of probable AD requires either (1) evidence of a causative genetic mutation from family history or genetic testing, or (2) clear evidence of decline in cognition, a steadily progressive course (i.e., without extended plateaus) and no evidence of mixed etiology. According to the criteria of McKhann et al. (2011), a diagnosis of probable AD can be given in the context of an insidious onset, clear-cut worsening of cognition, prominent cognitive deficits (amnestic or nonamnestic), and no evidence of mixed etiology. The level of certainty associated with the diagnosis is increased by documented decline in cognitive functions or evidence of a causative genetic mutation. In DSM-5, a diagnosis of possible AD is given when all conditions for probable AD are not met. According to the criteria of McKhann et al. (2011), a diagnosis of possible AD can be given when the course of decline is atypical or there is evidence of mixed etiology.

The typical early cognitive profile in AD is impairment of memory (particularly word-finding and episodic memory) and new learning that may co-occur with executive dysfunction. Visuospatial, perceptual–motor, and language impairment will emerge later, whereas social cognition (i.e., sensitivity to social standards, recognition of emotions) typically remains preserved until late in the course. It should be noted that social cognition has been defined far more broadly in other contexts and refers to how people make sense of themselves, others, and the social context (Hess & Blanchard-Fields, 1999). A growing body of social cognitive research focuses on the lived experience of people who have been diagnosed with dementia (Caddell & Clare, 2013; Clare, 2003) and examines the processes involved in adapting to and coping with changing life circumstances. This research goes beyond the limited conceptualization of social cognition presented in DSM-5 and focuses on the ways to assess and explore the social cognitive aspects of dementia, the impact of dementia on self and identity, and recommendations for interventions that support the social cognitive functioning of people diagnosed with dementia.

Summary of Factors Contributing to Initial Diagnosis and Differential Diagnosis

Table 8.4 summarizes the early key features that need to be taken into consideration when formulating differential diagnoses of dementia or a major NCD. The manner in which cognitive deficits initially present and evolve over time is particularly useful in making diagnoses. For example, PCA, the visual variant of AD, initially manifests with visuospatial and visuoperceptual impairments affecting reading, judging distances, or maneuvering stairs and escalators, with relative sparing of memory, executive functions, and linguistic skills (Charles & Hillis, 2005; Crutch et al., 2012). Features of Balint's syndrome (simultanagnosia, oculomotor apraxia, optic ataxia, environmental agnosia) and Gerstmann's syndrome (acalculia, agraphia, finger agnosia, right–left disorientation) may also be present (Crutch et al., 2012). These unusual deficits, taken in conjunction with a relatively young age at onset (i.e., mid-50s to early 60s), can lead to misdiagnosis (e.g., VaD) (Charles & Hillis, 2005). Similarly, individuals with SD, the semantic form of the language variant of FTLD, present with marked impairment in knowledge of word meaning with intact grammar and syntax, and relatively spared recent memories in relation to remote memories (Nestor, Graham, Bozeat, Simons, & Hodges, 2002). This is in contrast to the memory deficits seen in AD. Both SD and AD can show impairment in semantic memory (Libon et al., 2013), though those with AD are impaired in several other cognitive domains as well (Libon et al., 2013).

In addition to the types and temporal sequence of the emergence of cognitive impairments, the type of onset (i.e., sudden or gradual) and the course (i.e., rapid decline, fluctuating, progressive) can provide useful diagnostic information. Delirium and DLB appear similar in terms of early presentation: fluctuating cognitive impairments that primarily affect attention may be evident. Distinguishing between them is important for ensuring prompt treatment for an underlying medical disorder. Where no medical disorder is discernible, DLB may be considered. It is also imperative that the influences of other existing medical conditions on cognitive functions be carefully considered when formulating diagnoses. Treatment for some medical conditions (e.g., medication, chemotherapy) can also affect cognitive functions. In addition, undiagnosed medical conditions such as diabetes, hypothyroidism, and many others can present with cognitive symptoms. The behavioral presentation may be particularly useful when distinguishing major depressive disorders or major frontotemporal NCDs from other conditions such as AD. Differentiation between these conditions is of utmost importance for identifying all remediable sources of cognitive impairment and for establishing appropriate expectations concerning the present and future needs of the individual.

Dementia can also manifest in people with ID but may do so at younger ages (e.g., 40s and 50s), and the clinical presentation may be different than that seen in people without ID. While disturbances in cognition (e.g., memory, praxis) occur, behavioral and personality changes may be the first deficits to emerge and can compromise everyday functioning (Anderson-Mooney et al., 2016). The risk of developing dementia for people with ID is about the same or slightly higher than that for those without ID (Janicki & Dalton, 2000; Strydom et al., 2013; Zigman et al., 2004), except in the case of DS where the risk is substantially higher, with some suggesting that 50–70% of adults with DS will be affected with dementia by the age of 60 (Janicki & Dalton, 2000; McCarron, McCallion, Reilly, & Mulryan, 2014; Strydom et al., 2013). The genetic anomalies associated with DS are linked to the neuropathological changes characteristic of AD, and people with DS have a higher risk of developing AD than the general population (Nieuwenhuis-Mark, 2009).

For each of the disorders described, it must be noted that older adults often present with multiple medical conditions that can complicate the diagnostic process and influence the clinical course. This is particularly true for those with ID and for people over age 80 when multiple morbidities and multiple medications are the norm. It may not always be possible to clearly delineate a diagnosis. However, it is important that every effort be made to ensure that the comprehensive evaluation addresses those disorders that may compete with or confound the diagnosis of dementia, as some components of the presentation may respond to treatment (e.g., delirium, depression, other medical conditions).

Additional and Ongoing Assessment of Dementia

In practice, it is often difficulty with everyday functioning that brings older adults to the attention of clinicians and begins the diagnostic process. Difficulties performing everyday activities and work-related activities must be present for a diagnosis of dementia or major neurocognitive disorder to be made, and this condition must represent a decline from previous levels of functioning (DSM-5; McKhann et al., 2011). Once a diagnosis has been established, additional and perhaps ongoing assessments may be warranted to characterize the disorder more fully, particularly with respect to the extent of disability (World Health Organization, 1993) experienced by the person. At this point, the focus of the assessment process shifts from cause (i.e., diagnosis and etiology) to impact (World Health Organization, 2001). Here the emphasis in the assessment may be on care planning or capacity to manage.

While clear characterization of cognitive deficits is crucial for diagnostic purposes, the degree to which measures of cognition reflect how well a person will perform everyday tasks is often quite poor, particularly in the early stages of the disorder. Although measures of some cognitive domains, most notably executive functions, have been shown to be moderately related to global measures of everyday functioning (Tuokko & Smart, 2014), the relations between specific domains of cognitive functioning and the performance of everyday behavior are complex and multifactorial. Tasks encountered in everyday life (e.g., dressing, managing medications, driving a car) differ greatly in terms of requisite skills and draw on different cognitive domains to a greater or lesser extent. Moreover, different people can perform poorly on the same everyday task (e.g., driving) for very different reasons (i.e., attention, visuospatial perception, planning). The magnitude of the impact of cognitive deficits on specific everyday functions cannot be presumed, and information must be solicited through observation, self-report of the person with dementia, or the report of a knowledgeable informant such as a family member, friend, or other care provider.

The extent of disability experienced by the person with dementia can be influenced by other factors beyond cognition, such as physical health status and factors external to the individual such as the social context in which the person is situated. Older adults may experience many health problems, including chronic conditions, such as those affecting musculoskeletal (e.g., arthritis) and sensory (e.g., visual and auditory) functions. The symptoms (e.g., pain, stiffness, and numbness) associated with these disorders may limit a person's mobility and affect even simple everyday tasks such as dressing, shopping, or housework. Distinguishing disabilities due to cognitive deficits from those due to other influences can be challenging and will require clinicians to inquire beyond the mere presence of difficulties with everyday tasks and explore all relevant contributing factors.

Clarifying the factors affecting the performance of everyday tasks for people with dementia is important for finding ways to minimize the disability and maximize the functioning for as long as possible. Monitoring for changes in everyday competencies can yield valuable information of relevance for proactively altering care plans to best serve the needs of the person with dementia. Marked departures from what might reasonably be expected on the basis of existing impairments (i.e., excess disability) may be indicative of the emergence of comorbid conditions warranting further evaluation (e.g., depression, medical disorders).

While several measures are available for obtaining information about the everyday functioning of people with dementia, most emphasize what a person can do, not whether there are ways or situations in which the person can get things done. A person may not be able to carry out a task (e.g., remember to pay rent at the beginning of each month) but may be able to indicate the desire to have it done through another process (e.g., automatic withdrawal). Social and physical contexts can play a major role in facilitating the continued active engagement of a person with dementia in everyday tasks and can often serve as the foundation for interventions.

In any functional assessment of a person with dementia, it is necessary to obtain information about the person's environmental context. A clinical evaluation focused on enhancing the everyday functioning of a person with dementia is similar to the type of assessment required to address the legal capacity of the individual to engage in specific behaviors. Whenever possible, it is preferable for all concerned to address limitations in everyday decision making by engaging with the person with dementia and seeking the least intrusive alternatives for intervention. Only in exceptional circumstances may it be necessary for an individual with dementia to undergo a capacity assessment within the legal system where a finding of incapacity may result in the loss of a legally recognized right to perform a task or make a decision (American Bar Association Commission on Law and Aging & American Psychological Association, 2008).

Capacity Assessments

Questions about the legal capacity of older adults to engage in specific behaviors (e.g., financial decision making, driving, living alone in the community) can arise in a variety of circumstances, but these questions may become of particular concern when a diagnosis of major NCD (or dementia) has been made (American Bar Association Commission on Law and Aging & American Psychological Association Aging & Association, 2008). It is becoming more common for psychologists to be involved in capacity assessment, as they are well positioned to address complex cases requiring cognitive and functional evaluation. Capacity assessments may be part of a broad clinical assessment, or they may be requested in the context of legal transactions, including:

1. Decisions regarding personal care, including advanced directives, representation agreements, assigning power of attorney.
2. Health care, including consent to treatment and receipt of services.
3. Sexual consent.
4. Property transactions, including financial decision making.
5. Testamentary capacity (i.e., creating or altering a will).
6. Decisions to engage in contracts, including marriage.

A host of capacities are articulated within legal acts or regulations and differ across jurisdictions. Decision-making capacities can vary within an individual and can be conceptualized as a capacity continuum, with some decision-making activities requiring the demonstration of a higher level of skills and understanding than others. Some legal situations (e.g., making a will) require a more general understanding of the circumstances, whereas others (e.g., entering into a contract with financial implications) require knowledge of very specific and detailed information. When there is no evidence of diminished capacity, an individual has the right to make decisions that differ from those of others, even if those decisions place the person at increased risk.

When addressing a specific capacity in a specific legal context, it may be necessary to demonstrate the presence of:

1. An illness, disease, injury, or other condition that may affect decision making.
2. A functional impairment.
3. A lack of understanding/appreciation of the situation and the consequences of the decision.

The exact nature of the information requisite for capacity assessments may differ depending on the capacity in question and by jurisdiction. Familiarity with local state/provincial legal acts/regulations is essential. Here we will discuss general principles to take into consideration when providing a clinical judgment about the capacity of an older adult. An excellent resource, *Assessment of Older Adults with Diminished Capacity: A Handbook for Psychologists,* clearly describes the process of capacity assessment, taking into consideration that specific procedures may vary between jurisdictions (American Bar Association Commission on Law and Aging & American Psychological Association, 2008).

A capacity assessment will necessarily address the same components as a differential diagnostic assessment (e.g., description of the individual's background, determination of a diagnosis, articulation of cognitive strengths and weaknesses, recommendations for interventions) and will specifically address issues relevant to the specific capacity question. The mere presence of a cognitive impairment is not sufficient to indicate inability to engage in specific behaviors. Rather, additional assessment addressing the adaptive functioning of the individual will be required. This assessment must be tailored to the specific behavior in question and must go beyond a cursory assessment of activities of daily living or instrumental activities of daily living (for examples, see Appendix 8.1). The focus of this aspect of the assessment is on functioning and finding ways to adequately assess the specific capacity in question as directly as possible. Subsequently, practical accommodations may be recommended to improve capacity (i.e., treatment of an underlying condition) or provide supports to mitigate risk of harm using the least restrictive alternatives.

Whenever possible, it is preferable to observe and directly assess the person performing the specific behavior in question. In addition, questions concerning any difficulties performing the task can be asked of the individual and collateral informants (e.g., friends and family members).

Additional information can be gathered from the individual concerning the person's knowledge about the specific task. If knowledge is lacking, the opportunity to provide the information to the individual can be taken and his or her response to it evaluated. When evaluating whether a person can make decisions concerning the activity, self-report information sheds light on the person's awareness of his or her own limitations and possible risks. Discrepancies between the perception of the individual and the information obtained from collateral sources may indicate lack of awareness or lack of understanding/appreciation of the situation and the consequences of his or her behavior. For example, when the specific behavior in question is driving, a comprehensive assessment of cognition would be followed by an on-road assessment conducted by an authorized driving assessment agency (Korner-Bitensky, Gélinas, Man-Son-Hing, & Marshall, 2005). The individual can be asked questions about his or her driving (e.g., For what purposes, when, and where does he or she drive?), and collateral information can be collected from people who have been in the vehicle with the driver or who know his or her driving practices well (Has there been damage to the vehicle? Have there been changes in insurance rates?). The personal circumstance of the individual and his or her interpersonal context must be explored (e.g., Where does the driver live? Are there other drivers in the household? Does the person use other forms of transportation?). In many jurisdictions, the person can request his or her own driving record and may be requested to bring it to the assessment, or consent can be provided for others to access the record. The presence or absence of crashes and violations is not necessarily an indicator of performance. Rather, it is another source of information to be used when formulating an opinion concerning capacity to drive.

Other factors that may inform the clinician's opinion concerning an individual's capacity to engage in a specific behavior include psychiatric or emotional factors; values and preferences expressed by the individual (American Bar Association Commission on Law and Aging & American Psychological Association, 2008); and analysis of risk to the individual. Psychiatric disorders affecting mood or thought processes (e.g., depression, anxiety, psychosis), though not necessarily impairing capacity, may limit reasoning and judgment, and these limitations may be time-limited (i.e., improve with treatment). Possible improvement with treatment and timeline for reconsidering capacity are necessary elements to be addressed in a capacity assessment. Similarly, age cohort, gender, sexual orientation, culture, race, ethnicity, and religion may affect an individual's values (i.e., set of beliefs, concerns, and approaches that guide personal decisions) and/or preferences (i.e., various choices that inform values; American Bar Association Commission on Law and Aging & American Psychological Association, 2008). These must be addressed when conducting a capacity evaluation. The values of the individual being assessed will be taken into consideration when formulating a care plan for the individual and must be distinguished from those of the evaluator. That is, the values of the evaluator and the individual being assessed may differ, and the evaluator's opinion must be consistent with the values of the individual being assessed. The risk faced by the individual in his or her current situation will necessarily involve an assessment of the available environmental supports and demands. If the cognitive demands of the individual's life circumstances are high and environmental supports are low, the person is potentially at risk of harm. Here the social context of the individual is of particular concern, for the level of intervention or supervision recommended must match the risk of harm to the individual or others (e.g., inability to drive safely puts others at risk).

A capacity assessment within a legal context will culminate in a report describing the findings of the assessment as well as a clear opinion about the capacity in question. It may be clear in the case of a person with a dementia of profound severity that capacity is lacking with respect to decision making across a number of different specific behaviors. However, people in the early stages of a degenerative dementia may retain the capacity to engage in and make most decisions but may also lack the requisite awareness and/or capability to handle more complex decisions. All of the information obtained from the comprehensive cognitive evaluation, direct evaluation of the behavior in question, and information reported by the individual and others, taken together with information concerning the individual's values and preferences and personal/interpersonal circumstance, must be integrated into a reasoned opinion concerning the specific question at hand. Typically, a dichotomous "yes" or "no" opinion concerning a specific capacity is requested. In some cases, the capacity to engage in more than one behavior may be questioned, and separate opinions may be warranted. Under specific conditions based on the existing evidence (i.e., not clinician's reluctance to offer a clear opinion), a finding of "marginal capacity" may be warranted (American Bar Association Commission on Law and Aging & American Psychological Association, 2008).

The information contained in the report is used within the legal system to make a legal determination as to whether the individual has capacity to engage in the specific behavior in question (e.g., make a will, sell or acquire property). Such a determination cannot be made by physicians or psychologists. Instead, physicians or psychologists provide their professional opinions to those within the legal system for consideration in making a determination. Typically, the cases that come to the attention of the legal system are quite complex. Working with lawyers and judges requires some familiarity with the roles they play in capacity determinations; being cognizant of the specific requirements and procedures within a jurisdiction can facilitate the assessment process and improve communication and collaboration.

Assessing across the Trajectory of Dementia Decline

As indicated in Table 8.3, the temporal sequencing of the emergence of cognitive impairments over the developmental course of a dementia differs between the conditions underlying the disorder (Smits et al., 2015). As the most prevalent degenerative dementia, AD has received the most attention in terms of characterizing the associated evolution of cognitive and behavioral symptoms. To capture the emergence of symptoms, observational rating scales have been developed, including the Global Deterioration Scale (GDS; Reisberg et al., 2014), the Behavioral Assessment for AD (BEHAVE-AD; Reisberg et al., 2014), the Functional Assessment Staging (FAST; Sclan & Reisberg, 1992) in AD, and the Revised Memory and Behavior Problem Checklist (RMBPC; Teri et al., 1992). For example, the GDS describes seven levels of progressive changes seen in AD in terms of cognitive, functional, affective and behavioral disturbances (Reisberg et al., 2014). The final stage of severe dementia (GDS Stage 7), is described as the stage in which "verbal abilities are lost," "patients are incontinent," and the person can no longer walk. The FAST allows for a more detailed characterization of the final stages of dementia with six successive functional substages within GDS 7 and five functional substages within GDS Stage 6, moderate dementia (Reisberg et al., 2006). It is clear, then, that even when dementia is severe, there are differences between individuals in terms of functional capabilities that should not be overlooked. A clear understanding of the functioning of the individual when she or he is no longer able to communicate verbally has the potential to improve quality of care and reduce human suffering, neglect, and distress (Reisberg et al., 2014).

Many of the traditional, performance measures of cognitive functioning used for diagnostic purposes are not suited to ongoing cognitive evaluation into the later stages of the disorder. Typically, this is because the cognitive measure lacks sensitivity at the lower end of the scale where individuals with severe dementia are performing. While it is clear that the person is performing poorly, no information is provided about the types of cognitive function that are retained. Several instruments have been introduced to address this concern (see Table 8.5). Each of the measures in Table 8.5 was developed to assess multiple cognitive domains in the later stages of the disorder. All of the measures are suitable for use with severe dementia; some can also be used in moderate dementia. They vary in terms of the domains assessed, the amount of time for administration, and the degree to which verbal responses are required. All have demonstrated acceptable reliability and validity but differ in terms of the types of reliability (e.g., test–retest, interrater) and validity (e.g., discriminant, concurrent) examined. The measures differ with respect to the amount of training required for administration and the amount of equipment (e.g., stimulus materials) required. Some are particularly flexible and can easily be administered at the bedside. Some

TABLE 8.5. Performance-Based Measures of Cognition for Use in Advanced Dementia

Measure and authors	Description
Severe Impairment Battery (SIB) (Boller, Verny, Hugonot-Diener, & Saxton, 2002; Saxton, McGonigle-Gibson, Swihart, Miller, & Boller, 1990)	Forty items, six subscales assessing attention, orientation, language, memory, visuospatial, constructive abilities; brief evaluations of praxis and social interaction; 20–30 minutes to administer; acceptable for use with severe dementia; requires training to administer; reliability and validity established in multiple languages; longitudinal validity has been demonstrated; commercially available.
SIB—Short Form (de Jonghe, Wetzels, Mulders, Zuidema, & Koopmans, 2009; Saxton et al., 2005)	Assesses nine cognitive domains with items from SIB: Attention, Memory, Praxis, Concentration, Visuospatial Ability, Social Interaction, Language, Construction, and Orientating to Name; 10–15 minutes to administer; acceptable for use with severe dementia; requires training to administer; requires special equipment; commercially available.
Test for Severe Impairment (TSI) (Albert & Cohen, 1992; Appollonio et al., 2001)	Assesses well-learned motor performance, language comprehension, language production, immediate and delayed memory, general knowledge, conceptualization; 10 minutes to administer; requires verbal responses; acceptable for use with moderate and severe dementia; requires training to administer; requires special equipment; minimal language required.
Multi-focus Assessment Scale (MAS) (Coval, Crockett, Holliday, & Koch, 1985; H. Tuokko, Crockett, Holliday, & Coval, 1987)	Eight subscales including social behavior, receptive language (oral and visual stimuli), expressive language skills, orientation to person, place and time, mood, accessibility and sensory abilities; 45 minutes to administer; reliability .90 or better; discriminant validity demonstrated between groups differing in level of functioning; easily administered with little training; materials easy to create; minimal language required; availability uncertain.
Hierarchic Dementia Scale—Revised (Cole & Dastoor, 1987; Rönnberg & Ericsson, 1994)	Twenty items assessing orienting, prefrontal, ideomotor, looking, ideational, denomination, comprehension, registration, gnosis, reading, orientation, construction, concentration, calculation, drawing, motor, remote memory, writing, similarities, recent memory; hierarchically organized (success on an item implies success on "inferior" items based on Piagetian developmental model); scoring can reveal cognitive profile; 40–50 minutes to administer; requires training to administer; requires special equipment; commercially available.

(continued)

TABLE 8.5. *(continued)*

Measure and authors	Description
Modified Ordinal Scales of Psychological Development (Auer, Sclan, Yaffee, & Reisberg, 1994; Sclan, Foster, Reisberg, & Franssen, 1990)	Five subscales including object permanence, means-ends, causality, spatial relations, and schemes modified from Ordinal Scales of Psychological Development; hierarchically organized (success on an item implies success on "inferior" items based on Piagetian developmental model); 30 minutes to administer; requires training to administer; requires special equipment; unknown availability.
Baylor Profound Mental Status Examination (BPMSE) (Doody et al., 1999)	Requires special equipment; requires verbal responses.
Severe Cognitive Impairment Profile (SCIP) (Peavy et al., 1996)	Eight subscales assessing overall behavior, attention, language, memory, motor, conceptualization, arithmetic, visuospatial abilities; 30 minutes to administer; acceptable for use with severe dementia; inter-rater and test–retest reliability .96 or better; correlates well with other measures of global functioning; discriminant validity demonstrated between groups differing in level of functioning; requires training to administer; requires special equipment; only available in English; commercially available.
Severe Mini-Mental State Examination (SMMSE) (Harrell, Marson, Chatterjee, & Parrish, 2000)	Based on the Mini-Mental State Examination; assesses autobiographical knowledge, simple visuospatial function, executive function, simple language function, semantic fluency and spelling; less than 5 minutes to administer; requires verbal responses; requires no special equipment; requires no specialized training to administer.
Severe Cognitive Impairment Rating Scale (SCIRS) (Choe et al., 2008)	Eleven items assessing memory, language, visuospatial function, frontal function and orientation; less than 5 minutes to administer; requires verbal responses; acceptable for use with moderate and severe dementia; interrater reliability .90 or better; correlates well with other measures of severe dementia; easily administered with little training; only one-stimulus materials required; items available in source.
Clinical Evaluation of Moderate-to-Severe Dementia (KUD) (Ericsson, Malmberg, Langworth, Haglund, & Almborg, 2011)	Fifteen items assessing interaction, memory, verbal ability, visuospatial ability, overlearned activities of daily living, 20 minutes to administer; intact verbal ability not required for all items; acceptable for use with moderate and severe dementia; interrater reliability .92; correlates well with other measures of severe dementia; easily administered with little training; some tools available in most environments required; items available in source.

measures are available in the extant literature, while others are commercially available. Some are only available in English (SCIP), whereas others are available in many different languages (e.g., SIB, SMMSE).

The choice of measure will depend on the specific intent of the assessment. Some measures may lend themselves more to care (e.g., MAS), whereas others have been shown to be useful for monitoring change over time (e.g., SIB). Even though many of these measures were originally developed over two decades ago, there remains relatively little research on their utility for different purposes and their integration into care environments. Similarly, few studies have characterized the similarities and differences between major NCDs in the later stages of development.

Other more qualitative approaches to determining the retained cognitive functions of people in the moderate to severe stages of dementia can be taken. These may include the use of arts-based (e.g., visual arts, music, applied theater) approaches to engage the person with dementia and observation of functioning when opportunities of inclusion, occupation, comfort, and involvement are provided (Sabat & Lee, 2012). Similarly, opportunities to express social and cultural habits, movement, and other physical cues are important for social interaction and may reveal the breadth and depth of retained cognitive functions (Kontos, 2012), even after the use of language is limited.

Summary and Conclusions

In the context of dementia, neuropsychological assessment can contribute to the diagnostic process and, when applied over time, can characterize the trajectory of cognitive decline. Information concerning the temporal sequencing of changes in cognitive functions may provide confirmation of initial differential diagnosis. Conversely, marked departures from expected trajectories may be indicative of initial misdiagnosis or the emergence of a comorbid condition warranting further evaluation (e.g., medical disorders). Continued evaluation throughout the course of a dementing process can yield valuable information of relevance to care planning. The progressive characteristics of AD have been described (e.g., Global Deterioration Scale) thoroughly, though not all people manifest all features of a stage as described in the measure. However, similar descriptions of the expectations for decline are not available for most other forms of dementia. At best, anticipated trajectories are described in rather global terms. Research concerning these expected trajectories may prove informative and allow for unexpected deviations to be identified. This research may involve the development of assessment tools (e.g., performance measures, rating scales) appropriate for use with people in later stages of dementia. While some tools are already available, new tools may provide additional types of information concerning cognitive decline. Unexpected deviations may occur as a function of the protective (e.g., engagement in regular exercise) and predictive (e.g., emergence of a medical condition) factors identified earlier.

Recognition of the importance of finding ways to engage with and monitor the person with dementia across the trajectory of continued cognitive decline is growing. Providing and evaluating person-centered approaches to care that include active engagement of the person with dementia for as long as possible are becoming increasingly important in this context. Even people in later stages of dementia can benefit from engagement as arts-based programs like art and music therapy and continued research in this area of assessment will provide a solid foundation for developing future intervention programs.

KEY POINTS

✓ A diagnosis of dementia is considered when cognitive impairment and difficulties in everyday functioning co-occur.

✓ Key features for distinguishing among conditions that affect cognitive functioning include onset, course, and cognitive domains affected early in the course of the disorder.

✓ Spectrums of disorders affecting cognition occur that are characterized by distinct syndrome subtypes, possibly reflective of differences in distribution of pathology within the brain.

✓ Dementia may affect legal capacity to engage in specific areas of decision making, and a reasoned opinion may be requested from a psychologist by those within the legal system where a capacity determination is made.

✓ Assessment can continue across the trajectory of decline postdiagnosis, with measures specifically designed for this purpose.

Examples of Information Obtained
for Capacity Assessments

1. *Can the person perform the activity?*
   - *Assessment:* Observe the person performing the task
     - *Example (driving):* On-road driving assessment
     - *Example (financial management):* Assessment of skills (e.g., check writing, interpretation of bill statement, counting change)

2. *Does the person perform the activity?*
   - *Assessment:* Report from others as to daily behavior; evidence that tasks are not completed
     - *Example (Driving):* Report from family and others; damage to vehicle; traffic tickets; insurance rates increase; selective use of vehicle (specific purposes, times of day, weather permitting)
     - *Example (financial management):* Report from family and others; bills not being paid; taxes in arrears; money "missing"

3. *Can the person make decisions regarding the activity?*
   - *Assessment:* Understanding of own behavior (e.g., awareness of limitations, awareness of risk); understanding of alternatives
     - *Example (driving):* Understanding of own behavior (i.e., awareness of driving problems identified by others; awareness of medical conditions that may affect driving; awareness of the risk to self and others if driving unsafely); understanding of alternatives (i.e., knowledge of other forms of transportation; willingness to retrain)
     - *Example (financial management):* Understanding of own behavior (e.g., awareness of problems handling finances identified by others; awareness of the risk to self if finances are poorly managed); understanding of alternatives (i.e., knowledge of existing resources— e.g., willing family, trust officers, public guardian, trustee)

PART III

Interventions for Late-Life Cognitive Decline

CHAPTER 9

An Integrative, Developmental Approach to Intervention

This section of the book focuses on interventions for older adults at various stages of cognitive decline. This coverage is not meant to be exhaustive across the domain of older adult interventions, nor does it aim to be exhaustive within the particular domains discussed. Rather, the purpose of these chapters is to introduce the reader to the emerging research within a given area and to describe how to use this knowledge in developing a theoretically sound case conceptualization for the provision of intervention to individual clients.

Each chapter deals with a distinct area of focus—specifically, pharmacological approaches (Chapter 10), cognitive-behavioral approaches (Chapter 11), and psychological approaches (Chapter 12). These content areas are addressed separately for clarity and convenience. However, we believe that a holistic approach is likely to be the most effective, not only in terms of care provision, but also in how one thinks about the causes and conditions that give rise to problems warranting clinical attention. As such, the purpose of the current chapter is to present an overarching, integrative framework for care that respects the multiple determinants of clinical problems and the synergistic effect of interventions on one another. Our approach is broadly commensurate with the Pikes [sic] Peak model for training in professional geropsychology (Knight et al., 2009), which identifies six core competencies for providing interventions to older adults (pp. 213–214):

1. Apply individual, group, and family interventions to older adults using appropriate modifications to accommodate distinctive biopsychosocial functioning of older adults and distinct therapeutic relationship characteristics.
2. Use available evidence-based treatments for older adults.

3. Develop psychotherapeutic interventions based on empirical literature, theory, and clinical judgment when insufficient efficacy research is available on older adults.
4. Be proficient in using commonly applied late-life interventions such as those focusing on life review, grief, end-of-life care, and caregiving.
5. Use interventions to enhance the health of diverse older persons (e.g., chronic health problems, healthy aging, cognitive fitness).
6. Demonstrate ability to intervene in settings where older adults and their family members are often seen (e.g., health services, housing, community programs), with a range of strategies including those targeted at the individual, family, environment, and system.

To bring these ideas out of the abstract and provide some grounding for this discussion, we begin with an illustrative case study.

Sam is a 66-year-old, Italian Canadian, high school educated, right-handed gentleman who has been referred by his neurologist for assessment and treatment recommendations. Sam was diagnosed with PD 8 years earlier. His motor symptoms are relatively well managed using L-dopa and Sinemet, with minimal side effects at the current time.

Sam worked as a police officer but took early retirement at age 60. He has noticed a decline in his thinking abilities over the past 3 years, although, notably, his wife perceives even greater decline than Sam does himself, most evident in the past year. They are unsure whether his perceived decline is due to a lack of stimulation in retirement or to other causes. Since retirement, his daily routine has consisted of reading the newspaper, watching television, "tinkering in the garage" and socializing with his wife.

Sam has a prior history of depression and posttraumatic stress disorder (PTSD), associated with the many disturbing events he witnessed over the years working on the police force. He has had cognitive-behavioral therapy in the past and has learned some coping skills. As a result, he has improved his PTSD symptoms. However, he continues to report dissatisfaction with his life and fears about his future. Although his motor symptoms are relatively well managed, this change in physical status has negatively affected his self-concept, as he was once a physically active man whose physical abilities were a source of personal pride.

Sam also reports a longing for more meaningful social connection. He has a very loving relationship with his wife but has difficulty getting out to socialize and make new friends, in part owing to self-consciousness about his illness and his symptoms. He also has two adult sons both of whom live locally. He has a good relationship with one son, who is married and has children. His grandchildren are a great source of joy. However, his relationship with his younger son is conflictual, and he is uncertain how to resolve this conflict. Sam had a difficult relationship with his own father growing up, which he attributes to his father having been a survivor of World War II and likely dealing with his own issues of PTSD. Sam feels that he was never really able to make peace with his father before his death. As a result, he feels an impetus to have good relationships with his children and to make the most of what remains of his life ahead.

In terms of formal assessment results, neuropsychometric testing revealed that Sam is showing a decline in intellectual functioning. The most consistent pattern across cognitive testing was a marked decline in executive functions, including difficulty with set-shifting, adaptation to novelty, and problem solving, as well as self-monitoring and self-regulation. He also showed evidence of slowing across most testing. Memory, language, and visuoperceptual processing were relatively intact. Questionnaires reveal that, while Sam is aware of cognitive impairment, he seems to underestimate this deficit relative to his wife's report, suggesting he is experiencing some decline in self-awareness. He also reported moderate symptoms of depression and anxiety but denied suicidal ideation, plans, or intent.

Similar to the case of Deborah in Chapter 4, Sam illustrates the point that, even when an older adult presents for neuropsychological assessment and intervention, it is essential to situate the individual within the matrix of biopsychosocial factors that can affect current functioning and to recognize that these factors may extend back in time well before the immediate presenting complaints. Acknowledging Sam's complexity highlights his humanity and further reinforces the point that any intervention plan must strive to improve the client's overall quality of life and well-being rather than simply focusing on discrete symptoms.

The area of interventions for older adults provides exciting opportunities for both clinicians and researchers, a field that is in its infancy relative to assessment of late-life cognitive decline. Until relatively recently, pharmacological efforts have dominated the field, in the race to discover effective treatments for symptoms of AD and other dementias. While there is accumulating evidence that a variety of medications can palliate the symptoms of non-normal cognitive decline (see Chapter 10), the field has yet to find a pharmacological cure for dementia. There may have been a reticence in the past to pursue cognitive and behavioral interventions for older adults, assuming that they might not benefit or would keep declining, thus proving more costly than prescribing medication. However, emerging research using both animal and human models suggests that neuroplasticity is possible across the lifespan, including in older adulthood. These findings, in conjunction with the limited efficacy of pharmacological interventions, have led to a rapid uptick in research on nonpharmacological interventions, particularly cognitive and behavioral interventions (Chapter 11). Likewise, a relatively robust field of psychotherapy research is available, with attention being brought to the unique developmental concerns of older adults and to the potential need to modify traditional psychotherapy models or tailor them for an older clientele (Chapter 12).

The care of older adults is likely best served by taking a comprehensive, multimodal approach that includes both pharmacological and non-pharmacological interventions. An intervention designed for one domain of function may have additional therapeutic effects in another domain. For example, aside from targeting the underlying disease process, pharmacological treatments can attenuate symptoms that can otherwise interfere with engagement in nonpharmacological interventions. For example, an individual with severe major depression may benefit from an antidepressant medication to facilitate engagement with psychotherapy. Or use of a cognitive-enhancing medication may potentiate engagement in cognitive training or rehabilitation. Another example might be that improving symptoms of depression can ameliorate perceived or actual cognitive function, or alternatively, participating in cognitive rehabilitation can enhance self-efficacy and agency, which, in turn, improves mood. While the material in subsequent chapters is presented in isolation, we advocate for developing a sound case conceptualization for intervention that is informed by a biopsychosocial assessment of all relevant factors, with the express purpose of meeting the client's own goals and enhancing his or her overall quality of life. As discussed in Chapter 11, focusing on the client's own goals can promote intrinsic motivation to participate in intervention, as well as confer a sense of agency and autonomy, which may be diminishing in an older adult with cognitive impairment.

In an ideal world, an older adult would receive assessment and a comprehensive intervention program from the same provider, someone who knows them and can observe them in a variety of contexts and can contribute qualitative observations as well as objective test data to informing care. We acknowledge the practical reality that psychologists are often not equally trained in every intervention modality and may feel more or less skilled at one or another type of intervention. That said, it is an ethical mandate that psychologists only provide the care for which they are competent to deliver (American Psychological Association, 2002; Canadian Psychological Association, 2017). The aim of this section is to introduce the reader to a selection of interventions that are available and demonstrate how to weave these together within the context of a theoretically sound case conceptualization. Rather than attempting to "teach" psychologists how to provide every possible type of intervention, which other authors deftly accomplish in texts devoted solely to these interventions, we believe that taking a more integrative, holistic approach is a unique strength of this book. That is, we are more focused on teaching the clinician *how to think about older adult intervention,* rather than providing every detail on the dissemination of any given intervention. For psychologists seeking to pursue intervention work with older adults, it is incumbent on them to seek further training, where necessary, to effectively and ethically disseminate these interventions. In support of this requirement, resources for continuing education and training are appended to each subsequent intervention chapter.

An Applied Neuropsychological Approach to Intervention

The complexity of Sam's case illustrates the utility of the biopsychosocial approach to case formulation. While Sam has been referred for evaluation of current cognitive function, we see that there are a great many factors that could affect his cognitive function, as well as others that, while they may not influence, they nevertheless warrant clinical attention. In this chapter, we discuss factors that should be considered within any biopsychosocial formulation to intervention with older adults; these factors will provide context and foundation for the application of individual interventions as presented in Chapters 10–12.

A Client-Centered, Collaborative, Goal-Setting Approach

In Chapter 11, which focuses on cognitive and behavioral interventions, we discuss the differences between the treatment modalities of cognitive training, cognitive rehabilitation, and cognitive stimulation for older adults. This taxonomy is useful in informing the design and evaluation of various types of interventions within a research context (Clare & Woods, 2004). However, in clinical practice these boundaries are likely to be less sharply delineated. In this section of the book, we subscribe to rehabilitation not so much as a treatment method per se but as an overarching philosophical approach to treatment. That is, we view rehabilitation as a client-centered, collaborative process that is multimodal, holistic, ecologically relevant, and always situated within the client's own goals. This holistic approach follows the approach of other clinician–researchers, in both acquired brain injury (e.g., Cicerone et al., 2008) and older adulthood (e.g., Huckans et al., 2013). This also means being transparent at every step of the process about how the problem is being conceptualized, what the recommended course of intervention is, and how the intervention is expected to impact the client's life and everyday function.

As psychologists, we may develop a case formulation that focuses on symptoms, as these are measurable and inform the utility of our interventions. However, the meaningfulness of those interventions will vary as a function of how relevant this case formulation is to the achievement of outcomes directly salient in the client's life. For example, in Sam's case, his neuropsychometric test scores show evidence of executive dysfunction, including difficulties in self-monitoring and self-regulation. These symptoms may be amenable to intervention using methods such as metacognitive strategy training or mindfulness training. However, for clinicians, the goal of intervention would be to create meaningful improvement in Sam's life. As such, these interventions are likely to be beneficial only to the degree to which they meet Sam's goals, one of the most important of which is increased social connection. In this context, the clinician may want to incorporate self-monitoring activities and behavioral practice in a social context, as well as use social connection as an ecologically relevant outcome variable. Note that intervention itself becomes a source of data, as client and clinician understand more about a client's deficits, their origins, and their impact. This means that both client and clinician need to be alert to emerging data, and willing to revise goals and case formulations in a flexible and iterative fashion. This also speaks to the need for regular outcome assessment, which we will later discuss in more detail.

Ethical practice mandates prioritization of the client's autonomy, which would include generating his or her own desired outcomes for treatment. Moreover, goals that are ecologically relevant and salient are more likely to be motivating and will encourage persistence even in the face of difficulty (Kleim & Jones, 2008). Extant literature from cognitive and affective science indicates that older adults are more attuned to positive affect— the so-called positivity bias (Reed, Chan, & Mikels, 2014). In older adulthood, cognition and emotion may be experienced as competing processes; faced with a task that has both cognitive and emotional demands, an older adult may be more likely to devote available resources to maintaining positive mood, rather than performing well on the task (Peters et al., 2007). Furthermore, basic neuroscience literature demonstrates that activation of dopaminergic reward systems promotes motivation, which in turn supports new learning (Hamid et al., 2016). Building rewards and motivation can be intrinsic, such as for a client who sees him- or herself making measured progress toward some larger goal, or they can be extrinsic (e.g., token economy systems), such as for clients with more severe cognitive impairment. All of these factors support the notion that, to the extent that it is possible, intervention should be an inherently enjoyable or at least an engaging experience that progressively moves a client toward directly observable, meaningful change in his or her own life.

The willingness to work toward one's goals is related to a client's sense of *self-efficacy*. Self-efficacy pertains to the belief in one's ability to produce specific outcomes in events that will affect his or her life (Bandura, 1994). Evidence from the field of cognitive rehabilitation for acquired brain injury indicates that self-efficacy uniquely contributes to rehabilitation success and is a strong predictor of global life satisfaction (Cicerone & Azulay, 2007). Parallel findings from literature on the older adult indicate that memory self-efficacy has a small but reliable association with objective memory performance (Beaudoin & Desrichards, 2011). Early on, the client may report a goal that seems too large to obtain directly. In this instance, it is incumbent upon the clinician to help the client parse larger goals into smaller subgoals on which progress is directly measurable and self-efficacy can be enhanced. This parsing of goals can be done informally between the client and clinician, or it can itself be the focus of intervention, as exemplified in goal management training for executive dysfunction (Levine, Stuss, Winocur, & Binns, 2007; van Hooren et al., 2007).

Readiness for Change and Self-Awareness

Occasionally, a client will suggest a goal that seems highly unrealistic to attain, something that is more likely to occur with clients with anosognosia (Ernst, Moulin, Souchay, Mograbi, & Morris, 2016). One such example is a client with dementia who wants to start driving again after having his license revoked. Failed attempts to make progress on an unrealistic goal can undermine self-efficacy and therapeutic engagement, as well as involve tangible threats of harm to the client and others. The challenge is to discover how to work collaboratively with a client in this context, respecting wishes but not setting the client up for failure by clinging to an unattainable goal.

Although we support the use of both pharmacological and nonpharmacological interventions, the major difference between the two approaches is that the success of the nonpharmacological is heavily influenced by the client's level of readiness to engage in intentional change. The transtheoretical model (TTM) or "stages-of-change" model of Prochaska and DiClemente (Prochaska & DiClemente, 1983; Prochaska, DiClemente, & Norcross, 1992) provides one helpful framework to conceptualize a client's readiness to change. While there are many individual differences that could affect an individual's readiness for change, the stages-of-change model is unique in its integrative, biopsychosocial approach to change, in line with the overarching framework of this book. Although a current Cochrane review indicated limited evidence for the application of the TTM in lifestyle interventions for older adults (Mastellos, Gunn, Felix, Car, & Majeed, 2014), the findings seem to indicate a lack of high-quality studies rather than a statement about the lack of applicability of the model per se. In brief, there are six stages of change:

- *Precontemplation (denial).* The individual is not considering making any changes within the next 6 months and may be unwilling or unable to acknowledge the problem area.
- *Contemplation.* The individual is thinking about making change within the next 6 months. He or she is acutely aware of both pros

and cons to change, and such ambivalence can lead to behavioral procrastination and being stuck in this stage for long periods of time.
- *Preparation.* The individual is preparing to take action on the problem area within the next month (or immediate future). He or she may already have a plan in place and is highly motivated to benefit from structured intervention.
- *Action.* The individual has actively taken steps to address the problem within the last 6 months.
- *Maintenance.* The individual has been maintaining positive behavioral change for at least 6 months.
- *Relapse/Recycle.* The individual has temporarily stopped behavioral change and has returned to a prior behavioral state.

At the outset of intervention, it is useful to ascertain an older adult's stage of change, as this will inform what types of interventions, if any, are likely to be productive and feasible. A useful way to gauge this is by monitoring the client's response to neuropsychological assessment feedback. For example, individuals in the preparation stage may find the feedback as a source of information that motivates them to seek out concrete ways to change their behavior. Conversely, individuals in the precontemplation stage may seem defensive or dismissive, or minimize the real-world impact of feedback, particularly feedback suggesting clinically significant impairment. Broadly speaking, persons who are in the preparation–action–maintenance stages may be more immediately ready to take on structured interventions such as those discussed in the subsequent chapters. For individuals at the other stages, preparatory work may be needed to bring the individual to a point where he or she is willing to pursue intervention.

Anosognosia

A client may be at the precontemplation stage due to psychological reasons (i.e., defensive denial), neurogenic reasons (i.e., anosognosia, cognitive impairment), or some combination of both. As individuals decline from mild cognitive impairment to dementia, anosognosia may become more prominent (Ernst et al., 2016; Kalbe et al., 2005; Lehrer et al., 2015). Anosognosia can be particularly challenging to the extent that it prevents the older adult from engaging with interventions, particularly nonpharmacological interventions. In Chapter 11, we discuss principles of neuroplasticity as applied to cognitive and behavioral interventions; considering the principle of "use it or lose it," a failure to actively engage with the world could hasten the deterioration of neural and cognitive functioning. Thus, anosognosia in and of itself may need to take precedence as an intervention target before other modalities can be effectively engaged.

One intervention that holds promise for anosognosia in older adults is motivational interviewing (MI; Miller & Rollnick, 2002, 2009; Miller

& Rose, 2009). In brief, MI is a "client-centered, nondirective method for enhancing intrinsic motivation to change by exploring and resolving ambivalence" (Miller & Rollnick, 2002, p. 25). Every behavioral choice has pros and cons, even those that seem maladaptive. For example, while smoking is generally considered bad for one's health, it has short-term rewards in terms of making the smoker feel more relaxed and perhaps may promote socialization with other smokers. MI is based on the premise that, for adaptive behavior change to occur, one must address the underlying ambivalence about making that change, given that there will be costs and benefits to the change. The four guiding principles of MI are (1) expressing empathy, (2) helping the client to develop the discrepancy between present behavior and future goals, (3) rolling with resistance (i.e., avoiding logical argumentation about "right" and "wrong"), and (4) supporting self-efficacy. MI is nonconfrontational and collaborative, focused on developing the client's self-efficacy and autonomy with the understanding that long-term change will come from the client's own intrinsic motivation.

Although MI was initially developed for use in individuals with substance abuse disorders, it has been successfully applied in a wide variety of behavioral health contexts, including medication adherence, dietary changes, exercise, and gambling. In their review of cognitive rehabilitation therapies for AD, Choi and Twamley (2013) state that while the efficacy of MI for anosognosia has not yet been tested, it holds promise for helping clients find intrinsic motivation to engage in treatment. MI has tended to be applied in populations presumed to have relatively intact cognition. The authors note that it remains to be seen whether a certain level of cognitive function is required to engage individuals in MI, in terms of being able to self-reflect, follow what the therapist is saying, predict potential outcomes of behavioral choices, and hold those different choices in working memory. Interestingly, Medley and Powell (2010) produced a detailed conceptual review of the application of MI for anosognosia in individuals with acquired brain injury, including individuals who are expected to have significant cognitive impairment. They provide a useful model of how to apply MI in individuals at various levels of cognitive impairment, which the reader will find useful in conceptualizing how MI might be applied to older adults with anosognosia. For those who are seeking specific training in this modality, a list of training programs around the world are available online at *www.motivationalinterviewing.org*.

One final note on readiness for change: this may not be equally expressed across different problem domains. For example, in Sam's case, there is evidence that he has decreased awareness of his cognitive impairment, so he may be at the precontemplation stage and require help building awareness before further interventions can be implemented to enhance his cognitive function. Conversely, Sam seems to have greater awareness of psychological and emotional challenges and may be in the preparation stage in terms of making interpersonal changes in his life that will facilitate better relationships. It is incumbent upon the clinician to ascertain the client's readiness to make change in the different areas of his or her life and to apply the relevant interventions accordingly.

Socioeconomic and Cross-Cultural Factors

In subsequent chapters, we present empirical evidence for the various types of interventions. This evidence comes largely from controlled trials with homogeneous participant samples and tightly controlled dissemination of interventions. Controlled trials are important because they provide evidence on an intervention's *efficacy* based on the most experimentally rigorous, internally valid designs. However, as noted in Chapters 11 and 12, this does not necessarily mean that these treatments are *effective,* that is, translatable to a typical client with multiple comorbidities and a complex biopsychosocial history (Chambless & Hollon, 1998). We therefore caution the reader that, in implementing the interventions discussed, some *tailoring* is likely to be necessary to meet the needs of the individual client (Kreuter & Skinner, 2000).

Tailoring can occur along many dimensions, and in keeping with the focus of this book, Chapters 11 and 12 discuss the need to tailor according to a client's level of current cognitive function. In addition, from a biopsychosocial perspective, a clinician may need to tailor an intervention according to socioeconomic and cultural factors. For example, older adults often live on fixed incomes and have limited financial means, which of course affects their participation in intervention. An 8-week group psychoeducation program may not be feasible for an older adult who cannot drive and does not have the money to take taxicabs or mass transit on a weekly basis. Conversely, as telehealth rises in prominence (van den Berg, Schumann, Kraft, & Hoffmann, 2012), delivering interventions remotely via computer is becoming more common, but this, too, may be exclusionary to an older adult who either lacks the financial means to access a computer or has limited personal knowledge of computers. Moreover, as discussed in Chapter 11, available evidence suggests that electronically delivered cognitive and behavioral interventions provided in isolation have limited impact without additional therapist involvement.

Another important aspect of tailoring is cultural background. As a result of immigration and continued diversification of North America and Europe, neuropsychologists will, at some point in their careers, increasingly likely be asked to provide care for clients from cultural backgrounds different from their own. Perhaps the most obvious cross-cultural issue to address is language. Even a client who is conversant in English may miss certain nuances of expression or understanding if English is not the client's primary language. In Sam's case, we know that he has an Italian Canadian background, so it would be important to ascertain his preferred language for intervention, whether it is Italian or English.

Another example is in the meaning of intervention goals. For example, Western clinical neuropsychology is situated within a largely individualistic cultural context. This may translate to an implicit assumption that goals of assessment and intervention are related to the promotion of autonomous individual functions, with an emphasis on personal agency and peak performance. Such goals may hold less meaning for persons from collectivist cultures, where "function" is more socially and interpersonally grounded. For example, given Sam's growing up in an Italian family, intervention might entail greater involvement of the immediate family, as well as goal setting embedded within the needs and priorities of the family system. Cross-cultural differences further underscore the importance of a client-centered approach that prioritizes the client's own goals. It is incumbent on the clinician to "translate" the standard clinical-neuropsychological paradigm of assessment and intervention into terms that are meaningful for culturally different clients, in order to promote intrinsic motivation and transfer to everyday life.

Hays (1996) has proposed the ADDRESSING model of culturally responsive care of diverse older clients: that is, Age, Developmental and acquired disabilities, Religion, Social status, Sexual orientation, Indigenous heritage, National origin, and Gender. Neuropsychologists, in providing appropriate care to their clients, must consider each of these dimensions. Of course, it is unreasonable to expect a neuropsychologist to have equal expertise and experience in each of these areas. In following the mandates of professional ethics codes, where a neuropsychologist lacks particular expertise and experience, he or she must seek consultation and supervision in order to provide competent care. If the amount of training and experience is too great, then it may be necessary to refer a client to a provider with established competence in a particular area. The fields of cross-cultural neuropsychology and cultural neuroscience are growing rapidly, and there are many great resources on this topic. As starting points, we refer the reader in particular to Ferraro (2016) and Fujii (2017).

In sum, we encourage the reader to consider the material presented in subsequent chapters as a base of existing knowledge from which to develop a case formulation that is idiographic and respects the individual particularities of the client's life and background, applying appropriate tailoring where needed.

Staging of Intervention

In keeping with the theme of this book—a developmental approach to assessment and intervention—each subsequent chapter includes some discussion of the relative utility of different interventions as a function of current cognitive impairment (see Table 9.1). This staging of intervention is critical, as individuals at different stages of decline will have more or less manifest symptoms and more or less cognitive reserve available to support

TABLE 9.1. Conceptual Framework for Considering the Types of Interventions Most Likely to Benefit Older Adults at Various Levels of Cognitive/Neuropsychiatric Symptomatology

Clinical issue	Characteristics	Management approach	Intervention strategies	Considerations for consultation
Normal aging and SCD	Minor cognitive lapses within the scope and severity of other older adults of similar demographic background (e.g., word-finding). Significant concern about the meaning of such lapses, as in the case of subjective cognitive decline	Focus on prevention by providing information about expected changes with normal cognitive aging, as well as emphasizing taking active steps to boost cognitive reserve	• Psychoeducation on normal age-related cognitive failures, as well as the effect of situational variables such as mood, sleep, and blood sugar on cognitive performance • Provision of suggestions to offset failures (e.g., compensatory memory strategies, taking extra time to complete tasks) • Encourage physical, mental, and social engagement to increase cognitive reserve • Maintain physical health	Regular follow-up with general practitioner/geriatrician to monitor general health, particularly vascular risk factors (e.g., hypertension, type II diabetes)
MCI and variants thereof	Cognitive impairment that is beyond normal aging (i.e., >1.5 SD below performance of peers with similar demographics), yet instrumental activities of daily living remain intact. MCI in this instance includes the prodromes for AD and other dementias (e.g., VCI)	Continue focusing on enhancing cognitive reserve, as well as directed cognitive intervention to target deficits of interest	• Adaptation of existing, empirically supported cognitive rehabilitation protocols for older adults (e.g., Attention Process Training, Metacognitive Strategy Training, Mindfulness Training) • Use of procedural memory to train in use of assistive devices (e.g., smartphone) • Psychotherapy to assist with emotional reactions to cognitive impairment and changing life roles	Occupational therapy for in-home assessment to ascertain instrumental activities of daily living competence and need for relevant supports

192

Dementias (various types)	Cognitive impairment substantially below normal aging (i.e., >2 SD below peers) with impairment in one or more instrumental activities of daily living	Maintain safety and independence in home as long as feasible; transition to full-time supervised care, when appropriate	• Training in task-specific routines using preserved procedural memory (e.g., self-care/hygiene) • Maintain optimal mental and social stimulation and engagement congruent with the individual's previous interests (e.g., music, dance, art, movies)	Social worker for care planning assistance (e.g., homecare, transportation, formal care facilities); Eldercare attorney for consultation on medicolegal and financial decisions (e.g., health care proxy designation, financial power of attorney)
Neuropsychiatric syndromes	Recurrence of premorbid psychiatric syndromes (e.g., major depression, anxiety disorders), as well as those that may be part of an underlying neurological disease process (e.g., depression associated with vascular dementia, hallucinations associated with DLB, and Capgras syndrome associated with certain dementias or traumatic brain injury	Minimization of symptoms, particularly those that lead to agitation or cause safety concerns; Balancing symptom management with allowing the individual to experience normative feelings of grief or sadness associated with the developmental challenges of late life (e.g., partner loss, retirement)	• For mood/anxiety disorders, provision of psychotherapy appropriate to the source of symptoms (e.g., cognitive-behavioral therapy for situational stressors; existential therapy for developmentally appropriate end-of-life concerns) • For psychotic symptoms (i.e., hallucinations and delusions), providing psychoeducation to the patient, as well as working with caregivers to minimize agitation (e.g., avoiding directly challenging delusional beliefs)	Neuropsychiatrist or behavioral neurologist for medication consultation

193

intervention efforts (Stern, 2009, 2012). For example, in terms of cognitive and behavioral interventions, significant restoration of cognitive function may be unrealistic in an individual already experiencing dementia owing to the degree of cognitive loss already sustained. Conversely, without longitudinal follow-up, improvement in the instrumental activities of daily living function may go unnoticed in currently cognitively normal individuals who are yet to show impairment in this area of function. In terms of psychotherapy, cognitive-behavioral therapy for various conditions is a popular and well-validated evidence-based intervention with younger and middle-aged adults. However, an older adult with difficulties in memory or abstract reasoning may struggle with the cognitive demands of this intervention. Likewise, for an individual whose primary concern is coming to terms with grief and finding meaning in life, targeting automatic thoughts may seem irrelevant.

Being clear about the individual's current level of function and the kinds of goals that are attainable will likely lead to more fruitful application of intervention. Regardless of stage, any intervention should serve the individual's dignity, autonomy, and independence to the greatest degree possible. It goes without saying that, for any intervention, informed consent (or assent, in the case of persons who lack capacity) should always be sought (American Psychological Association, 2002; Canadian Psychological Association, 2017).

Maintenance of Physical Health

With advancing age, older adults are more likely to face chronic medical comorbidities. Coping with so many health issues can negatively impact cognitive performance (McConnell, 2014), as well as psychological functioning and quality of life. Lifestyle factors comprise an important part of overall health and well-being for older adults, and evidence suggests that these are an efficacious and complementary approach to formal cognitive/behavioral and psychological interventions (Jak, 2012). In Sam's case, even though his PD is currently well managed, it has already affected his self-concept, and as the disease progresses, it may create further stress and negative effects on his quality of life (Salive, 2013). Thus, an important intervention goal for Sam may be to optimize his physical health to the greatest degree possible.

In Chapter 2, we reviewed some of the available literature on nutrition and physical activity in healthy aging and non-normal cognitive decline. For physical exercise in particular, there is accumulating literature to support its utility in older adults, not only in terms of physical health but also cognitive benefits—literature that we discuss further in Chapter 10. Recent work by Lauenroth, Ioannidis, and Teichmann (2016) suggests that the combination of exercise and cognitive interventions has a synergistic effect on cognition that is greater than either intervention in isolation. Based on their review, Lauenroth et al. provided some recommendations regarding the adequate amount of exercise: they suggested that training sessions should range between 60 and 180 minutes per session, at a frequency of three times per week, over a period of 3 to 4 months, or longer. They further recommended that physical training be stimulating and engaging, include both cardiovascular and strength-training components, and be conducted with constant monitoring of heart rate. This mirrors the basic neuroscience research indicating that it is not the mere repetition of rote activities that promotes neuroplasticity, but rather activities that challenge and stimulate the individual. (We discuss neuroplasticity in detail in Chapter 10.) It is recommended that older adults work with professionals who have expertise in exercise programs for older people, particularly those with health conditions such as PD, which may affect mobility.

Aside from physical health difficulties occurring in late life, as already discussed in Chapter 4, chronic stress has been shown to create immunosenescence, or accelerated aging of the immune system. Recent research has examined the deleterious effects of stressful early life experiences and childhood adversity on immunosenescence and immune dysregulation in middle and older adulthood (Fagundes, Glaser, & Kiecolt-Glaser, 2013; Miller, Chen, & Parker, 2011). Considering particular cohorts of older adults may have survived major wars as well as geographic displacement through war or immigration, in addition to socioeconomic stressors such as poverty, these intriguing studies emphasize the need to consider how early life history may have influenced an older adult's unfolding developmental trajectory. In Sam's case, he has his own history of PTSD through repeated exposure to trauma associated with his job. Considering his father was a war survivor, he may bear an additional biological burden: emerging research demonstrates the epigenetic transmission of intergenerational trauma (Bowers & Yehuda, 2016). The chronic effects of stress may or may not place upper limits on how much response an older adult will show to intervention, as well as influence the type of therapeutic approach that may be indicated in someone with long-standing stress and early-life adversity.

Any intervention plan should begin with a comprehensive medical assessment. This assessment should include an evaluation of factors that can cause reversible cognitive impairment, such as vitamin and hormone levels, liver and thyroid function, as well as infectious disease processes such as HIV/AIDS, syphilis, and Lyme disease (American Academy of Neurology, n.d.). Diagnosis and management of these conditions can improve an older adult's cognitive and psychological functioning, as well as further clarify which cognitive changes may be associated with underlying neurodegenerative disease processes. In order to monitor the person on an ongoing basis, ideally an older adult should be followed by a provider with whom the client has an ongoing relationship (e.g., a general practitioner or geriatrician). Additionally, if pharmacological approaches are warranted (see Chapter 9), additional referral to a geriatric psychiatrist, neuropsychiatrist, or neurologist can be fruitful.

Outcome Measurement

While research studies are a critical source of information, time and economic limits mean that they may lack comprehensiveness in outcome measurements. This is particularly true of outcomes that are most relevant to the client but are much more difficult to operationalize, such as living independently or improving one's social network. While we revisit this point in subsequent chapters, here we remind the reader to consider the following points regarding appropriate outcome measurement:

- Standardized measures should be *psychometrically robust*. This means that, minimally, they are reliable and valid for the construct under study, ideally designed for (and tested in) an older adult population, and scored according to older adult norms;

- Measures should be matched to the purported *goal of intervention*. For example, mindfulness training is alleged to improve self-regulation of attention, emotion, and self-awareness (goal) through training in being able to attend to the present moment. Appropriate outcome measures would be self-reported mindfulness, as well as objective measures of self-regulation of attention, emotion, and self-awareness;

- Measures should be relevant for the presumed *mechanism of action* of intervention. This issue is particularly true of the field of cognitive and behavioral interventions and is a weakness we observed time and again in our review of that literature. For example, if the goal of memory strategy training is to improve compensatory strategy use, then following intervention, we would not necessarily expect cognitive or neural changes, but rather an improvement in ecologically relevant outcomes. Conversely, a working memory training program may show near-transfer to other working memory tasks, but not produce far-transfer to real-world behaviors. Ideally, where time and resources permit, the clinician would use multimodal outcomes to have the best chance of capturing intervention effects, including ecologically oriented outcome measures;

- In an older adult population, "no change in outcome measures" does not necessarily mean that no change has occurred. For example, in the context of psychotherapy, many self-report scales are symptom-oriented. This type of measure might make sense for a symptom-focused form of treatment such as cognitive-behavioral therapy, but less so for more existentially oriented therapy such as life-review. In terms of cognitive and behavioral interventions, most of the empirical evidence is based on short-term follow-up, yet ground-breaking research studies such as the ACTIVE trial (discussed in Chapter 10) show that meaningful change may not occur until 2–3 years after the active intervention period is complete. Plasticity and change in brain, behavior, and self-report measures can all occur on differing time-scales and take longer than in younger or middle-age adults. Moreover, maintenance of current function may be as reasonable a goal as objective "improvement" or enhancement of function, in which case one is more concerned about the presence of declining test scores over time than about the absence of improved test scores. The clinician faces the challenge of balancing the need to evaluate the impact of the intervention with the fact that change is a complex variable that may occur on longer-range time-scales with older adults than with other clientele.

The Single-Case Experimental Design as a Guiding Approach to Intervention

Most trainees in graduate clinical psychology programs—as well as psychologists—are familiar with between-subjects research designs exemplified by the randomized controlled trial (RCT) approach. However, an equally powerful methodology is the single-case experimental design approach, which may be less familiar to trainees and practitioners (Kazdin, 2011). While this approach is typically considered a form of clinical research design, ideally the scientist–practitioner approach to clinical psychology exemplifies this model in routine clinical practice. In other words, the psychologist uses available assessment data to make reasonable clinical hypotheses about how a certain intervention or interventions would ameliorate current difficulties. Then outcomes are systematically measured in order to demonstrate that the intervention is more effective than doing nothing.

Using this type of approach to inform the application of intervention has many benefits. For one, it facilitates translation and application of group-based research findings to individual clients, allowing for tailoring to that individual client. In addition, one can ascertain the overall effectiveness of an intervention plan for a particular client, even when multiple approaches have been used simultaneously. This is more naturalistic than the strict experimental designs that are often published in the literature. Likewise, following this type of methodology means that a treatment suc cess could be submitted for later publication. For disorders with a lower base rate or where it is difficult to access a large number of clients with the same diagnosis simultaneously (e.g., frontotemporal dementia), publishing a series of case studies is a viable means of building the evidence base in a particular population or for a particular type of intervention.

The Chambless criteria (Chambless et al., 1998) provide guidance on what should be considered an efficacious psychological treatment; they note that nine well-controlled case studies are considered sufficient evidence for efficacy. The appeal of this approach is that clinicians in routine practice, who do not have access to the time and economic resources required to conduct RCTs, can nevertheless contribute to the evidence base in this field, providing commentary on how these interventions work in the real world for typical clients.

A recent consensus statement was published on the conduct and subsequent publication of single-case experimental designs, the so-called Single-Case Reporting Guideline in BEhavioral Interventions (SCRIBE) guidelines (Tate et al., 2016). This expert group outlined several key points illustrating how to set up and conduct such case studies, including the specific type of design (e.g., withdrawal/reversal, multiple-baseline, alternating treatments), the use of blinding and randomization, control conditions, and maintenance of treatment fidelity. Even if a psychologist has no direct intent to publish a particular case study, these guidelines provide useful support for deriving a theoretically and empirically supported case conceptualization for a given client, along with robust means to evaluate the impact of the interventions contained therein.

In concluding the case of Sam for this chapter, in Appendix 9.1 we provide an example of a psychoeducation handout we created for him, discussing his assessment results in the context of his goals and an agreed-upon treatment plan. Creating such a handout is a place to weave together each aspect of intervention we will discuss in Chapters 10, 11, and 12—something that has utility for both the client and the clinician. Being transparent about treatment will also facilitate the client's "buy-in" and provide a useful point of reference for clients, particularly those with significant memory impairment. (The use of a therapy journal is discussed further in Chapter 12.)

Summary and Conclusions

This chapter provides an overview of the integrative, developmental approach to intervention that is articulated further in this summary section. In Chapter 10, we discuss the use of medications in persons at all stages of cognitive decline, although the evidence base focuses primarily on persons with MCI and dementia. Under certain conditions, medications can provide some symptom relief and improvement in cognitive function. However, their true utility may lie in their combination with other non-pharmacological interventions: medications provide a stable foundation on which to build, using other interventions that require more active engagement from the individual. Chapters 11 and 12 are notably longer than most other chapters, which is expected given the sheer volume of literature covered in these areas of practice. That said, we have still taken a rather broad approach to the material in these chapters, again focusing on providing a higher-level view for practitioners who then want to dive more deeply into a given area.

Chapter 11 provides an overview of the rapidly expanding area of cognitive and behavioral interventions for older adults at every stage of cognitive decline, focusing particularly on cognitive training, cognitive rehabilitation, and cognitive stimulation. A review of the current state of evidence is provided, along with specific guidance about how to conceptualize the implementation of such intervention methods. We also discuss the important distinction between restitution and compensation, and how certain mechanisms of action may call for different outcome measures, in order to ensure the most meaningful assessment of outcome.

Chapter 12 provides an overview of some of the more commonly used or most empirically supported interventions to improve psychological function in older adults. As is true of the material in Chapter 11, the literature in this area is formidable. As such, we focus on providing a high-level summary of available evidence, again coupled with conceptual guidance on how to implement these interventions. With certain clinical presentations, such as psychosis, medications may be contraindicated entirely; this underscores the utility of psychological approaches in affected individuals. Having been introduced to these three major modalities of medication, cognitive and behavioral interventions, and psychological interventions, the reader can then return to this chapter to consider how one or more of these interventions may be integrated into a holistic treatment plan for a given individual.

In reviewing the material for Chapters 10–12, we see an emphasis in the literature on proof-of-principle, RCT intervention designs that seek to establish efficacy and focus on internal validity. This provides a solid evidence base across a variety of interventions, particularly nonpharmacological interventions, under the most well-controlled conditions. In terms of future directions, while this research is important and worthwhile, we feel that it is time for the field to consider other complementary approaches as well. Given the very real and pressing need to provide effective care to older adults, effective knowledge translation and dissemination with regard to what already exists is essential, and we would even go as far as to say, an ethical imperative. More research needs to be conducted on effectiveness designs, including single-case experimental designs, to ascertain the conditions under which these interventions are successful in routine clinical practice and to suggest where tailoring needs to occur to make interventions accessible. Moreover, RCT designs are based on a medical model of intervention, which uses pharmacological terminology such as "active ingredients" and "dose response." While such terminology can help to bring precision to the study of psychological phenomena, there are limitations. For example, we will review literature in a variety of intervention contexts, suggesting that multicomponent interventions, as well as those that are personalized and tailored to the individual, are ultimately more beneficial than those that take a "one-size-fits-all" approach or are focused on isolating specific ingredients. The difference between medication and nonmedication trials is that thought, feeling, and behavior are part of a matrix of biopsychosocial influences that are difficult to study in isolation. That is, we caution the field against taking an overly reductionist approach to the study of psychological phenomena, particularly as they apply to clinical samples and clinical interventions. With that said, even pharmacological trials could benefit from better biopsychosocial characterization of their participants, as medications may only modify one specific contributor to an older adult's current cognitive function.

KEY POINTS

✓ Cognitive function in older adulthood is multiply determined, including concurrent factors such as health and mood, as well as historical factors such as interpersonal functioning and early-life stress and adversity.

✓ Given the multiplicity of contributing factors, we advocate for a holistic and integrative approach that considers different intervention approaches consecutively or concurrently.

✓ The single-case experimental design is a useful heuristic for developing an intervention plan that is grounded in solid clinical hypotheses with a clear means to test outcome. This also provides a rigorous way to implement and test the findings of group-based research studies in individual clients.

✓ While many intervention studies focus on discrete symptoms, in clinical practice we advocate for a client-centered, collaborative approach that is grounded in the client's goals. Focusing on the client's desired outcomes will enhance intrinsic motivation, particularly when tasks become challenging.

✓ As opposed to medications, nonpharmacological interventions require active engagement in intervention activities (e.g., homework exercises). Thus, the client's readiness for change should be considered, and different levels of readiness will indicate different approaches to intervention. This is particularly true for clients who have anosognosia, or diminished self-awareness.

✓ The client's current level of cognitive decline should be taken into consideration in terms of which interventions are likely to be beneficial or not, and will help shape expectations about the scope of improvement that can be expected.

Example Psychoeducational Handout for Sam
Prior to Initiating Treatment

This handout is to provide you with information on what we have learned about you thus far and how we can use that information to support your care going forward.

As you may remember, your neurologist referred you for a neuropsychological assessment, given concerns about a decline in your thinking abilities. In an assessment, the neuropsychologist is asking three main questions:

1. Does the client have impairment in his or her thinking abilities, more than normal aging?
2. If there is evidence of impairment, can we determine the most likely cause?
3. What can be done to help minimize the impact of this impairment and/or prevent it from getting worse in the future?

In the evaluation, we determined that there was evidence of impairment in your thinking abilities that was more than just normal aging. This was most obvious in the domain we refer to as *executive functions*. You can think of executive functions like the "CEO of your brain"—they are responsible for functions such as planning, organization, time management, being able to switch from one task to another, problem solving, and also regulating your behavior from one moment to the next. We also found evidence that your *speed of processing* is lower than we would expect for your age and education. In terms of what is causing these impairments, these are consistent with the effects of Parkinson's disease and may be a manifestation of your illness. We also found that you were experiencing symptoms of depression and anxiety, which may be in part due to dealing with your illness, as well as some of the relationship stressors you have going on in your life right now.

In terms of what we can do to help you deal with these challenges, there are different options. Despite the difficulties described, your evaluation showed us that you have many cognitive functions that remain in good shape, including your memory, your ability to communicate and understand language, and your visual-perceptual abilities. These are positive signs that you could benefit from learning skills and strategies to actively manage your difficulties in speed of processing and executive functions. We discussed a trial of intervention where we would work together to help your thinking abilities, and we will put this in the context of helping you achieve your goals of improving your relationship with your son and improving your quality of life. We will start with a trial of 6 weeks, and at that point we will reevaluate and see how you are doing.

(continued)

Another thing we are recommending is that your neurologist consider putting you on a trial of an antidepressant. Aside from helping your mood, this type of medication might also improve your processing speed, something that can be affected not only by Parkinson's disease but also depression. If your neurologist does not feel comfortable prescribing this type of medication, then you may need to see a behavioral neurologist or a neuropsychiatrist, medical doctors who specialize in prescribing medications to people who have neurological conditions such as Parkinson's disease. I will be in contact with your neurologist so that together we can coordinate the best care possible for you.

As a psychologist, it is my ethical obligation to provide you with access to psychological treatments that have been shown to be effective for people like you. It is also my obligation to be as upfront with you as I can each step of the way. This is so that you can be informed about how we are working together, and so we can collaborate together on helping you reach your life goals. If at any point you feel that the treatment is not going the way you had hoped, or you want to change direction, it is your right to tell me about this and request that a different approach be taken. I also encourage you to ask me any questions that come up and I will do my best to answer them.

CHAPTER 10

Pharmacological Interventions

In this chapter, we review pharmacologically based intervention strategies for older adults with cognitive/behavioral and emotional symptoms at the various stages of cognitive decline. Medications can be an important part of a holistic treatment plan for older adults with cognitive and emotional symptoms. Moreover, older adults are likely to present with multiple medical comorbidities that may require pharmacological management that in and of itself could impact cognitive and emotional functioning (i.e., iatrogenic effects). Although a neuropsychologist would not typically be the person prescribing medication, nonetheless it is important to have a basic working knowledge of psychopharmacology, the major classes of drugs that might be prescribed in older adults, the reasons for medication use, and knowledge of how to monitor the potential impact on cognitive, behavioral, and emotional functioning.

The purpose of this chapter is to provide a broad introduction to how and when medications may be used in older adults at various stages of cognitive decline. The knowledge base regarding medication efficacy and safety changes rapidly, and information can quickly become obsolete. As such, clinicians and researchers working in this field would be advised to avail themselves of continuing education to ensure that their knowledge and understanding is based on the most contemporary evidence available. In Appendix 10.1, we provide resources for further education and training on this topic.

Medications as Part
of the Biopsychosocial Framework of Intervention

As we have discussed throughout this text, the biopsychosocial framework is the major organizing principle of the work of neuropsychologists. Ideally, patients are viewed holistically, and a successful clinical outcome is one in which the person's overall functioning is improved or enhanced by the care we provide. Just as there are multiple contributors to current cognitive and emotional functioning, likewise there are multiple pathways to pharmacological intervention that could improve an older adult's overall functioning.

Medications are typically provided by a physician, which in the case of an older adult might be a general practitioner, geriatrician, neurologist, or psychiatrist, for example. However, depending on regulations of the particular jurisdiction, other health care providers may be involved, such as nurse practitioners or even psychologists who have prescription privileges. It is beneficial for the neuropsychologist, when possible, to establish a relationship with the professional providing pharmacological care in order to provide the greatest continuity of care.

Neuropsychologists should be educated on basic principles of psychopharmacology such as how medications work, what classes of medications are available, how these are used in an older adult population, and evidence for efficacy, benefits, and potential side effects. Knowledge of this information can enhance the creation of a biopsychosocial treatment plan for the individual that will best address current cognitive, behavioral, and emotional needs while minimizing potential harm caused by side effects or drug interactions.

Basic Principles of Psychopharmacology

For the purposes of this chapter, the reader is introduced to basic principles of psychopharmacology that may be useful as part of the biopsychosocial framework and understanding of the potential impact and utility of pharmacological interventions in older adulthood. For those seeking more detailed information on psychopharmacology, we direct the reader to the end of this chapter, where we provide resources for continuing education, including Preston, O'Neal, and Talaga's (2017) *Handbook of Clinical Psychopharmacology for Therapists* (8th ed.), which is an excellent reference text from which much of the current discussion is drawn.

Basic Principles of Neurobiology

The human brain is composed of approximately 100 billion neurons, or nerve cells. Neurons communicate with one another through dendrites (which deliver information to the cell body) and axons (which conduct information away from the cell body). Each neuron produces and secretes specific neurotransmitters, or messenger molecules. When neurons are activated at a critical level, the neurotransmitter is released into the synapse, the space between the neurons. Some of the molecules bind to appropriate receptors on the adjacent cells, thereby influencing their function. Other neurotransmitter molecules are chemically destroyed by enzymes in the extracellular fluid, and still others are reabsorbed by the presynaptic neuron. Several mechanisms of neuronal malfunction can give rise to psychiatric—and likely cognitive—symptoms (Preston et al., 2017). These symptoms include the following:

- Deficient synthesis of neurotransmitters.
- Excessive degradation of neurotransmitters via enzymes (e.g., monoamine oxidase or cholinesterase).
- Facilitation or inhibition of neurotransmitter release associated with certain biologically based disorders.
- Altered reuptake absorption (e.g., accelerated reuptake of serotonin in clinical depression).
- Abnormal upregulation or downregulation of receptors (e.g., due to stress).
- Pathological alterations in gene expression that can cause a wide range of abnormal cellular responses.

Different mental disorders are theorized to be based on one or more of these mechanisms of neuronal malfunction, and thus various classes of medications are designed to address these mechanisms of malfunction.

Pharmacodynamics and Pharmacokinetics

These two terms refer to the basic mechanisms by which a medication exerts its impact. More specifically, pharmacodynamics refers to the physiological effects of medications on cellular systems and their presumed mechanism of action. By contrast, pharmacokinetics refers to how the body impacts the medication through absorption, distribution, metabolism, and excretion of said medications (American Society for Pharmacology and Experimental Therapeutics, n.d.).

The pharmacodynamics of a medication can be influenced by a variety of physiological changes, including aging, changing factors such as receptor binding, the level of binding proteins, or receptor sensitivity. For example, in older adults, using the same medication concentration at the site of action (i.e., sensitivity) may exert greater or smaller effects compared to a similar concentration in a younger person. The *Merck Manual* provides a comprehensive review of how aging can affect the responsiveness of certain drugs (Ruscin & Linnebaur, 2014). Of note is the fact that older adults are particularly sensitive to so-called anticholinergic effects, such as blurred vision, constipation, dry mouth, and—particularly relevant to older adults—memory impairment. Older adults, including those already presenting with cognitive impairment, are particularly sensitive to adverse central nervous system effects, including drowsiness and confusion. Some classes of medications, particularly antipsychotic medications, carry such an elevated risk of morbidity and mortality in the elderly that they often come with a "black box warning" and should only be prescribed with caution (Greenblatt & Greenblatt, 2016).

There are four principles of pharmacokinetics: absorption, distribution, biotransformation, and excretion (Preston et al., 2017). *Absorption* pertains to how a medication is absorbed by the stomach, or how and when it can transit across the blood–brain barrier. Once absorbed, *distribution* determines to which sites of action the medication is made available. Certain classes of medication have characteristic distribution patterns, such as distribution of tricyclic antidepressants in fat and muscle cells. Once distributed, the body responds to the medication as a foreign substance. In *biotransformation,* medications are chemically altered into chemical by-products, referred to as metabolites. Some of these metabolites have the desired therapeutic effect (i.e., reduction in symptoms), whereas others may affect bodily tissues and organs and cause side effects. If metabolism is impaired, significant drug toxicity may build up. By contrast, *excretion* occurs when medications are eliminated from the body, typically via the kidneys but also through other routes such as the gastrointestinal tract and respiratory system. The main contributors to age-related changes in pharmacokinetics include age-related changes in certain organs, blood circulation, and body composition (Davies & O'Mahony, 2015). For example, liver size has been found to decrease by 25–35% in normal aging (Schmuker, 2001), and hepatic blood flow to decrease by 40% (Wynne et al., 1989; Le Couter & McLean, 1998), both of which can decrease medication clearance. Moreover, kidney mass and blood flow have likewise been found to reduce through the adult lifespan, resulting in a 40% reduction in nephrons by the eighth decade of life (Fliser, Zeier, Nowack, & Ritz, 1993).

Understanding the principles of pharmacodynamics and pharmacokinetics and their interaction helps explain the dose–response relationship (i.e., how much of a medication is needed to exert a therapeutic effect) (Moroney, 2013a). The dose–response relationship is determined as a function of both potency and efficacy. *Potency* refers to the dose of a drug required to bind to a particular class of receptor, while *efficacy* pertains to the ability of the drug to activate a conformational change in said receptors) (Moroney, 2013b).

A basic grasp of neurobiology, pharmacodynamics, and pharmacokinetics can provide a foundation for appreciating the mechanism of action of certain classes of drugs, purported therapeutic effects, as well as potential side effects and other factors that could affect their impact in an older adult population. Some of the major classes of medications that can affect cognition/behavior and psychological state, relevant to a geriatric population, are discussed in detail in this chapter. Before this discussion, however, we consider the ways in which neuropsychologists can contribute to the care of older adults who are undergoing psychopharmacological intervention.

Neuropsychologists' Contributions to Psychopharmacological Interventions

Although neuropsychologists are not typically responsible for direct prescription of medications, in concert with a treatment team, they can fulfill a valuable role in helping to ascertain who may be a good candidate for such an intervention, as well as monitoring outcomes, both positive and negative.

Providing Comprehensive Assessment of Current Function

A neuropsychologist's primary activity centers on comprehensive assessment of an older adult's current cognitive/behavioral and emotional function. The outcome of such an assessment can include identifying clinically significant symptoms (both cognitive and psychological) that could benefit from pharmacological intervention. For example, an older adult (e.g., with late-life depression) might be a candidate for psychological intervention but would also benefit from an appropriate medication (e.g., an antidepressant) to enhance treatment effects.

Establishing Possible Barriers to Adherence

Regardless of the reason for medication usage, an older adult's ability to adhere to a treatment regimen may be affected by a variety of factors, including psychological reasons (e.g., apathy associated with depression, worry about side effects) as well as cognitive reasons (e.g., forgetting to take medication, accidentally taking extra doses, not being able to follow complex regimens) (Davies & O'Mahony, 2015). In working with older adults being prescribed medication, it is important that plans are in place to support the appropriate use of those medications, whether it be through using timers and pill boxes or having a family member or other caregiver dispense the medication on their behalf. Having provided a comprehensive assessment of current cognitive and emotional functioning, neuropsychologists can supply important information to support an older adult in effectively adhering to a medication regimen that will maximize the likelihood of therapeutic effects.

Monitoring Response to Intervention

A unique feature of neuropsychological assessment is the use of standard-ized neuropsychometric tests to assess cognition, in addition to standard-ized clinical measures of psychological functioning. These standardized test scores can establish an important pretreatment baseline in order to moni-tor subsequent response to intervention. For example, a neuropsychologist might determine that an older adult has amnestic MCI and refer back to a neurologist who institutes a 6-month trial of a cognitive-enhancing medica-tion. After several months of treatment (or at other clinically relevant inter-vals), neuropsychological assessment can be repeated to ascertain whether the medication has had a meaningful impact on the individual's cognitive function. Given that certain medications may have significant side effects, severe enough to warrant discontinuation, a neuropsychologist can provide information about the magnitude of apparent benefit so that the patient can weigh the pros and cons of continuing with medication usage.

Several measures can be used to provide broad screens of cognition. For example, the MMSE (Folstein, Folstein, & McHugh, 1975) is a well-known measure to both researchers and clinicians, and can be quickly and easily administered by neuropsychologists as well as physicians. However, it is a rather gross tool and may lack the fine discrimination to see enhance-ments—or declines—in persons with early MCI. Conversely, the Dementia Rating Scale, 2nd Edition (DRS-2; Jurica, Leitten, & Mattis, 2001) is a slightly longer measure but provides more in-depth screening of current cognitive function across multiple domains. Again, this measure and asso-ciated scores are well known in research and clinical practice across vari-ous disciplines. Ideally, if time permits, the neuropsychologist can provide a more tailored neuropsychometric screening to assess cognitive function before and after institution of a medication trial. In repeating these tests, the neuropsychologist is advised to compute RCIs in order to ascertain whether change has clinical relevance as well as statistical significance (see Chapter 5; Duff, 2012; Frerichs & Tuokko, 2005). If alternate forms of a test are available (e.g., for certain list-learning tasks), this is another alter-native to using RCIs. Note that, in an older adult population, evidence in support of a medication-related "improvement" might not necessarily mean an absolute improvement in test scores, but rather stability of performance and absence of further decline between assessments. Conversely, appar-ent improvement on repeat administration could be a function of practice effects (Calamia, Markon, & Tranel, 2012). RCIs are typically believed to account for clinically meaningful change that occurs over and above the impact of practice effects (Goldberg et al., 2015).

Another aspect of monitoring response to intervention is ascertain-ment of whether medications have iatrogenic side effects that are negatively impacting cognitive/behavioral and psychological function. For example, an older adult may be experiencing cognitive difficulties associated with chronic pain. Prescribing a medication for pain may help ameliorate the symptoms of pain; however, the medication itself could have deleterious effects on cognition, for example, through causing sedation (Pickering & Lussier, 2015). Again, the neuropsychologist is best served by educating him- or herself on the various medications that an older adult may be taking and on any potential effects on cognition, mood, and behavior.

Classes of Medications and Their Potential Influence on Cognitive/Behavioral and Emotional Functioning in Older Adults

General Considerations

The American Geriatrics Society has created the Beers criteria for potentially inappropriate medication use in older adults. This is a list of certain medications that should be avoided in older adults in general, as well as medications whose doses should be altered when used in populations with certain diseases or syndromes. The Beers criteria list is updated by the American Geriatrics Society on a regular basis (most recently in 2015) and can be accessed at *http://onlinelibrary.wiley.com/doi/10.1111/jgs.13702/ full*. Neuropsychologists should review this list and become familiar with the types of medications typically contraindicated in older adults.

Unquestionably, a variety of medications can enhance the physical, cognitive, and emotional health of older adults. That said, medication use in the geriatric population is complicated by several factors. For one, older adults are likely to have multimorbidity (i.e., multiple diagnoses). This increases the likelihood of polypharmacy, which in turn raises the possibility of adverse drug reactions both individually or multiplicatively (Davies & O'Mahony, 2015). Moreover, as noted earlier, medication use is further complicated in older adults with manifest cognitive impairment, regardless of the context in which the medication is being prescribed. Because of declines in memory, particularly prospective memory (van den Berg et al., 2012), older adults may forget when it is time to take medications and will miss doses, leading to subtherapeutic dosing. Conversely, a decline in episodic memory or even attention may mean that an older adult does not attend to or remember having taken a particular dose and then takes extra doses, which increases the risk of serious side effects and drug toxicity.

Depending on his or her role, a neuropsychologist may have more frequent contact with an older adult than the medication provider, for example, through the provision of regular psychotherapy or cognitive rehabilitation. This provides further opportunities to observationally monitor an individual's response to treatment and gather anecdotal evidence suggestive of an adverse response to medication. In an ideal scenario, an older adult's providers would form a team that works collaboratively to provide multimodal, holistic care where decisions to institute interventions—pharmacological and otherwise—are theory- and evidence-based, and their efficacy is monitored through reliable and valid measurements.

Cognitive-Enhancing Medications

The coming of age of the "baby boomer" population has meant not only greater proportions of older adults living in our societies, but also increasing numbers of older adults who may experience non-normative cognitive decline (Versijpt, 2014). Major research and clinical efforts have been directed toward finding disease-modifying agents to slow or delay the rate of progression from normal cognitive aging to dementia, yet no intervention has been found to cure or even reliably affect the course of AD (Jiang, Yu, & Tan, 2012). The development, testing, and prescription of pharmacological interventions has been a major focus for aging research, if not to cure the underlying disease, then at least to slow the course of decline from MCI to dementia, palliate the major symptoms of cognitive decline, and improve associated quality of life. Moreover, to the extent that medication use could slow or delay decline, this has tangible implications for cost savings to the individual and the health care system (Versijpt, 2014).

In the following section, we review the major classes of medication and indications for their efficacy in persons with MCI and dementia. The preponderance of evidence is available on AD, although evidence for other dementias is increasing over time. In persons with SCD, the issue of cognitive-enhancing medication has not yet been fully explored; given the heterogeneous etiologies of SCD, it is unclear what the target of such medication might be (Smart et al., 2017). The use of cognitive-enhancing medication should be pursued with caution in healthy older adults, given that the side effects of these medications must be weighed against the uncertainty of any preventative benefits.

Acetylcholinesterase Inhibitors and N-Methyl-D-Aspartate Receptor Antagonists

These are the two classes of drugs most frequently prescribed for older adults with various stages of cognitive decline. Sometimes they are prescribed in isolation, and other times in combination. Many of the trials available compare these medications to one another for efficacy and safety within a given patient population.

AD is associated with a depletion of acetylcholine, a neurotransmitter that is implicated in smooth muscle movement as well as memory function.

Cholinesterase is the enzyme that accelerates the breakdown of acetylcholine in the synapse. Accordingly, acetylcholinesterase inhibitors (AChEIs) cause a net increase in cholinergic transmission in the central nervous system and periphery by inhibiting the action of cholinesterase (Birks, 2006). The major examples of these drugs include tacrine (Cognex), donepezil (Aricept), rivastigmine (Exelon), and galantamine (Razadyne). Tacrine has such a severe side-effect profile that it is no longer currently prescribed (Winslow, Onysko, Stob, & Hazlewood, 2011). By comparison, the other three agents have similar side effects; these are less frequent and severe than tacrine but by no means completely benign. A recent meta-analysis considering the efficacy and safety of the AChEIs indicated that the most frequently reported side effects were gastrointestinal (i.e., nausea, vomiting, diarrhea, and anorexia). Compared to placebo, donepezil, rivastigmine, and galantamine all showed significantly higher risk of adverse effects, as well as study dropout, compared to placebo-treated individuals (Tan et al., 2014). The Beers criteria (American Geriatrics Society, 2015) note that AChEIs should not be prescribed to individuals with a history of syncope, due to increased risk of orthostatic hypotension or bradycardia.

N-Methyl-D-aspartate (NMDA) receptor antagonists function by blocking excess glutamatergic activity, as glutamatergic toxicity is known to negatively impact memory (McShane, Areosa Sastre, & Minakaran, 2006). The main NMDA receptor antagonist available for prescription is memantine (Namenda), as well as Namzaric, a newer drug combining memantine with donepezil. Whereas the AChEIs tvend to be favored with mild to moderate stages of AD, memantine tends to be more frequently prescribed—and apparently is more effective—in the more severe stages of the disease (Di Santo, Prinelli, Adorni, Caltagirone, & Musicco, 2013). A recent meta-analysis examined the efficacy and safety of the three major ACheEIs and memantine. This study suggested that memantine has the most benign side-effect profile and, compared to placebo, was not associated with increased risk for adverse events such as those typically reported for the AChEIs (Tan et al., 2014).

Next we discuss available evidence for the use of AChEIs and NMDA receptor antagonists in the major dementia subtypes. While a plethora of individual trials have examined the impact of specific medications, there are too many to review and summarize individually here. Rather, we have chosen to present evidence primarily from recent systematic reviews and meta-analyses. In particular, where possible, we included *Cochrane Database Reviews*. These are systematic reviews of primary research in health care and health policy, typically based on RCTs, conducted under rigorous analysis and reporting guidelines and internationally recognized as the highest standard in evidence-based health care (Evidently Cochrane, 2016).

Mild Cognitive Impairment

The rationale behind using cognitive-enhancing medications is that, if implemented early enough, they could delay or slow the rate of decline to dementia. As such, the impact of these medications on persons with MCI has been a topic of great research and clinical interest. Unfortunately, however, the literature from two recent reviews has not made a compelling case for the use of pharmacological treatments for MCI. Russ and Morling (2012) conducted a *Cochrane Review* on the efficacy and safety of AChEIs for MCI. Nine double-blind, placebo-controlled studies were included, comprising well over 5,000 participants with MCI, broadly defined. The authors noted that it was difficult to pool results due to variance in trial length across studies. Results indicated no strong evidence of a beneficial effect on risk of progression to dementia at one-, two-, or three-year follow-up, with little evidence of the effect of AChEIs on tests of cognition. Fitzpatrick-Lewis, Warren, Ali, Sherifali, and Raina (2015) conducted a more recent systematic review and meta-analysis, with findings that were comparable to those of Russ and Morling (2012). Seventeen studies between 2010 and 2014 were included that involved community-dwelling adults diagnosed with MCI broadly defined. They included not only AChEI trials, but also one behavioral study and one study using vitamin E. Of the pharmacological studies, there was no significant benefit from AChEIs compared to control on either the Alzheimer's Disease Assessment Scale-Cognitive Subscale (ADAS-Cog) or the MMSE.

In a way, the lack of compelling results in these two recent reviews is not surprising, as several methodological issues are evident in this research. Presumably, the rationale for prescribing AChEIs, medications targeted for AD, would be based on the premise that MCI inevitably involves a decline to AD. However, MCI is a very heterogeneous condition in terms of its presentation, its potential etiology, and also risk of subsequent decline to dementia. Both of the aforementioned reviews included participants with MCI broadly defined, not specifying that participants had to have MCI associated with preclinical AD, such as in the Albert et al. (2011) criteria. With a highly heterogeneous sample of persons with MCI, one would expect the findings to be mixed at best. Moreover, although persons with amnestic MCI seem to have greater risk of decline to AD, this is not necessarily a 1:1 association. With regard to the biopsychosocial model, there are a large number of factors that moderate the association between underlying brain function (including integrity of neurotransmitter systems) and current cognitive function, including cognitive reserve, cognitive and social activity, and physical health. Finally, using measures such as the ADAS-Cog and MMSE may be insufficiently sensitive and/or specific to truly detect MCI from a psychometric perspective. Thus, it is easy to see why there might be mixed results at best evaluating the impact of AChEIs and other drugs to slow or avert decline to dementia.

Based on these results, we would say that while there is a lack of compelling evidence to date, the various methodological issues at play suggest that further work is needed to definitively say that AChEIs and other drugs do not help persons with MCI. In Chapter 7, we discussed some of the ways in which persons with MCI could be more rigorously characterized in both research and clinical samples. Perhaps with more precise operational definition of the type of MCI and presumed etiology, as well as more in-depth psychometric characterization, there could be more focused targeting of medications. Moreover, in the future, it will be worthwhile to examine whether concurrent participation in cognitive/behavioral or even psychological interventions (discussed in subsequent chapters) potentiates the impact of pharmacological interventions.

Alzheimer's Disease

Tan and colleagues (2014) have conducted a meta-analysis to examine the efficacy and safety of the three major AChEIs and memantine for the treatment of AD at various stages of disease severity. They note that, while many region-specific guidelines promote the use of these drugs for various stages of AD, their usage is not without controversy, and the clinical utility with regard to cost effectiveness has been called into question. Their systematic review yielded 23 RCTs on AD comprising over 11,000 participants. Significant effects on cognition were observed for all active drugs in all eleven studies using the ADAS-Cog to measure cognitive function; all participants had mild to moderate dementia. The authors note that these findings may in part have been due to worsening in the placebo group, rather than to explicit improvement in the active drug groups. The observed efficacy of these drugs on cognitive function did not seem to vary as a function of disease severity. However, this may have been a statistical artifact rather than an actual clinical observation. That is, the authors state that they chose the ADAS-Cog as their primary measure of cognitive function. Yet as they observe, this measure was only used in trials of participants with mild to moderate dementia, not severe dementia. Thus, the lack of significant findings may be due to the exclusion of trials and participants with the most severe dementia, which could lead to a range restriction of symptoms against which to track differential drug effects.

For global assessment of change, 12 out of 17 studies reported an improvement on the Clinician's Interview Based Assessment of Change scale, nine of which included persons with mild to moderate dementia and three with severe dementia. Therapeutic effects were observed for the three AChEIs but not for memantine. Eleven studies (seven with mild–moderate severity of dementia) measured behavioral symptoms using the Neuropsychiatric Inventory (Cummings et al., 1984), and no benefits were observed except for 10 mg donepezil and 24 mg galantamine. Finally, twelve studies reported change in functional outcome based on the Alzheimer's Disease Cooperative Study-Activities of Daily Living scale, five of which included participants with mild to moderate severity, and the remainder, persons with severe dementia. All drugs and doses had a significant effect on functional outcome except for 5 mg donepezil. Based on these findings, the authors concluded that the AChEIs and memantine are relatively safe and efficacious for individuals with a range of severity of dementia symptoms.

In order to be effective, AChEIs require the residual availability of adequate amounts of endogenous acetylcholine. As such, the efficacy of these medications is expected to diminish with disease severity, which likely explains why AChEIs have been favored in mild to moderate AD. The aforementioned Tan et al. (2014) meta-analysis failed to differentiate drug effects as a function of disease severity. However, Di Santo et al. (2013) conducted a meta-analysis of placebo-controlled RCTs of AChEIs to address the question of whether differing drug effects are observed as a function of disease progression. Data were pooled across clinical trials to examine the effects of AChEIs and memantine separately for cognition, functional status (i.e., activities of daily living), and behavioral and psychological disturbances. Dementia severity was indexed using the MMSE in order to investigate possible differential effects as a function of disease severity.

Thirty-four RCTs of AChEIs and six studies of memantine were included in the meta-analysis. Effects on cognition (available in all forty studies) were generally small to medium. These were independent of dementia severity for the AChEIs; only memantine showed a tendency to be more effective for participants with more severe dementia. In twenty-three studies assessing functional outcomes, all but one trial (using memantine) showed improvement (small effect sizes), again with memantine tending to be more effective in those with more severe dementia. Eighteen studies on behavioral and psychological outcomes were heterogeneous in methods and outcomes, making it difficult to draw firm conclusions.

The authors note some limitations to their findings. First, the comparatively lower number of trials on memantine ($n = 6$) may mean an incomplete picture of the efficacy of this drug, particularly at varying stages of the disease process. Second, within the AChEIs, most data were available on donepezil, so one cannot exclude the possibility that significant findings for AChEIs are primarily attributable to the effects of this drug as compared to rivastigmine or galantamine. Third, most trials lasted 6 months, so the data cannot speak either to long-term efficacy or to the conditions under which drug discontinuation is warranted. The major take-home point is that both AChEIs and memantine may be effective in enhancing cognition and functional status regardless of disease severity. This conclusion runs counter to prevailing guidelines in many countries which advise that AChEIs are effective in milder disease states and that memantine should be reserved for those with more severe dementia.

In summary, available empirical data suggest that AChEIs and memantine are relatively safe in persons with AD at various levels of severity. Based on the measures used in the various studies, these medications are associated with generally small effects on cognition and functional status. However, further data are required to ascertain whether these medications slow the rate of decline in milder cases of dementia. Moreover, it would be worthwhile to assess whether medications plus nonpharmacological interventions such as cognitive rehabilitation have synergistic effects on preserving current cognitive function or delaying the rate of subsequent decline.

Vascular Cognitive Impairment and Vascular Dementia

After AD, VaD is the second most prevalent form of dementia. Aside from "pure" cases of VaD, there are also a large number of older adults who show both Alzheimer's and vascular pathology, presenting with mixed dementia (Birks, McGuinness, & Craig, 2013). VCI and VaD can arise from a variety of distinct vascular pathologies, including (but not limited to) multiple small strokes, a single stroke, or ischemic white matter disease (i.e., subcortical dementia). Given the variety of etiologies, it has been difficult to identify specific treatment targets in the same way that AChEIs were designed to address purported acetylcholine deficiencies in AD (O'Brien & Thomas, 2015). As such, there are currently no established pharmacological treatments for VCI and VaD.

Birks and colleagues (2013) conducted a *Cochrane Review* of placebo-controlled RCTs of rivastigmine for vascular cognitive impairment, VaD, and mixed dementia. This study was based on the notion that reductions in acetylcholine and acetyltransferase are common to both AD and VCI, and AChEIs such as rivastigmine are beneficial in AD. The authors reviewed three trials, with 40, 50, and 710 participants, respectively. In the first trial on persons with subcortical dementia (mean MMSE scores of 13.0 and 13.4 in drug versus placebo), 26 weeks of rivastigmine treatment provided no significant benefit over placebo on neuropsychiatric symptoms, functional status, or global rating. In the second trial, participants with VCI (mean MMSE scores of 23.7 and 23.9 in drug vs. placebo), following 24 weeks of rivastigmine, showed no improvement in cognitive abilities, neuropsychiatric symptoms, functional status, or global rating. In the third and largest trial, participants with both cortical and subcortical forms of VaD (mean MMSE score of 19.1 for drug and placebo groups) were given 24 weeks of rivastigmine. The researchers observed a statistically significant advantage in cognitive response for rivastigmine but no effect on global impression of change or on noncognitive measures. Also, significantly more participants randomized to rivastigmine (odds ratio [OR] = 2.02) experienced adverse gastrointestinal effects and were likely to withdraw from treatment (OR = 2.66). Thus, there is tentative evidence for the use of rivastigmine in persons with various forms of VCI based on only one large clinical trial; this should be considered within the likelihood of adverse drug effects so significant as to prompt withdrawal from treatment.

More recently, Chen, Zhang, Wang, Yuan, and Hu (2016) conducted an updated meta-analysis on the efficacy of AChEIs in vascular dementia. Based on the results of twelve studies, both donepezil versus placebo and galantamine versus placebo were associated with significant improvement in the ADAS-Cog at 5-mg and 10-mg daily doses, with no such improvement seen on the MMSE. Interestingly, in contrast to the findings from the previous study on VCI, rivastigmine was not found to relate to significant improvement on the ADAS-Cog, although admittedly this was based on only two studies. Overall, treatment with AChEIs was associated with a twofold increase in the likelihood of discontinuation due to adverse events (pooled OR = 1.966), numbers similar to those reported in the Birks and colleagues (2013) review.

In summary, the evidence for AChEIs and NMDA receptor antagonists in persons with cognitive impairment of vascular etiology is limited in scope and of mixed efficacy at best. Moreover, there is concern about the rate and severity of adverse drug reactions in this population. As noted, given the diverse manifestations of VCI and VaD, the lack of compelling results is perhaps not surprising. In contrast to AD, however, vascular risk factors can be managed proactively through lifestyle changes and other medications (e.g., antihypertensives); this may be a more productive avenue for pharmacological intervention until more precise targets for cognitive-enhancing medication are ascertained.

Parkinson's-Related Cognitive Impairment, Parkinson's Disease Dementia, and Dementia with Lewy Bodies

Loss of dopaminergic neurons is the key neuropathology believed to underlie PD, and as such, most drugs used to manage symptoms of PD include a mechanism of action that increases dopaminergic availability. Several systematic reviews and meta-analyses have been conducted in this area in the last 5 years. In 2011, the Movement Disorder Society provided an updated evidence-based review of treatment of nonmotor symptoms in PD (Seppi et al., 2011). Treatment of these symptoms may be more challenging than that in other dementia subtypes, given the likely concurrent use of dopaminergic medications to control motor symptoms. This evidence-based review examined fifty-four RCT studies, both pharmacological and nonpharmacological RCT, published between 2002 and 2010. The only drug that was considered efficacious for PD dementia was rivastigmine; the evidence was insufficient for donepezil, galantamine, and memantine. Notably, this evidence-based review provided other recommendations for the treatment of depression and psychosis in this population specifically. Trials were typically only 6 months in duration, and as such any long-term benefits could not be observed.

Rolinski, Fox, Maidment, and McShane (2012) conducted a *Cochrane Review* of AChEIs in PD-related cognitive impairment, PD dementia, and DLB. They reviewed six RCT studies that included a variety of measures of cognitive, neuropsychiatric, and activities of daily living. In terms of global cognitive function, no data were available for DLB or PD-related cognitive impairment. Of the three trials on persons with PD dementia, AChEIs were superior to placebo on global cognitive function, with no difference between medication types (i.e., rivastigmine versus donepezil). There were several indicators of improved cognitive function in persons with PD dementia and PD-related cognitive impairment, but not DLB. Pooled data indicated a treatment effect on behavioral disturbance, specifically in trials of rivastigmine lasting 18 weeks or longer, again not including persons with DLB. There was a combined positive effect of AChEIs on activities of daily living. In terms of safety and tolerability, there were more dropouts and more adverse events in the treatment groups, including increased tremor and other Parkinsonian symptoms but not falls. These effects were observed in trials of rivastigmine but not donepezil. However, the number of severe adverse effects did not differ between drug and placebo, and the number of deaths was actually lower in the groups receiving drug versus placebo. In sum, the evidence seems to support the use of AChEIs in persons with PD-related cognitive impairment and PD dementia, but with only one study conducted on persons with DLB, evidence is lacking to make firm recommendations in this area.

A further systematic review and meta-analysis were conducted by Pagano and coworkers (2015) to examine the efficacy and safety of AChEIs for PD. Four double-blind RCTs were eligible for inclusion, with a total of 941 patients included, indicating that these drugs improve cognitive function and delay the rate of cognitive decline but do not improve the risk of falls. No difference was observed between donepezil and rivastigmine. Conversely, AChEIs did seem to increase tremor and other adverse drug effects, which seems to have been driven primarily by the one study using rivastigmine, suggesting that perhaps this drug contributes to more side effects.

In summary, there is some evidence to suggest that AChEIs in persons with PD-related cognitive impairment and PD dementia is effective, although some studies point to a possible increased risk of worsening in tremors. Moreover, there is a lack of available evidence for DLB, and anecdotally this condition is difficult to treat given the concomitant neuropsychiatric symptoms. Managing the underlying disease process through dopaminergic medications may contribute to maintenance of cognitive function, although these medications can also lead to iatrogenic effects over time, including impulse control disorders.

Less Frequently Occurring Dementias

Li, Hai, Zhou, and Dong (2015) conducted a *Cochrane Review* on the efficacy and safety of AChEIs for rarer dementias associated with various neurological conditions. They included dementias associated with HD, cerebral autosomal dominant arteriopathy with subcortical infarcts and leukoencephalopathy (CADASIL), FTLD, multiple sclerosis, and PSP. They reviewed eight RCTs, all double-blind and placebo-controlled, including a total of 567 participants. Half of the trials (i.e., 4) were conducted on patients with multiple sclerosis, with two on HD, one each on FTLD and CADASIL, and none on PSP. Taken together, the data suggest that AChEIs are associated with improvement on discrete neuropsychometric tests for persons with multiple sclerosis, HD, and CADASIL (e.g., recognition memory, verbal fluency, cognitive flexibility), although no significant impact was observed for improving overall cognitive level, activities of daily living, or quality of life, raising questions about the ecological relevance of these discrete cognitive test improvements. With such small trials and limited data, no clear conclusions can be made about the efficacy of AChEIs for rarer forms of dementia, although in terms of safety, these drugs were associated with more gastrointestinal side effects as compared to placebo.

Interpreting Clinical Trial Data on the Impact of Cognitive-Enhancing Medications

Available reviews suggest that AChEIs and certain NMDA receptor antagonists can be helpful for various stages of AD and PD, with mixed evidence at best for vascular-related etiologies and insufficient data on DLB and other less frequent dementias. Conducting pharmacologic trials on persons with late-life cognitive decline is challenging. Even when certain variables are controlled for such factors as disease severity/chronicity, there may be variability in medical and psychiatric comorbidities, as well as other moderator variables such as cognitive reserve. Alternative approaches to the usual RCT designs may have to be explored, such as rigorously controlled $n = 1$ case series where individual patient effectiveness of these medications can be investigated, including more ecologically relevant assessments of daily function in response to these medications.

Table 10.1 provides a summary of evidence regarding the three main AChEIs and memantine in older adults with different etiologies of cognitive impairment, including observed benefits as well as any risks.

TABLE 10.1. Application of AChEIs and NMDA Receptor Antagonists for Cognitive Decline

Clinical issue	Benefits	Risks
MCI	Minimal evidence to support the use of AChEIs or other cognitive-enhancing medications in persons with MCI.	Similar side effects to those observed in persons with more severe cognitive impairment.
AD dementia	Both AChEIs and memantine have positive effects on cognition and functional status, regardless of disease severity. Less data available for behavioral and functional outcomes, although appears favorable. Most evidence available for donepezil.	Gastrointestinal effects in drug versus placebo. Insufficient evidence regarding when to discontinue (i.e., when risks outweigh benefits).
VCI and VaD	Mixed findings regarding the beneficial effects of rivastigmine on cognition but not global change or noncognitive measures.	Gastrointestinal side effects severe enough to warrant drug discontinuation with rivastigmine.
PD dementia, PD-related cognitive impairment, and DLB	Best evidence for rivastigmine in PD dementia; evidence insufficient for other medications. AChEIs effective for PD dementia, improving cognition, behavioral disturbance, and daily function. Impact in DLB is unclear, and evidence lacking to support use in PD-related cognitive impairment. Donepezil and rivastigmine found to improve cognition, delay rate of cognitive decline, and decrease behavioral disturbance in PD dementia.	AChEIs and memantine have acceptable risk without specialized monitoring. Increased risk of tremor and other adverse effects but not falls, particularly with rivastigmine. Increase in tremor in persons with PD dementia. Insufficient evidence regarding impact on risk of falls in persons with PD dementia and PD-related cognitive impairment.
Less common dementias	Some evidence of benefit on discrete cognitive tests in multiple sclerosis, HD, and CADASIL; no clear evidence of benefit on overall cognitive function, activities of daily living, or quality of life.	More gastrointestinal side effects as compared to placebo.

Medications Designed to Enhance Current Mood and Psychological Function

Older adults may experience any number of psychiatric disorders. These conditions can appear for the first time later in life, or they may have initially manifested many years prior to older adulthood. Some of the more common disorders include depression and anxiety, as well as bipolar disorder and psychosis. Neuropsychological evaluation can contribute vital information regarding the diagnosis of psychological disorders in older adults. Estimates of the prevalence of psychological disorders in late life are likely to vary considerably depending on the sample, particularly differences between community samples, inpatient units, rehabilitation settings, and residential care facilities. As such, the neuropsychologist should consider the setting in which they are evaluating an older adult, to take into account base rates of certain mental disorders as well as their likely antecedents and consequences.

There is compelling evidence that certain mental disorders have a strong biological basis and therefore would benefit from pharmacological intervention. Thus, neuropsychologists are likely to work with older adults with psychological disorders who are already taking psychotropic medication or have been referred for an evaluation for such treatment. *Psychotropics* is the term used to refer to medications specifically designed to alter mood and psychological function. Within this general designation, there are several types of medications designed to target specific symptoms or disorders, the most common of which are antidepressants, anxiolytics (antianxiety drugs), and mood stabilizers. Each of these is discussed as follows, with example medications and available evidence for efficacy and side effects.

Antidepressants

Late-life depression can negatively impact cognition, as well as increase risk for development of dementia. As such, comprehensive management of depression—which may include both psychotherapy and medication—is essential to the overall health and well-being of older adults. One caveat to this statement is the presence of disturbance in mood that is normative or part of normal existential concerns of late life. For example, grief is a common part of older adulthood (Malkinson & Bar-Tur, 2014). As a normative experience, grief should typically not be treated with medication. The exception is prolonged grief or complicated bereavement associated with a sudden or traumatic loss (Hartz, 1986; Horowitz et al., 1997), which could evolve into a major depression. Approximately 25–30% of individuals who have encountered a major loss develop clinical depression (Preston et al., 2017), and in these cases it may be worthwhile to consider the use of medication, in conjunction with psychotherapy. Additionally, older adults may face existential concerns or go through a "life review" (Bhar, 2014) that leads to negative mood states. Again, this is not necessarily a context in which medication is necessary, but rather appropriate psychotherapy to help the individual make meaning and come to terms with late-life concerns. This underscores the need for comprehensive psychological and psychiatric assessment to best understand the nature of any mood disturbance with which an older adult presents and to consider whether medications are an appropriate part of the treatment plan.

There are several major classes of antidepressants based on their targeted neurotransmitter system. These include selective serotonin reuptake inhibitors (SSRIs), those that target norepinephrine (NE) or dopamine (DA), serotonin–norepinephrine reuptake inhibitors (SNRIs), tricyclic antidepressants (TCAs), and monoamine oxidase inhibitors (MAOIs). Of these medications, the SSRIs are considered a frontline treatment for late-life depression, given their low profile of adverse events, which include nausea and headache (Taylor, 2014). Examples of SSRIs are fluoxetine (Prozac), sertraline (Zoloft), and paroxetine (Paxil). Taylor (2014) reviewed RCT evidence for SSRIs in late-life depression, finding that larger studies tend to find significant effects favoring SSRIs over placebo. Rates of SSRI response (i.e., >50% reduction in symptoms) range from 35 to 60%, as compared with placebo response rates ranging from 26 to 40%. Likewise, available data on remission rates ranged from 32 to 44% for SSRIs as compared with 19 to 26% with placebo. SNRIs such as venlafaxine (Effexor) and duloxetine (Cymbalta) may be used as second-line agents when a satisfactory treatment response is not achieved with SSRIs. While studies suggest that their efficacy does not differ, adverse effects may be more frequent with SNRIs (Oslin et al., 2003; Schatzberg & Roose, 2006). Finally, TCAs such as amitriptyline (Elavil) or imipramine (Tofranil) have comparable efficacy to SSRIs and SNRIs, and so may be considered if neither of these classes of medications is effective. However, the Beers criteria include TCAs—as well as paroxetine—as being potentially inappropriate for older adults due to the likelihood of adverse effects such as anticholinergic effects as well as orthostatic hypotension (American Geriatrics Society, 2015).

The U.S. Centers for Disease Control and Prevention (CDC) in the United States estimate that approximately 80% of older adults have at least one chronic health condition (e.g., chronic pain, cardiovascular disease), which further elevates the prevalence of depression (CDC, 2015). Medication management of depression in the context of medical comorbidities can pose significant challenges, including drug interactions that alter medication efficacy, as well as increased likelihood of serious side effects (Davies & O'Mahony, 2015; Taylor, 2014). In addition, regardless of class of medication, a recent meta-analysis found that antidepressants contributed to a 1.68 increase in the OR of falls in older adults (Woolcott et al., 2009). Thus, antidepressant use, though important, should be closely monitored for the possibility of adverse events, particularly when medications other than SSRIs are being prescribed.

Anxiolytics

Anxiety disorders are relatively common in older adults, though less common than in younger adults, and highly comorbid with depression (Wolitzky-Taylor, Castriotta, Lenze, Stanley, & Craske, 2010). Older adults may have premorbid histories of anxiety disorders or experience new onset of worry or anxiety associated with declining physical health or even perceived cognitive decline (Rabin et al., 2017). Recent research has revealed complex interrelationships between anxiety and late-life cognitive impairment, possibly moderated by dysfunction of the hypothalamic–pituitary–adrenal axis (Joshi & Pratico, 2013; Pietrzak et al., 2015a, 2015b). Despite the prevalence of anxiety disorders in older adults, compared with depression, relatively less empirical literature is available regarding the effective management of anxiety disorders in the elderly, including the use of psychopharmacological interventions (Hendricks, 2014). Likewise, there is limited data to speak to the relative efficacy of certain medications or the utility of long-term treatment (Gonçalves & Byrne, 2012; Pinquart & Duberstein, 2007).

The major classes of medications associated with anxiety treatment are benzodiazepines (both short and long-acting), as well as atypical and nonbenzodiazepines and other miscellaneous agents that have anxiolytic properties, such as certain beta-blockers, antihistamines, and antidepressants. Benzodiazepines interact with benzodiazepine receptors, which have a high density in the limbic system, the region of the brain intimately associated with expression of emotion, including fear (Preston et al., 2017). Gamma-aminobutyric acid (GABA) neurons are also directly associated with fear circuitry and anxiety (Möhler, 2013); benzodiazepine receptors are co-located with GABA receptors, which usually function as presynaptic inhibiting receptors. In general, benzodiazepines are considered an effective choice for short-term management of anxiety symptoms, although long-term use is discouraged due to the strong potential for abuse and dependence (Preston et al., 2017).

While benzodiazepines may be a viable treatment choice for younger and middle-aged adults, older adults are particularly vulnerable to adverse effects with this class of medication, including sedation (Preston et al., 2017). Benzodiazepines have been associated with a 1.57 increased OR for falls (Woolcott et al., 2009), as well as a threefold increase in the odds of delirium (Clegg & Young, 2011). The Beers criteria list notes that all benzodiazepines increase risk of cognitive impairment, delirium, falls, fractures, and motor vehicle accidents, although some long-acting agents (e.g., clonazepam, diazepam, flurazepam) may be acceptable in specific contexts such as severe generalized anxiety disorder, ethanol withdrawal, and rapid-eye-movement sleep disorders. They further advise that benzodiazepines not be used in persons with dementia or cognitive impairment due to the incidence of adverse central nervous system effects (American Geriatrics Society, 2015).

Available evidence from several reviews suggests that antidepressant medication may be a viable alternative for the management of certain anxiety disorders in older adults (Pinquart & Duberstein, 2007; Wolitzky-Taylor et al., 2010). In a systematic review and meta-analysis of treatments for late-life anxiety, Gonçalves and Byrne (2012) found that both benzodiazepines (OR = 0.19) and antidepressants (OR = 0.46) exhibited statistically significant treatment effects. The greater treatment effect for antidepressants, in addition to their safer side-effect profile, supports them as the favored treatment for older adults. Similar to prior studies, a more recent review by Hendricks (2014) highlights SSRIs as the preferred choice of antidepressant over other classes. The author also suggests a more nuanced approach to prescribing based on the chronicity and severity of anxiety. More specifically, it was suggested that cognitive-behavioral therapy is preferred in either late-onset anxiety disorders or in those with mild–moderate anxiety symptoms, whereas early-onset/chronic anxiety that is more severe and comorbid with depression is better managed with SSRIs. It stands to reason that the same concerns regarding adverse drug effects with antidepressants prescribed for depression should be considered in the management of anxiety. In general, it is recommended that medications be prescribed at 50% the typical dose for younger adults, with a similarly slow increase of the dose over time as needed.

Mood Stabilizers

Bipolar disorder is a condition that that may be diagnosed early in life but persist into later adulthood and is typically managed with mood-stabilizing agents. The first-line treatment for bipolar disorder is lithium; yet its mechanism of action remains incompletely understood. It has a narrow therapeutic window, and as such, blood levels must be continuously monitored for toxicity that can be fatal. Lithium is associated with a range of other side effects, including gastrointestinal disturbance, hypothyroidism, rash and acne-like lesions, and minor changes in cardiovascular function (Preston et al., 2017). Three other medications commonly used for bipolar disorder include divalproex (Depakote), carbamazepine (Equetro), and lamotrigine (Lamictal), all anticonvulsant agents. Carbamazepine is associated with gastrointestinal and central nervous system effects (e.g., sedation, dizziness, drowsiness, blurred vision, and incoordination), whereas divalproex has similar side effects to a lesser frequency and severity. Again, blood levels should be monitored for potential toxicity. Lamotrigine has similar dose-related side effects, with the addition of a potentially life-threatening dermatological reaction known as Stevens–Johnson syndrome (Preston et al., 2017).

A recent meta-analysis of population-based prevalence rates of mental disorders in older adults estimated the rates of bipolar disorder at 0.53% for current illness and 1.10% for lifetime illness, notably lower compared to lifetime prevalence of depression (16.52%) and generalized anxiety disorder (6.36%) (Volkert, Schulz, Härter, Wlodarczyk, & Andreas, 2013). Diniz, Nunes, Machado-Vieira, and Forlenza (2011) provided a comprehensive review of available evidence for management of geriatric bipolar disorder, with several points that warrant mention. First, they note that available evidence to guide management of geriatric bipolar disorder is generally lacking, and due to differences in pharmacokinetics, one cannot assume that management of the disorder for younger and midlife adults will safely translate to older adults. Second, the use of mood stabilizers in older adults can cause or exacerbate cognitive impairment, particularly with polydrug use, although effects do seem to be reversible upon drug discontinuation. Interestingly, mood stabilizers were associated with increased risk of dementia, but only using the anticonvulsants; lithium was actually associated with lower risk, and there is some suggestion that lithium may have neuroprotective effects. Third, mood stabilizers are associated with increased risk of MetS (i.e., risk for cardiovascular disease, diabetes mellitus, and premature mortality), which increases with age. This would be an issue of concern for any older adult, but particularly for older adults who already have vascular risk factors (e.g., hypertension) or VaD. Olanzapine and clozapine in particular seem to be associated with the highest risk for MetS. Finally, older adults with bipolar disorder are at elevated risk for suicide; this is most concerning because older adults in general are less likely to seek mental health treatment than younger and middle-aged adults.

The Beers criteria list again provides guidance on potential contraindications in the use of mood stabilizers in older adults. They advise that carbamazepine should be used with caution due to an increased risk of the syndrome of inappropriate antidiuretic hormone secretion and hyponatremia. Olanzapine and clozapine, antipsychotic medications that may be prescribed for bipolar disorder, can both lower the seizure threshold and are associated with strong anticholinergic properties; as such, physicians advise against their use (American Geriatrics Society, 2015). Diniz et al. (2011) noted that lithium might have neuroprotective effects; however, the Beers criteria list advises that lithium toxicity may be potentiated by concomitant use of AChEIs, which may be prescribed for someone with MCI or dementia, as noted above (American Geriatrics Society, 2015). In this case, then, one should weigh the risks and benefits of managing cognitive symptoms versus bipolar symptoms, in order to avoid serious adverse drug reactions. Divalproex and lamotrigine are not explicitly mentioned by the criteria.

Antipsychotics

Psychosis can be a particularly challenging phenomenon to manage in older adults. Aside from individuals who are aging with lifelong primary psychotic disorders (e.g., schizophrenia) and schizoaffective disorders, psychosis can also arise in older adulthood in conjunction with delirium, dementia, substance abuse, and PD (Broadway & Mintzer, 2007). Reinhardt and Cohen (2015) note that, while the prevalence of late-life psychotic disorders is rather high—an estimated lifetime risk of 23%—there is a striking paucity of evidence available regarding effective treatments for these disorders, both pharmacological and nonpharmacological.

The so-called first-generation antipsychotic medications include well-known agents such as chlorpromazine (Thorazine), thioridazine (Mellaril), and haloperidol (Haldol). These medications are potent blockers of dopamine D2 synaptic receptors, and the degree of receptor blockade predicts their clinical potency. These medications are also referred to as neuroleptics, given their potent neurological side effects, which include extrapyramidal symptoms such as Parkinsonism, dystonia, and akathisia (intense restlessness), the last-named of which is associated with increased risk of suicide (Preston et al., 2017). Other miscellaneous effects of neuroleptics include anticholinergic effects (to which older adults are already sensitive) and antiadrenergic effects, which can lead to orthostatic hypotension and increased risk of falls. The second generation or "atypical" antipsychotics have greater serotonin blockade and produce varying degrees of dopamine D2 blockade. Their side-effect profile is considered more favorable than that of the older generation medications, with a lower likelihood of extrapyramidal symptoms. However, these medications can cause anticholinergic and antiadrenergic side effects, severe sedation, and significant metabolic effects such weight gain, blood sugar dysregulation, and altered lipid metabolism. Common examples of atypical antipsychotics include clozapine (Clozaril), aripiprazole (Abilify), olanzapine (Zyprexa), quetiapine (Seroquel), risperidone (Risperdal), and ziprasidone (Geodon) (Preston et al., 2017).

It is not uncommon for younger and middle-aged adults to safely be prescribed an antipsychotic medication to help manage their symptoms. However, most of these medications are clearly contraindicated in older adults according to the Beers criteria list (American Geriatrics Society, 2015). For one, many of these drugs have strong anticholinergic properties, to which older adults are known to be more sensitive in general (Ruscin & Linnebaur, 2014). More significant, perhaps, are the clear risks of elevated morbidity and mortality with these medications. For example, while agitation and psychosis can be sequelae of delirium, the list strongly recommends against the use of antipsychotics in this context, given the mixed evidence for their effectiveness, as well as potential for adverse drug effects. Moreover, for individuals with dementia and severe behavioral disturbance, both first-generation and newer atypical antipsychotics are contraindicated unless all behavioral interventions have failed and the older adult is at serious risk of harm to self or others. This is due to the elevated risk of cognitive decline, stroke, and overall mortality associated with these medications (Greenblatt & Greenblatt, 2016). The clear indication is to avoid such medication if at all possible except in persons with schizophrenia, bipolar disorder, or for short-term use as an antiemetic (i.e., antisickness) during chemotherapy (American Geriatrics Society, 2015).

Finally, antipsychotics are not advised for persons with PD, given their potential to worsen extrapyramidal symptoms. This makes for a particular challenge in the treatment of persons with DLB, who may simultaneously present with both movement disorder symptoms and psychotic symptoms. Overall, antipsychotic medications should only be prescribed with extreme caution and ideally only when other options have already been explored and exhausted.

Summary and Conclusions

Psychopharmacology can play an important role in a biopsychosocial formulation of current cognitive/behavioral and emotional functioning in older adults at various stages of cognitive decline. It behooves the neuropsychologist to be as well informed as possible about the various medications that can influence cognitive and emotional functioning in older adults. Pharmacological interventions offer certain benefits, including ease and efficiency of administration (and possible short-term cost effectiveness) as compared to nonpharmacological interventions (Versijpt, 2014). Moreover, for individuals whose symptomatology is so severe that it impacts their function, medications can provide a foundation on which to build using nonpharmacological interventions such as cognitive rehabilitation or psychotherapy. There are risks and limitations, however, in relying primarily on pharmacological interventions. For example, many of the medications discussed would be prescribed on a long-term basis; this can create significant costs for the individual, caregivers, and the health care system (Bond et al., 2012; Pouryamout, Dams, Wasem, Dodel, & Neumann, 2012). In addition, many of the cognitive-enhancing or psychotropic medications have significant side-effect profiles; for individuals with certain medical conditions, use of such medications may be directly contraindicated (Winslow et al., 2011). In routine clinical practice, the application of pharmacological intervention should be highly individualized; any given patient should be fully informed of the potential risks and benefits and able to actively participate in making informed choices about their care.

For many years, the primary focus of intervention for persons with cognitive decline was pharmacological. Significant time and financial resources have been allocated to the development and evaluation of medications, primarily for AD but also applied to other types of late-life cognitive decline. There is some evidence that medications such as AChEIs can be beneficial in persons with AD as measured by cognitive screening measures, but the impact on everyday behavior remains open for debate. As we noted in earlier chapters, one of the purported benefits of identifying individuals earlier in the spectrum is to be able to implement interventions that could slow or even avert the course of decline toward dementia. However, there is a relative paucity of evidence in support of the use of drugs such as AChEIs for persons with MCI.

There are many methodological issues in this literature, the most salient being how persons with MCI are classified and characterized. Taking MCI at the broadest and most heterogeneous definition, it is perhaps not surprising that there is a dearth of significant findings. In order to improve future research in this area, more precise neuropsychometric characterization of study participants will be necessary. Given the biopsychosocial influences on cognition, a variety of factors may moderate any given person's response to intervention (e.g., some of the various risk and protective factors already discussed), and these should be systematically measured in future studies. Another worthwhile future endeavor would be to ascertain the impact of combined pharmacological and nonpharmacological (i.e., cognitive/behavioral or psychological) interventions in persons with MCI. In the broader clinical psychology realm, many studies have indicated that, for example, people with major depression who receive combined medication and psychotherapy benefit more than those receiving either modality in isolation. Likewise, while pharmacological agents might not in and of themselves improve cognition, they may improve more basic functions such as drive and motivation, which in turn promote engagement in cognitive/behavioral or psychological interventions, leading to an overall therapeutic effect.

The use of cognitive-enhancing medications in SCD is controversial: not only is it a condition that is etiologically heterogeneous, but unlike MCI, participants present with normal neuropsychological function, thus raising ethical issues about which symptoms would actually be targeted by pharmacological interventions. This is not to say that all medications should be ruled out for persons with SCD. For those who have comorbid mood, anxiety, and physical health concerns, treatment-as-usual, which may include pharmacological care, should be pursued and may again lead to ascertaining different subtypes of SCD that do or do not experience later decline.

Finally, many medication trials use limited outcome assessment or are restricted to gross screening measures that may lack the sensitivity to detect subtle changes in cognition or in functional abilities. While it is understood that clinical trials are extremely time- and resource-intensive, it would be a worthwhile investment for future studies to use measures that are more likely to detect response to intervention. In individual clinical practice, different measures may be more or less appropriate for individual clients. We refer the reader back to Chapter 9 and our discussion of the single-case experimental design, which provides some guidance on how medication impact could be ascertained in individual clients as part of this research design.

KEY POINTS

✓ Medications are an important part of the biopsychosocial conceptualization of treatment of older adults. Psychologists should be aware of the different classes of medications that can have either direct or indirect effects on cognition and mood and psychological functioning.

✓ It is essential for psychologists to understand basic pharmacology, how medications might work differently in this population, as well as being aware of those medications that could cause iatrogenic effects or be contraindicated more generally.

✓ While neuropsychologists do not prescribe medications, they can provide comprehensive assessment of function that allows for determination of which medications might be appropriate to prescribe. They can also determine barriers to adherence, such as motivation and memory, as well as measure response to intervention using a variety of tests sensitive to clinically meaningful change

✓ The AChEls and NMDA receptor antagonists are the most frequently prescribed cognitive-enhancing medications. The strongest evidence of efficacy is for individuals already diagnosed with dementia, particularly individuals with AD and PD dementia. The literature is mixed on vascular-related cognitive impairment and DLB, with insufficient evidence on less common dementias. Little evidence exists to support the use of these medications in persons with MCI, although methodological issues may hamper the ability to detect significant effects in these studies.

✓ Empirically supported treatments exist for psychological function, particularly geriatric depression, which may have secondary benefits on cognition. However, some medications should be used with great caution in older adults (e.g., anxiolytics), while some others are largely contraindicated (i.e., antipsychotics).

Resources for Continuing Education on Psychopharmacology

Suggested Articles and Texts

American Geriatrics Society Beers Criteria Update Expert Panel. (2015). American Geriatrics Society updated Beers Criteria for potentially inappropriate medication use in older adults. *Journal of the American Geriatrics Society, 63,* 2227–2246.

Preston, J. D., O'Neal, J. H., & Talaga, M. C. (2017). *Handbook of clinical psychopharmacology for therapists* (8th ed.). Oakland, CA: New Harbinger.

Other Continuing Education Resources

Several professional organizations serving psychologists provide continuing education resources relevant to the topic of clinical psychopharmacology. Some of these are prerecorded courses, while others are ongoing, time-limited courses (e.g., 14 weeks) completed online with assigned reading and interactive discussion boards. Each country likely has professional organizations that provide such continuing education; a sampling of these is listed as follows.

American Psychological Association (APA)

Currently offering a video on-demand course on "Basics in Psychopharmacology."

www.apa.org/education/ce/ccw0005.aspx

Canadian Psychological Association (CPA)

Currently offering a course on "A Psychologist's Guide to Psychopharmacology."

www.cpa.ca/professionaldevelopment/webcourses

National Academy of Neuropsychology (NAN)

Currently offering semester-long (i.e., 14-week) courses on clinical psychopharmacology and clinical neuroanatomy, both of which would provide up-to-date information relevant to the topic of psychopharmacology in older adulthood. More information on NAN's resources can be found at *http://nanonline.org/nan/Continuing_Education/NAN/Continuing_Education.aspx?hkey=dcd8fb99-079a-4093-9aeb-7bc667c7a98a.*

CHAPTER 11

Cognitive and Behavioral
Interventions

In this chapter, we review cognitive and behavioral intervention strategies for older adults across the spectrum of cognitive decline. We begin with a review of theoretical principles relevant to this topic, followed by a review of contemporary empirical literature in this burgeoning field. Finally, we present a practical model and illustrative examples of application of cognitive interventions at various stages of cognitive decline, as well as a case example.

First, a note to the reader about our use of the term *cognitive and behavioral interventions:* we chose this term because we felt it was the most representative of the material in this chapter. Given the possible confusion with cognitive-behavioral therapy (an empirically supported intervention for mood and psychological disorders, discussed at length in Chapter 12), we considered omitting the term *behavioral.* However, to say that the interventions covered in this chapter are only cognitive is not accurate, given that, for example, some rehabilitation strategies target the changing of one's behavior, not necessarily the changing of cognition. We also considered the broader term *nonpharmacological interventions* (NPI), which has been used elsewhere (Smart et al., 2017). However, NPI includes potentially any intervention that is not medication-based, including nutrition and complementary/alternative medicine, which we did not cover here. As such, we felt that *cognitive and behavioral interventions,* while imperfect, was the best terminology to capture the scope of material discussed in this chapter.

Theoretical Foundations

We contend that holistic care of older adults with cognitive decline would optimally include a combination of the various intervention modalities discussed in this book—pharmacological, cognitive/behavioral, psychological, and caregiver support. As such, although this chapter specifically discusses the use of cognitive and behavioral interventions and available evidence for their efficacy, ideally these methods would not be used in a vacuum, but rather implemented within the context of one or more of these other interventions. In practice, clinicians are advised to use the same scientist–practitioner, biopsychosocial case conceptualization process they would normally apply in routine clinical care.

Neuroplasticity in Later Life

The last decade in particular has seen a rapid proliferation in the literature on cognitive and behavioral interventions for older adults with cognitive decline. Two major advances have set the stage for this proliferation of research. The first is the literature on neuroplasticity, particularly experience-dependent plasticity (EDP). Kleim and Jones (2008) define EDP as "the remarkable ability [of neurons] to alter their structure and function in response to a variety of internal and external pressures, including behavioral training . . . [it is] the mechanism by which the damaged brain relearns lost behavior in response to rehabilitation" (p. 225). Until relatively recently, it was believed that the brain was most malleable and adaptive early in life and that damage to the brain in middle and older adulthood offered limited capacity for recovery of function (Jellinger & Attems, 2013). Clinicians and researchers may have been reticent to pursue cognitive and behavioral interventions in older adults, or they may have had modest goals regarding likely improvement. However, both animal and human models indicate that the brain can continue to change in adaptive ways in response to training, even in older adulthood (Greenwood & Parasuraman, 2010). This finding has led to increased optimism about the potential for nonpharmacological intervention. In fact, the field of dementia research is beginning to orient itself toward primary and secondary prevention of pathological cognitive impairment at earlier stages of the decline trajectory, even before clinical symptoms are evident (Imtiaz, Tolppanen, Kivipelto, & Soininen, 2014).

Neuroplasticity takes at least two major forms—structural and functional—and there is accumulating evidence that both can occur in older adulthood in response to structured intervention. *Structural plasticity* pertains to changes in the underlying structure of the brain in response to training. Neurogenesis—or the growth of new neurons—was once thought to be a feature only of the developing nervous system (Jellinger & Attems,

2013). However, animal models indicate that hippocampal neurogenesis can occur following physical exercise (Foster, Rosenblatt, & Kuljiš, 2011; Yau, Gil-Mohapel, Christie, & So, 2014), an important finding given that Alzheimer's disease, for example, is associated with neurodegeneration in hippocampal cells (Winner, Kohl, & Gage, 2011). These findings underpin the accumulating literature examining the cognitive benefits of physical exercise in older adults (e.g., Karr, Areshenkoff, Rast, & Garcia-Barrera, 2014). By contrast, *functional plasticity* means changes to the functional organization of the brain with or without any concomitant change in brain structure. One example of functional plasticity is the "posterior–anterior brain shift" in response to aging (Davis, Dennis, Daselaar, Fleck, & Cabeza, 2008). Neuroimaging studies indicate that, when comparing healthy older adults to younger adults, both groups often show comparable performance on cognitive tasks; yet older adults demonstrate greater recruitment of frontal brain regions to maintain the same task performance (Park & McDonough, 2013; Reuter-Lorenz, 2013). This is thought to be associated with deployment of executive control abilities to allow older adults to compensate for losses in other areas, such as episodic memory retrieval (Bouazzaoui et al., 2013).

Nuanced investigation of the potential for neuroplasticity in the human brain has been supported by a parallel increase in the sophistication of (and access to) advanced neuroimaging methods. For example, structural magnetic resonance imaging (sMRI) has demonstrated evidence of increased cortical thickness and volume in response to training such as meditation (Luders, 2014; Smart, Segalowitz, Mulligan, Koudys, & Gawryluk, 2016). Conversely, methods such as functional magnetic resonance imaging (fMRI) can show the function of the aging brain in real time in response to various task demands, allowing confirmation or disconfirmation of existing theories of cognitive aging (Park & McDonough, 2013). The time-scales and mechanisms of neuroplasticity in aging may differ from those of younger and middle adulthood (Jellinger & Attems, 2013). Moreover, structural and functional neuroplasticity may occur on different temporal orders and take place prior to change in manifest behavior (Valkanova, Rodriguez, & Ebmeier, 2014). This underscores the value of a multimodal approach to assessment of intervention outcomes, which we advocate for in this chapter.

Neuroplasticity becomes further relevant in considering the concept of *cognitive reserve,* that is, the notion that there are individual differences that moderate the impact of underlying brain pathology on manifest cognitive and behavioral function (Stern, 2009, 2012). Several factors that contribute to cognitive reserve have been identified, including greater years of formal education, greater occupational attainment, better physical health, and social engagement. Compared to those with lower reserve, individuals with higher cognitive reserve tend to withstand the impact of brain pathology for longer before demonstrating significant cognitive impairment.

More importantly, rather than being a static individual difference, one can make contributions to cognitive reserve even in older adulthood, allowing one to take active steps to buffer the onset or rate of cognitive decline. This finding is supported by animal models showing that enriched environments and physical activity positively influence hippocampal neurogenesis in adult animals (Kent, Oomen, Bekinschtein, Bussey, & Saksida, 2015). Together, these findings suggest that boosting cognitive reserve is one mechanism by which neuroplasticity is realized, and encourages the active engagement of older adults at all levels of cognitive decline.

Cognitive Rehabilitation for Acquired Brain Injury

The second major advance that supports the proliferation of older adult interventions is the field of cognitive rehabilitation for acquired brain injury. While research on neuroplasticity provides evidence of underlying neurobiological mechanisms that support restoration and recovery of function, cognitive rehabilitation provides information on how such restoration and recovery occurs in practice. Here, we refer to cognitive rehabilitation as a holistic and integrative intervention approach that can include both restorative and compensatory approaches to improving cognitive and psychological function, with an emphasis on translation to everyday function and adaptive behavior (Sohlberg & Mateer, 2001). While still a comparatively young subdiscipline within the field of clinical neuropsychology, the last two decades have seen the accumulation of a substantial body of literature in support of the application of cognitive rehabilitation for acquired brain injury (Cicerone et al., 2011; Mateer & Smart, 2013). There is often confusion in the older adult literature with regard to the nomenclature of various cognitive and behavioral interventions, with the terms *cognitive rehabilitation, cognitive training,* and *cognitive stimulation* often being used interchangeably, despite pertaining to quite different methodological approaches and anticipated outcomes (Clare & Woods, 2004; Gates & Sachdev, 2014). In this chapter, we clarify these terms and offer a clinical model about when and where these approaches may be more or less useful. Although cognitive rehabilitation is beginning to be implemented in older adults, we also advance the position that much is to be learned by considering the extant literature on cognitive rehabilitation for acquired brain injury, where the evidence is most robust.

Empirical Evidence for Cognitive and Behavioral Interventions

To date, pharmacological interventions alone have been unable to reliably delay progression to dementia. Over the last decade, there has been a formidable increase in the amount of empirical work focused on nonpharmacological approaches, particularly cognitive and behavioral interventions. In general, we believe that older adults are well served by a holistic care program that includes both pharmacological and cognitive/behavioral and psychosocial interventions. At the same time, nonpharmacological interventions, including cognitive and behavioral interventions, have distinct advantages. While many studies show stabilization or improvement in cognitive function with medication use, the tangible impact on everyday behavior remains an open question. The cost of clinical trials for medications is high, as are the ongoing costs of prescribing to the individual and the health care system (Bond et al., 2012; Pouryamout et al., 2012). While limited work has been done in the way of formal economic analysis of nonpharmacological interventions (Davis, Bryan, Marra, Hsiung, & Liu-Ambrose, 2015), it would be fair to assume that these are less costly to develop and implement compared to medications. For one, many existing interventions can be tailored to and tested in an older adult population, rather than having to reinvent the wheel. Additionally, unlike medications, a greater range of appropriately trained personnel can implement these interventions, including psychologists, as well as some allied health care professionals such as speech–language pathologists and occupational therapists. Finally, cognitive and behavioral interventions, even when ineffective, rarely produce significant side effects, unlike cognitive-enhancing medications that may have significant side effects. These many benefits, as well as theory and evidence for neuroplasticity in older adulthood, all provide encouragement for the implementation of cognitive and behavioral interventions, rather than a reliance on pharmacological interventions in isolation.

The literature in this area is prolific, and providing an exhaustive review of primary studies is beyond the scope of this book. Rather, here we provide a review of recent systematic reviews and meta-analyses for the major types of cognitive intervention (i.e., cognitive training, cognitive rehabilitation, and cognitive stimulation) at the various stages of cognitive decline (i.e., healthy aging, SCD, MCI, and dementia). This evidence-based review, in concert with the aforementioned theoretical principles, provides context for a discussion of how these methods might be applied in an idiographic fashion with individual clients.

Different Theoretical Approaches to Intervention

Before exploring the literature in detail, it should be noted that interpreting this literature can be challenging due to inconsistencies in intervention terminology. Three main types of intervention have been used in the older adult population—cognitive training, cognitive rehabilitation, and cognitive stimulation—which, as traditionally conceived, have different mechanisms of delivery and expected outcomes (Gates & Sachdev, 2014; Tuokko & Smart, 2014). Clare and Woods (2004) proposed specific definitions for these interventions in the context of older adults. *Cognitive training* involves guided practice on a set of standardized tasks designed to impact specific cognitive functions with a range of difficulty levels. These can be offered to individuals or groups, using paper and pencil or computerized formats (e.g., computerized working memory training). *Cognitive stimulation* is typically applied in persons with diagnosed dementia. This approach is derived from earlier work in reality orientation therapy (Taulbee & Folsom, 1966) and refers to a range of pleasurable activities that provide general stimulation for thinking, concentration, and memory, and typically occur in a social context. Finally, *cognitive rehabilitation* has a greater focus on the individual needs and goals of the client. According to Clare and Woods (2004), the emphasis is on enhancing everyday function rather than improving cognitive test performance, and it incorporates the use of compensatory practices rather than focusing on restitution of function as seen in cognitive training.

This nomenclature lends methodological clarity to the empirical literature, particularly for clinical trials attempting to establish the efficacy of any of these interventions in isolation. While we generally agree with these definitions, we would note that in clinical practice, these definitions may be less sharply delineated. For example, in the field of acquired brain injury rehabilitation, both early and concurrent proponents have advocated for a holistic, multicomponent approach (e.g., Ben-Yishay & Gold, 1990; Cicerone et al., 2008, 2011). In other words, what may be broadly considered as "cognitive rehabilitation" in fact involves a blend of restorative activities (e.g., attention training), compensatory strategy use (e.g., memory book training), and cognitive stimulation (e.g., group socialization, art therapy). Even in the field of older adult intervention, it has been acknowledged that these three intervention types may occur in tandem at any particular level of cognitive decline (Gates & Sachdev, 2014). Bahar-Fuchs, Clare, and Woods (2013) state that the overarching orientation of cognitive rehabilitation is one that is client-centered and collaborative, and based on ecologically relevant goals.

Cognitive and Behavioral Interventions for Healthy Older Adults

As the field of dementia research moves toward primary prevention, before clinical symptoms are manifest (Imtiaz et al., 2014; Thal, 2006), there is burgeoning interest in cognitive and behavioral interventions for healthy older adults. Accordingly, the preponderance of this literature focuses on various forms of cognitive training as opposed to rehabilitation or stimulation, a sampling of which we provide in the subsequent section.

Computerized Cognitive Training

In recent years, the literature has reflected an explosion of interest in computerized cognitive training (CCT) interventions, or "brain training." This interest has been spurred in part by the ready availability of commercially marketed programs such as Lumosity and Nintendo BrainAge. CCT interventions are appealing for several reasons, including standardization of training exercises, the ability for use in one's own home, and visually stimulating methods of delivery. In the field of cognitive interventions, this is perhaps one of the most controversial topics of study. Conflicting reviews have been published on the relative efficacy, or lack thereof, of brain-training programs (Simons et al., 2016). Recent estimates of sales of commercial CCT programs suggest as much as U.S. $1 billion per annum, indicating that CCT is a booming business (The Economist, 2013). Accordingly, there has been concern that commercial companies with a vested financial interest may overstate or misinterpret the empirical evidence in support of the cognitive benefits associated with these programs. This is exemplified by the recent class-action lawsuit against Lumosity (Federal Trade Commission, 2016). Given that older adults are often a prime target for these programs, many of which claim to stave off or prevent cognitive decline, it is important to critically review the available literature and consider the specific benefits, if any, of such training programs.

Lampit, Hallock, and Valenzuela (2014) conducted a systematic review and meta-analysis of CCT programs in cognitively healthy older adults. This review was novel insofar as CCT was narrowly defined and did not include pooled data from other cognitive interventions, and only included RCTs. Eligible studies had to involve healthy older adults >60 years of age, and include >4 hours of practice on standardized computer tasks or video games with a clear cognitive rationale, as compared to an active or passive control condition. After removal of one outlier, fifty-two trials including 4,885 participants were eligible for inclusion, with one study finally excluded as an outlier. Meta-analysis indicated an overall effect size that was small but statistically significant for CCT versus control (Hedges's g = 0.22, 95% confidence interval [CI] = 0.15–0.29). Small to moderate effects were observed for specific cognitive domains, with the greatest effects for processing speed (Hedges's g = 0.31, 95% CI = 0.11–0.50) and visuospatial skills, Hedges's g = 0.30, 95% CI = 0.07–0.54), modest effects for nonverbal memory (Hedges's g = 0.24, 95% CI = 0.09–0.38), and smallest effects for verbal memory (Hedges's g = 0.08, 95% CI = 0.01–0.15). Although working memory as an outcome variable yielded modest effects (Hedges's g = 0.22, 95% CI = 0.09–0.35), working memory training per se was deemed likely to be ineffective. CCT did not produce any significant effects for attention or executive functions.

The analyses of verbal memory and executive functions were considered adequately powered, and outcome measures appropriate to the interventions. Thus, the authors felt confident in determining that the negligible efficacy of these interventions is truly due to the training itself and not a lack of power. Sufficient data were available to examine treatment moderators, indicating that home-based interventions were ineffective compared to group-based interventions. This may be due to inability to maintain treatment fidelity (i.e., following predetermined treatment protocols) in unsupervised conditions, and/or the lack of positive reinforcement from an *in vivo* interventionist. Interestingly, greater than three training sessions per week was less effective than three or fewer sessions, although sessions of less than 30 minutes seem likely to be ineffective because synaptic plasticity is more likely after 30–60 minutes of training (Lüscher, Nicoll, Malenka, & Muller, 2000). Finally, the studies only reported on immediate postintervention effects. This is an important limitation, given the fact that, if the goal of CCT is primary prevention, then the preventive benefits may not be seen for months or even years after the active intervention period.

The review of Lampit and colleagues (2014) indicates that the short-term benefits of CCT are modest at best. This echoes a very recent and extensive review by Simons and colleagues (2016) that similarly finds that CCT tends to improve performance on trained tasks, with limited evidence of near-transfer to related tasks and very little evidence of far-transfer to ecologically relevant behaviors. However, while these rigorous systematic reviews and meta-analyses are important commentaries on the state of evidence for CCT, there is one major caveat that remains unaddressed. For the goal of primary prevention to be realized, this means delaying or averting altogether the progression to non-normal cognitive decline (Thal, 2006). For the potential preventative benefits of CCT to be established, studies necessarily require long-term follow-up. For example, the hypothesized time-course of conversion from SCD to MCI and dementia has been estimated to be as long as 15 years (Reisberg et al., 2008). Understandably, few studies have this type of follow-up due to time and economic constraints. As such, what appear to be null results in the short term could translate to positive benefits much later in time, particularly where participants continue to actively engage with material provided in interventions.

One example of a study with long-term follow-up is the Advanced Cognitive Training for Independent and Vital Elderly (ACTIVE) study, a large-scale, multicenter RCT investigating the longitudinal impact of cognitive training in healthy older adults. In this study, 2,832 participants ages 65–94 years were assigned to one of four intervention groups where they received ten 60- to 75-minute sessions over 5–6 weeks: verbal episodic memory, reasoning, speed of processing, or a no-contact control. A four-session booster training was administered to the three intervention groups at 11 months following the active intervention period. Initial outcome results of this study (included in the Lampit et al., 2014, review) indicated that training in specific cognitive domains resulted in immediate enhancement of that cognitive domain (based on specific neuropsychometric tests), with highest rates of improvement for processing speed (87% of participants) and reasoning (74% of participants) as opposed to memory (26% of participants). The booster sessions enhanced gains for only the processing speed and reasoning groups, and these were maintained at 2-year follow-up. No changes in everyday function were observed at 2 years, although for healthy older adults, this may be too short of a window to see significant benefits (Ball et al., 2002).

Recently, the ACTIVE group published results from a 10-year follow-up of their participants (Rebok et al., 2014). Forty-four percent of the original sample was retained at 10-year follow-up. Of the original group that received booster sessions in the Ball et al. (2002) report, 60% of these received further booster sessions at 3 years postintervention. Neuropsychometric tests were used to reassess cognitive function, and self-report and performance-based measures of instrumental activities of daily living were also included. Immediate postintervention gains in reasoning and processing speed were maintained at 10-year follow-up, but not for memory. Likewise, the reasoning intervention had a small effect size (0.23) on the reasoning outcome, and the speed intervention had a medium-to-large effect size (0.66) on the speed outcome at 10 years. In terms of maintenance of cognitive function, 73.6% of reasoning participants and 70% of speed participants were performing at or above their respective cognitive ability levels compared to 61.7% and 48.8% of control participants. In terms of performance in self-reported instrumental activities of daily living, declines were seen in all groups from year 2 onward; declines were less in the intervention versus control groups between years 3–5, and this difference was maintained until year 10. Interestingly, there was no direct effect of training on actual performance-based measures of instrumental activities of daily living. In terms of the disparity between self-report and performance-based measures, the authors note that objective everyday behavior is likely multifactorial in its influences, including overall health, social class, gender, as well as specific cognitive factors not targeted in this study. Nevertheless, this large-scale RCT suggests that the effects of cognitive training for certain domains can be maintained over time, exerting protective effects on cognitive decline, as well as maintaining perceived everyday function.

Cognitive Training plus Physical Exercise

The literature on physical exercise per se was discussed in Chapter 9 in the context of overall maintenance of physical health. Some studies compared or examined the interactive effects of physical versus cognitive training. For example, Karr et al. (2014) examined the impact of cognitive training in older adults. "Cognitive training" was broadly construed, including cognitive training, rehabilitation, exercise, and remediation. All older adults over the age of 65 were included, that is, those with and without pathologic cognitive impairment. The overall effect size for cognitive training was small and positive (0.26; 95% CI = 0.13–0.39). This was not significantly different from that obtained for physical exercise alone (0.12; 95% CI = 0.04–0.20), although it did trend toward cognitive training being more effective. This difference may have been driven by benefits experienced by healthy participants, as cognitive training was found to be effective for them but not for those with MCI and dementia. The limitation of this analysis is the very broad and all-encompassing definition of cognitive training, which precludes identifying specific types of cognitive intervention that may be preferentially effective in healthy older adults.

In a recent review, Lauenroth, Ioannidis, and Teichmann (2016) compared the multiplicative effects of cognitive training and physical exercise to either modality alone. Compared to the Karr et al. (2014) review, cognitive training was more narrowly defined and appeared consistent with the Clare and Woods (2004) definition. Twenty articles met inclusion criteria—controlled trials or RCTs that included a condition of combined cognitive training and physical exercise, thirteen of which employed these interventions concurrently and seven consecutively. Eighteen of the reviewed studies showed a positive impact on cognition (typically, attention and/or executive function/working memory), seventeen of which included aerobic or strength training or a combination of both. Notably, positive benefits seem limited to trained cognitive functions, with little evidence of near-transfer to untrained tasks and no specific assessment of everyday functional abilities. Of the two studies that specifically examined everyday function, one study reported a generalized improvement for both intervention and control groups, and the second study reported specific benefits for the concurrent cognitive/physical exercise groups and the physical exercise/psychoeducation conditions, but not single physical exercise or single cognitive training. Overall, this review suggests that multicomponent interventions combining physical exercise with cognitive training may have additional benefits for cognition beyond either intervention alone. Moreover, exercise is an important aspect of overall physical health and is an appropriate recommendation for most older adults regardless of cognitive status.

Cognitive Rehabilitation

Cognitive rehabilitation is typically employed when a client already has manifest deficits in cognitive function and/or everyday behaviors. As such, less of this literature is available in healthy older adults compared to individuals with MCI and dementia. That said, a recent review by Mowzowski, Lampit, Walton, and Naismith (2016) examined the impact of strategy-based cognitive training (SCT) for improving executive functioning.

Although their review was focused on "training," their portrayal of SCT appears to be much more akin to rehabilitation under the Clare and Woods (2004) nomenclature. Mowzowski et al. describe SCT as inherently involving more emphasis on supervised and guided practice, focused on more compensatory as opposed to restorative methods and providing clients with alternative means to achieve their goals (cf. Sitzer, Twamley, & Jeste, 2006). The main target of SCT is typically executive functioning (EF). Given that so much of the intervention literature focuses on memory, the examination of training for EF is salient, particularly since it is the cognitive domain most closely linked to everyday behaviors and instrumental activities of daily living (Tuokko & Smart, 2014). Moreover, in light of the fact that so much of the cognitive training literature is hampered by negligible evidence of transfer of training, methods to improve EF—and ergo everyday behaviors—provide promise as ecologically relevant forms of intervention.

The review by Mowzowski et al. (2016) included any controlled trial involving adults >50 years where SCT was delivered at home or in person, and any aspect of EF was the main target of training. Computerized interventions were allowed only when the computer provided a platform for strategy instruction (as opposed to drill-and-practice training) and, again, where EF was targeted. The review yielded thirteen studies of healthy older adults, of which eleven were RCTs. Eleven studies targeted inductive reasoning, while the other two studies focused on goal-directed behavior related to everyday problems and tasks. Dosage of sessions varied from 5 to 24, with an average of 10.4 sessions across studies. Studies also varied in terms of delivery method (i.e., group versus individualized, research center versus home). In terms of intervention effects, ten of eleven studies showed near-transfer to untrained tasks of EF, with moderate effect sizes (i.e., Hedges's $g > 0.3$). Four of eight studies that measured long-term follow-up found that those gains were maintained over time, specifically in the area of inductive reasoning. For far-transfer, only one of six studies that measured it found immediate posttest benefits, although two other trials that did not show immediate benefit did show gains at longitudinal follow-up. Analysis of transfer effects is important as (1) finding any evidence of transfer is significant, given that declining instrumental activities of daily living are associated with the transition from MCI to dementia, and (2) findings suggest that there may be some delays in ascertaining transfer to everyday behavior. Overall, results inform the utility of SCT in healthy older adults as a primary prevention strategy against declines in EF (and potentially a decline in instrumental activities of daily living) and speak to the importance of longitudinal follow-up to truly understand the impact of the intervention. While the evidence obtained is promising, limitations of the review include the well-established difficulty in assessing EF, as well as the great methodological heterogeneity in approaches used. Moreover, although the authors also set out to find evidence on persons with MCI, the quality of the evidence was too limited in amount and quality, precluding any meaningful synthesis. Given that persons with MCI are at elevated risk for decline in instrumental activities of daily living and dementia, this area of secondary prevention intervention warrants further investigation.

Cognitive and Behavioral Interventions for SCD

Compared to the other stages on the trajectory of late-life cognitive decline, comparatively less is known about the phenomenon of SCD, including the fact that some but not all affected persons show subsequent non-normal decline. Not surprisingly, then, the literature on cognitive and behavioral interventions for this group of individuals is notably less than that available for persons with MCI and dementia. The first proposed operational criteria for SCD were published in 2014, the Jessen criteria (Jessen et al., 2014). Prior to this, two systematic reviews had been conducted on healthy older adults with cognitive complaints. The first of these reviews, by Metternich, Kosch, Kristen, Härter, and Hüll (2010), included a meta-analysis of fourteen RCTs of any nonpharmacological intervention for individuals with subjective memory complaints. Along with the fourteen studies, Metternich et al. included various approaches ranging from psychoeducation to standard memory training and cognitive restructuring (such as that used in cognitive therapy). The primary outcomes were self-report of memory, mood, and well-being, as well as objective measures of memory. Cognitive restructuring was found to reduce self-reported memory complaints, while memory training did not reduce complaints. Conversely, only memory training improved objective memory function. These results speak to the specificity of mechanism of action in influencing specific outcomes. In terms of study limitations, while the rationale for the systematic review seemed to focus on the impact of nonpharmacological interventions for subjective memory complaints in older adults, the authors did not specify an age range for participants in the systematic review criteria, nor did they separate persons with significant concern about cognitive function from typical healthy older adults.

　　Canevelli and colleagues (2013) conducted the second systematic review, which included six studies that targeted individuals with subjective cognitive complaints. Each intervention was structured as a cognitive training program, most commonly focusing on episodic memory, although other cognitive domains (e.g., attention and executive function) were occasionally considered. Likewise, follow-up assessment tended to focus on memory, while one focused exclusively on executive function. While each study reported some improvement in cognitive function in their samples, the studies varied widely in terms of characteristics and feasibility of implementation. A strength of the review was that it focused only on persons with subjective cognitive complaints (as opposed to healthy older adults).

However, the authors included clinical trials of any nonpharmacological intervention, not specifying whether they limited the review to RCTs or even controlled trials of any kind, raising questions about the rigor of the studies on which their conclusions are based. In addition, similar to Metternich et al.'s (2010) review, the authors did not specify that there was an age range for participants or that studies were confined to older adults.

Many of the studies included in these prior two systematic reviews provided limited specification of their participants, and it was unclear how many would actually be classifiable as having SCD. The Jessen criteria for SCD (Jessen et al., 2014) were only recently published. It is possible that, with stricter operational criteria for classification of SCD, a reanalysis of existing studies might reveal different effects of cognitive and behavioral interventions in this group. Accordingly, Smart et al. (2017) conducted an updated systematic review and meta-analysis of controlled trials of nonpharmacological interventions and their effects on cognitive, behavioral, and psychological functioning in persons 55+ with SCD broadly construed based on the Jessen criteria. After review for eligibility, only those that involved cognitive and behavioral intervention were ultimately included, for a total of eleven studies. Given the limited available information for self-report outcomes, the meta-analysis (n = 9 studies) was restricted to cognitive outcomes. There was a small effect size for cognitive outcomes for all studies (Cohen's d = 0.22), but the effect was larger when focused only on studies with cognitive interventions as opposed to other types of intervention (Cohen's d = 0.37).

Because of the limited amount of data available, the study had some limitations. First, it was necessary to take cognitive outcomes as a global indicator rather than being able to ascertain individual effects for specific cognitive domains. Second, it was not possible to test for the moderating effects for variables such as age and gender. Third, with a greater focus on efficacy, outcome measures tended to focus on cognitive and neuropsychometric outcomes and did not assess ecologically relevant measures to ascertain transfer of training. Finally, trials tended to focus on immediate posttest outcomes only, so the primary preventive effects of these interventions remains unknown. These limitations notwithstanding, this analysis provides preliminary evidence that cognitive and behavioral interventions have efficacy in persons with SCD and are worth further investigation in terms of effectiveness and long-term preventive benefits. The available evidence was insufficient to test the relative benefits of training versus rehabilitation, which offers another area for future investigation.

Cognitive and Behavioral Interventions for MCI

Individuals with MCI are a unique group, insofar as some persons decline to dementia, others remain stable, and still others actually revert to cognitive health (Albert et al., 2011). This highlights the importance of multiple types of intervention at this stage—both restitution and compensation—which we explore in the context of available evidence.

Cognitive Training

Hill and colleagues (2017) conducted a meta-analysis of CCT interventions for persons with MCI and dementia, a study which, to their knowledge, is the first of its kind. Seventeen studies on persons with MCI were included, comprising 686 participants (CCT = 351). Studies were required to utilize CCT solely, or if combined with another intervention type, this had to be accounted for in the control condition. Results indicated that, for persons with MCI, the overall efficacy of cognitive outcomes was moderate and statistically significant (k = 17, g = 0.35, 95% CI = 0.20–0.51), which the authors note is actually larger than the effect sizes previously reported for healthy older adults and for PD. This was true regardless of whether the study involved an active control group (k = 11, g = 0.40, 95% CI = 0.17–0.63) or a passive control group (k = 6, g = 0.32, 95% CI = 0.09–0.55). Specific effects were found for attention, working memory, and verbal learning and memory, but not processing speed, language, executive function, visuospatial skills, or instrumental activities of daily living. Positive effects were also seen on psychosocial functioning (k = 8, g = 0.52, 95% CI = 0.01–1.03). Despite the positive findings, studies tended to have small sample sizes, thus potentially underestimating the clinical effects of these interventions. Moreover, most studies focused exclusively on short-term, postintervention outcomes; therefore, whether CCT slows the rate of decline (or rates of conversion) to dementia remains an open question.

Cognitive Rehabilitation

Huckans et al. (2013) provided a comprehensive theoretical model of MCI and conducted an evidence-based review of RCTs of various cognitive rehabilitation therapies (CRTs) for the specific symptoms of MCI. The scope of the review was to evaluate the efficacy of CRTs for older adults with MCI in terms of short-term (i.e., <1 month postintervention) and long-term (i.e., >1 month postintervention) impact on objective cognitive performance, as well as subjective cognitive complaints, everyday functioning, quality of life, neuropsychiatric symptom severity, and other related constructs. They also sought to ascertain whether CRTs fulfill the role of secondary prevention (Thal, 2006) by examining the impact on conversion rates to dementia. Although the review was reported to be on CRTs, the search parameters for the review included studies within the class of cognitive training, consistent with their theoretical model that restorative training can comprise an aspect of cognitive rehabilitation (Huckans et al., 2013).

Fourteen RCTs were included in the final review. Overall, the seven life-style interventions showed a positive impact on objective cognitive performance. Specifically, aerobic exercise enhanced executive functioning, with longer interventions impacting multiple cognitive domains. Nonaerobic exercise (i.e., resistance training and tai chi) was associated with significant improvements in attention, memory and executive function. Other interventions included a low-fat/glycemic index diet (improving visual memory) and practicing calligraphy as a cognitively stimulating activity (improving global cognition). One study on restorative attention training showed limited effects on untrained tasks, whereas a study on compensatory memory training showed improved memory self-efficacy and daily functioning, the latter of which was maintained at 6 months postintervention. Two comprehensive interventions focused on memory. For both studies, the biggest impact seems to have been from the provision of psychoeducation and compensatory strategies, which led to endorsement of better memory abilities, as well as greater knowledge and increased use of strategies. However, neither group showed improved objective memory performance. Finally, three studies reviewed multimodal interventions. These had mixed findings; studies with greater sample sizes seemed to have increased power to detect significant effects on objective cognition, with additional benefits seen in knowledge and use of compensatory strategies and neuropsychiatric symptoms. Overall, the authors consider the evidence encouraging but inconclusive, owing to several methodological limitations in the literature reviewed. These limitations include questionable classification methods for MCI, questionable intensity or "dose" of interventions employed, low power to detect significant effects, measures potentially lacking in sensitivity, limited long-term follow-up, and often a narrow focus on global cognition to the exclusion of other important outcomes such as neuropsychiatric symptoms, daily function, and quality of life.

Functional Impact of Interventions for MCI

A recent systematic review and meta-analysis by Chandler, Parks, Marsiske, Rotblatt, and Smith (2016) had the express purpose of examining the everyday impact of controlled trials of cognitive interventions in MCI, as opposed to only focusing on objective cognitive performance. Given the fact that everyday function begins to erode as individuals transition from MCI to dementia, interventions that can preserve everyday function are ecologically relevant and could serve as important means of secondary prevention (Thal, 2006). Of the thirty articles included in this analysis, fourteen were therapist-based, ten were multimodal, and six were computerized interventions. Similar to other reviews, overall conclusions are difficult to draw, based on a limited amount of empirical evidence as well as significant heterogeneity in methods and outcomes. That said, the overall meta-analysis for the viable studies ($n = 24$) suggested a small, positive effect on everyday outcomes. Significant effects were seen in mood, activities of daily living, and metacognition. Computerized interventions (typically, restitution-based) tended to improve mood, whereas therapist-led interventions did not. Conversely, effects on performance of activities of daily living were most commonly observed in therapist-based interventions, whereas computerized interventions showed no such effect. In terms of multimodal interventions, combining physical activity and cognitive intervention seemed to be particularly beneficial. Quality of life was not impacted by any intervention. Chandler and colleagues speculated that this could be due to several factors, including the complexity of quality of life, as well as the fact that it could be negatively impacted by the time and effort needed to participate in intervention, particularly if transfer of training to everyday life was not explicitly emphasized.

Cognitive and Behavioral Interventions for Dementia

A sizeable evidence base has accumulated for cognitive and behavioral interventions for persons with dementia, including separate systematic reviews and meta-analyses for each of the three main types of intervention: training, rehabilitation, and stimulation.

Cognitive Training

Bahar-Fuchs, Clare, and Woods (2013) conducted an updated *Cochrane Review* on cognitive training and cognitive rehabilitation for mild to moderate AD and VaD. The intent was to examine impact on cognitive and noncognitive outcomes on affected individuals as well as primary caregivers, in the short, medium, and long term. Eleven RCTs were identified that involved cognitive training. There was significant heterogeneity in the types of intervention employed, their duration, and delivery format (e.g., individual versus group; paper-and-pencil vs. computer). Likewise, there was a wide variety of targeted cognitive processes, including attention and concentration, memory, language, executive function, and perceptual and motor skills. Primary outcomes were cognitive and noncognitive outcomes for those with dementia; secondary outcomes pertained to the course of dementia, disease biomarkers of dementia, and outcomes for the family caregiver. Meta-analysis indicated no beneficial effects of cognitive training versus control conditions on any of the primary or secondary outcomes identified. The studies reviewed were adjudicated to be of low to moderate quality.

Overall, results did not support the use of cognitive training for persons with dementia. However, Bahar-Fuchs, Clare, and Woods (2013) noted that this might be in part due to use of inadequate outcome measures, particularly the use of standardized neuropsychometric tests. Use of such tests implies transfer of training to untrained tasks, evidence for which is highly equivocal (Owen et al., 2010). Instead, future studies should incorporate measures of everyday behavior, particularly tasks that mimic those involved in training, which may be more sensitive to training effects. Moreover, none of the studies included in this review assessed the impact of cognitive training on long-term outcomes related to the trajectory of dementia (e.g., rates of subsequent admission to residential care). Given that neuroplasticity in the older adult brain likely takes longer than in younger individuals, it is possible that training effects need longer periods of time (and perhaps greater doses of treatment) to show therapeutic effects. Overall, findings suggested the need for a greater variety of outcome measures, including those with a more ecological focus, as well as longer-term follow-up to ascertain whether cognitive training interventions alter the trajectory of cognitive decline in persons with dementia.

As noted in the review of interventions for healthy older adults, there has been a massive expansion in the field of CCT. At least two major reviews have been conducted examining the impact of these interventions in persons with dementia. The first of these reviews provided a separate analysis of persons with MCI and dementia (Hill et al., 2017). Hill et al. included twelve studies on persons with dementia, comprising 389 participants (CCT = 201). Unlike prior reviews, these studies used CCT alone rather than multicomponent interventions that used CCT with cognitive stimulation or rehabilitation. Despite the encouraging findings for persons with MCI, computerized cognitive training was deemed unlikely to be beneficial for individuals already diagnosed with dementia. The only studies that found clinically meaningful effects used nontraditional approaches to CCT, including virtual reality and Nintendo Wii. This suggests that more immersive computerized approaches are more stimulating and personally engaging than traditional CCT. This finding is consistent with the overall cognitive stimulation approach found beneficial in dementia and is worth pursuing in future research.

The second study, by García-Casal and colleagues (2017), involved a systematic review and meta-analysis of computer-based cognitive interventions specifically for persons with dementia. Their search included cognitive recreation, cognitive rehabilitation, cognitive stimulation, and cognitive training. Dementia diagnoses included AD, FTLD, VaD, and mixed AD-VaD. Twelve studies were included in the final review, with acceptable methodological quality according to Downs and Black (1998) criteria; these criteria were chosen to provide an assessment of external validity (i.e., generalizability). As with other studies, there was great diversity in dose and modality (i.e., individual versus group) of each intervention. Outcome measures included cognition (e.g., ADAS-Cog, MMSE), depression, anxiety, and generalizability (e.g., activities of daily living and improvements in everyday life). Meta-analytic results indicated that computer-based interventions had moderate effects on cognition (standardized mean difference [*SMD*] = −0.69, 95% CI = −1.02 to −0.37), depression (*SMD* = 0.74; 95% CI = 0.31 to 1.17), and anxiety (*SMD* = 0.55; 95% CI = 0.07 to 1.04). Significantly greater benefits were observed for computerized versus noncomputerized interventions for cognition (*SMD* = 0.48; 95% CI = 0.09 to 0.87) and depression (*SMD* = 0.96; 95% CI = 0.25 to 1.66). However, no significant effects were found on activities of daily living, a finding that mirrors that of other studies, calling into question transfer of training following computerized cognitive interventions (Owen et al., 2010).

Cognitive Rehabilitation

The intent of the aforementioned *Cochrane Review* by Bahar-Fuchs and colleagues (2013) was to include trials of both cognitive training and cognitive rehabilitation for dementia. However, only one RCT on cognitive rehabilitation was identified and subsequently reviewed. In this single study by Clare et al. (2010), sixty-nine participants with either AD or mixed AD-VaD were randomized to the active intervention, relaxation therapy, or no intervention. Cognitive rehabilitation was delivered in eight 1-hour, weekly sessions, conducted in participants' homes. The purpose of the intervention was to address personally meaningful goals that were collaboratively identified, based on which, individualized interventions were developed. Participants were given compensatory aids and strategies, practice in maintaining attention and concentration, as well as techniques for stress management. Caregivers participated in the final 15 minutes of each session to facilitate between-session home practice. Results indicated that cognitive rehabilitation resulted in short-term benefits in terms of self-rated competence and satisfaction in performing personally meaningful goals, memory capacity, and overall quality of life. Compared to the control condition, caregivers in cognitive rehabilitation also had improved social relationships following intervention. A subset of participants underwent functional MRI pre- and postintervention, which suggested functional brain changes in support of selective effects for the rehabilitation group. This high-quality study, in conjunction with the cognitive rehabilitation trials included in the review provided by García-Casal and colleagues (2017), suggests that cognitive rehabilitation for dementia warrants further research and clinical investigation.

Cognitive Stimulation

Woods, Aguirre, Spector, and Orrell (2012) conducted a *Cochrane Review* on the effects of cognitive stimulation to improve cognitive functioning in persons with dementia. Participants were primarily diagnosed with AD,

VaD, or mixed AD-VaD. The review was based on any RCT that incorporated some measure of cognitive change (including tests of memory and orientation), with a minimum intervention duration of one month. Cognitive stimulation was defined based on the operational definition of Clare and Woods (2004), whereby interventions were required to provide exposure to generalized cognitive activities, rather than training in any particular modality. Fifteen studies were included in the final review, incorporating 718 participants (407 receiving active intervention, 311 in control groups). Methods were relatively heterogeneous, with participants coming from a variety of settings, as well as interventions that varied significantly in their intensity and duration. Interventions were typically delivered in groups to enhance social functioning, as well as those including family caregivers.

Meta-analytic results indicated that cognitive stimulation produced clear benefits to cognitive function (SMD = 0.41, 95% CI = 0.25–0.57), which persisted at 1- to 3-month follow-up after the completion of intervention. The most commonly used measure was the ADAS-Cog, followed by the MMSE and the Clifton Assessment Procedures for the Elderly (CAPE) Information/Orientation scales. Secondary analyses were conducted on noncognitive variables (and smaller sample sizes). Benefits were found for self-reported quality of life and well-being (SMD = 0.38, 95% CI = 0.11–0.65) and staff ratings of social interaction and communication (SMD = 0.44, 95% CI = 0.17–0.71). However, no improvements were found for mood, activities of daily living, general behavioral function, problem behavior, or family caregiver outcomes. Despite the small number of studies of variable quality and small sample sizes, this review provided evidence from multiple trials that cognitive stimulation has a beneficial effect on persons with mild to moderate dementia above and beyond medication effects. With this preliminary support for the efficacy of these interventions, further evidence is needed to investigate the effectiveness and clinical meaningfulness of changes in cognition following cognitive stimulation.

Interpretive Caveats in Reviewing the Extant Literature

A review of available contemporary evidence shows promise for various types of cognitive and behavioral interventions at the various stages of late-life cognitive decline. While available evidence is encouraging, some interpretive issues should be considered in reviewing this literature as a whole; these issues provide further considerations for future research and clinical practice in this area.

The first concern relates to the measurement of outcomes, which are often limited to cognitive outcomes and specifically to neuropsychometric test scores. Given the time-scales of neuroplasticity in older adulthood (Jellinger & Attems, 2013), changes may be seen in direct brain measurements before manifest behavior (Valkanova et al., 2014). Yet these measurements either were not a focus of the systematic reviews/meta-analyses or were not collected by the individual research studies. Moreover, restitution of cognitive function is not a primary objective of many types of intervention, including compensatory training in the context of cognitive rehabilitation. This can lead to false-negative outcomes or underestimation of therapeutic effects (Chandler et al., 2016). In this instance, neuropsychometric tests may be less appropriate outcome measurements than ecologically oriented instruments, which are infrequently used. These two factors suggest that many null results may be due to inappropriate instrumentation, rather than ineffective interventions per se.

The second issue relates to the time-scale of follow-up. The goal of most interventions—particularly those for healthy older adults, as well as those with SCD and MCI—is prevention. However, for prevention to be ascertained, this necessarily implies comparing the rates of decline over time in those receiving intervention as opposed to control groups. Most studies are conducted in a prototypical RCT fashion, focused on internal validity and short-term, postintervention follow-up. While this type of design is helpful to establish proof-of-principle, it cannot speak to the utility of long-term prevention. In fact, more than one study mentioned in this literature review indicated that intervention benefits were not evident until months or even years after the active treatment was completed. This is another factor that may account for null results in the short term and also speaks to the need to shift toward longer-term outcomes in assessing the true therapeutic impact of these interventions.

Another significant issue is what we consider to be the evidentiary standard for empirical evidence. Clinical-psychological research places a heavy emphasis on the medical model approach to outcome research, focusing on RCTs as the most internally valid form of empirical evidence. RCTs and other forms of controlled trials are typically the primary source of evidence included in systematic reviews and meta-analyses. However, gaining access to participants with clinical diagnoses is more challenging than healthy participants, which means that intervention studies may often have small sample sizes and be underpowered to detect significant group-level effects. This can result in the file drawer problem whereby promising interventions go unreported due to a lack of significant findings (Franco, Malhotra, & Simonovits, 2014). Moreover, RCTs favor treatments in which interventions are homogeneous and outcomes are strictly specified and easily measured. This means that cognitive training, with cognitive outcomes, is likely easier to evaluate using RCTs than other intervention methods that are more complex or multifaceted or have multiple targets of outcome (i.e., cognitive rehabilitation and stimulation). Consequently, the effects of these interventions may be underestimated in typical RCT designs.

One final and related point about RCTs is that they focus primarily on establishing the efficacy of an intervention using the most homogeneous samples under the most well-controlled conditions (Chambless & Hollon, 1998). This focus has been an appropriate one in this relatively early phase of building an evidence base. However, it remains uncertain how well, if at all, these interventions would translate to routine clinical practice where clients typically have multiple comorbidities and other biopsychosocial factors that could systematically affect the impact of intervention. Moreover, real-world application of intervention often involves multiple modalities simultaneously (as we advocate in this book), the impact of which can be difficult to ascertain using strict RCT designs. For this field to advance, more attention needs to be directed to effectiveness designs with a greater emphasis on real-world application and ecologically relevant outcome assessment (Chambless & Hollon, 1998). One alternative to RCTs could be to encourage the compilation and publication of more $n = 1$ case–control study designs (Bahar-Fuchs et al., 2013), also referred to as single-case experimental designs (Tate et al., 2016) and discussed in detail in Chapter 9.

Practical Application of Cognitive and Behavioral Interventions

An understanding of the theoretical literature, as well as existing empirical evidence, provides a foundation on which to build an individualized case conceptualization for cognitive and behavioral intervention with older adults. Here we provide guidance on how to implement such a case conceptualization in routine clinical practice. Our focus will naturally be on implementation specific to cognitive and behavioral interventions. At the end of this chapter, we provide further resources on how to implement some of the specific therapeutic protocols discussed. Of course, any intervention plan should begin with, and be grounded in, a comprehensive assessment of cognitive and psychological function, following the recommendations provided in the first half of this book. Such assessment will not only provide targets for intervention but also bring to light variables that may moderate the impact of intervention (e.g., premorbid and psychosocial functioning).

Derivation of Clinically Meaningful Goals

In keeping with the theme of this book, it is important to consider the stage of cognitive decline in ascertaining the most appropriate cognitive and behavioral intervention. The stage of decline likely interacts with intervention type, that is, training, rehabilitation, and stimulation (Gates & Sachdev, 2014), and a mismatch between the two may set a client up for unnecessary failure. In broad terms, the purpose of cognitive and behavioral intervention is to enhance current cognitive function and/or prevent or slow the rate of further decline, also referred to as primary, secondary, and tertiary prevention (Thal, 2006). Cognitive training, rehabilitation, or stimulation may be more or less emphasized, depending on the stage of cognitive decline and the client's intervention goals. In the following we provide a broad overview of how clinical goals may be conceived as a function of the client's level of functional decline, further summarized in Table 11.1.

Healthy Older Adults and SCD

Clients at the very earliest stages of cognitive decline have minor lapses in cognitive function that may or may not cause concern and have little to no appreciable impact on everyday functioning. The overarching goal of intervention for these clients is to maintain them at this level for as long as possible. Before beginning cognition-focused intervention, psychoeducation on cognitive aging is a worthwhile place to begin treatment. Many concerns that older adults have about current function could be due to a lack of accurate information about cognitive aging; conversely, evidence suggests that both metamemory and memory self-efficacy have a small but reliable association with objective memory performance (Beaudoin & Desrichards, 2011; Crumley, Stetler, & Horhota, 2014). Provision of accurate information about how the brain changes with age, as well as compensatory strategies, can lead to significant psychological benefits. Psychoeducation can be provided informally or through a manualized treatment protocol such as the Memory and Aging Program from the Rotman–Baycrest Center (Troyer, 2001; Vandermorris et al., 2016; Wiegand, Troyer, Gojmerac, & Murphy, 2013). Having accurate information about cognitive aging can empower older adults to make informed choices about how to maintain cognitive health, including ways to boost cognitive reserve.

Based on the literature reviewed, although cognitive training may not transfer to everyday behaviors, it could serve as a form of mental engagement. In brief, any cognitive training program should be sufficiently challenging, of high intensity and frequency, and intrinsically enjoyable for the client. The evidence reviewed also highlights the importance of the appropriate dose (i.e., at least 60 minutes per session), administered with therapist support rather than at home and client-led. In order to promote motivation, it may be worthwhile to explain to clients the concept of cognitive reserve (Stern, 2009, 2012) and how engaging in challenging mental exercises is one way to contribute to reserve. Cognitive rehabilitation in the form of metacognitive strategy training may provide compensatory support for older adults who perceive challenges in everyday behaviors (even if these are not currently evident). Within the context of primary prevention, learning metacognitive strategies may promote "good habits" that can attenuate the rate of any future decline in everyday function.

TABLE 11.1. Theoretical and Conceptual Framework for the Application of Cognitive and Behavioral Interventions as a Function of Stage of Cognitive Decline

Clinical issue	Characteristics	Management approach	Intervention strategies
Normal aging and SCD	Minor cognitive lapses within the scope and severity of other older adults of similar demographic background (e.g., word-finding); significant concern about the meaning of such lapses, as in the case of SCD	Maintain current function. Focus on primary prevention by providing information about expected changes with normal cognitive aging, as well as emphasizing taking active steps to boost cognitive reserve	• Psychoeducation on normal age-related cognitive failures, as well as the effect of situational variables such as mood, sleep, and blood sugar on cognitive performance • Cognitive training to promote mental engagement • Compensatory strategies to create "good habits" • Encourage physical, mental, and social engagement to increase cognitive reserve • Maintain physical health
MCI and variants thereof	Cognitive impairment that is beyond normal aging (i.e., >1.5 SD below performance of peers with similar demographics), yet instrumental activities of daily living remain intact. MCI in this instance includes the prodromes for AD and other dementias (e.g., VCI)	Slow further decline; continue focusing on enhancing cognitive reserve, as well as a combination of cognitive training and compensatory training to offset current deficits	• Psychoeducation on normal versus non-normal cognitive change • Cognitive training to promote mental stimulation • Adaptation of existing, empirically supported cognitive rehabilitation protocols for older adults (e.g., memory strategy training, metacognitive strategy training, mindfulness training) • Continue activities to build cognitive reserve • Psychotherapy to assist with emotional reactions to cognitive impairment and changing life roles (see Chapter 11)
Dementias (various types)	Cognitive impairment substantially below normal aging (i.e., >2 SD below peers) with impairment in one or more instrumental activities of daily living	Slow further decline; maintain safety and independence in home where feasible; facilitate subsequent transition to full-time supervised care	• Cognitive rehabilitation focused on realistic yet meaningful goals • Training in task-specific routines using preserved procedural memory (e.g., self-care/hygiene) • Maintain optimal mental and social stimulation and engagement, congruent with the individual's previous interests (e.g., music, dance, art, movies)

Although no formal evidence review was provided on this topic, cognitive stimulation may further support contributions to cognitive reserve in healthy older adults, and clients should be encouraged to remain as mentally, physically, and socially engaged as possible. This could include any activities such as learning to play a musical instrument, learning a new language, or attending dance classes. For example, novel research by Park and colleagues (e.g., Park et al., 2013) assigned healthy older adults to 3 months of engagement with high-demand cognitive activities, specifically, quilting, learning digital photography, or a combination of both. Social groups and low-demand cognitive tasks with no social contact were used as comparison conditions. At posttest, the researchers found that, compared to the control conditions, episodic memory was improved for participants who engaged in the cognitively demanding activities. In a follow-up study, the same group of researchers (McDonough, Haber, Bischof, & Park, 2015) found that participating in such cognitively demanding activities promoted neural efficiency, as evidenced by performance on a semantic classification task with two levels of difficulty. Specifically, the cognitive stimulation group showed increased modulation of neural activity in medial frontal, lateral temporal, and parietal cortex compared to the control conditions. Some of these activations were maintained at one-year follow-up. These novel findings suggest that remaining engaged in mentally challenging activities can promote cognitive reserve in healthy older adults, and they are consistent with animal models showing that enriched environments positively influence hippocampal neurogenesis in adult animals (Kent et al., 2015).

The lack of significant findings for the social groups was surprising to the researchers, given that the benefits of social relationships have been documented elsewhere in the aging literature. Perhaps it is not socialization per se that influences cognitive reserve, but rather how one is engaged with others. This notion would be supported by the findings from the literature suggesting that social dancing, for example, contributes to cognitive reserve (e.g., Kshtriya, Barnstaple, Rabinovich, & DeSouza, 2015). Dance is a complex activity that involves motor coordination and regulation, procedural learning, as well as interpersonal skills. Participants enjoy the social aspect and often the associated music, both of which could promote learning through activation of dopaminergic reward systems (Hamid et al., 2016).

In general, when making recommendations to clients, we suggest advising them to engage in activities that are mentally stimulating and challenging, but also enjoyable. Again, following the principles of experience-dependent plasticity, benefits are likely to be seen to the extent that the activity is sufficiently challenging, of sufficient intensity/duration, and enjoyable.

Finally, an important part of any care plan for cognitive health, but certainly for currently cognitively normal older adults, is maintenance of good physical health. In particular, cardiovascular health should be attended to, given that vascular cognitive impairment is recognized as the second most common etiology of dementia and that vascular risk factors are largely modifiable (Alzheimer's Association, n.d.).

Individuals with MCI

Clients with MCI are already showing demonstrable cognitive impairment, beyond normal aging, and may or may not be showing subtle difficulties in higher-order functional activities (e.g., difficulties in maintaining finances). The overarching goal for these clients is secondary prevention, that is, to attenuate the rate of further decline. The previously discussed study by Huckans et al. (2013) provided a comprehensive theoretical model of MCI that yields multiple targets for nonpharmacological intervention. The four main components of their CRT model are: (1) restorative cognitive training, (2) compensatory cognitive training, (3) lifestyle interventions, and (4) psychotherapeutic interventions. While Clare and Woods (2004) provided a sharp delineation between cognitive training, rehabilitation, and stimulation, the model of Huckans and colleagues (2013) is more comparable to the approach of holistic cognitive rehabilitation for acquired brain injury (Ben-Yishay & Gold, 1990; Cicerone et al., 2008). Based on the evidence reviewed and clinical practice, we believe that this model provides a useful clinical heuristic and foundation for case conceptualization in persons with MCI.

Several studies reviewed indicated the benefit of psychoeducation for persons with MCI, which can provide compensatory strategies, promote a healthy lifestyle, and provide psychological support. Similar to currently cognitively normal older adults, psychoeducation can empower individuals with MCI to make proactive choices and learn ways to compensate for their difficulties. That said, in the MCI population in particular, psychoeducation should be provided judiciously. Many persons with MCI may continue to retain awareness of their difficulties (Kalbe et al., 2005; Lehrer et al., 2015). This awareness of cognitive impairment can lead to depression, anxiety, and fears of the future, particularly development of dementia. This is further exacerbated by the fact that MCI is a diagnosis with an uncertain outcome and course of progression (Albert et al., 2011). Psychological effects of cognitive impairment can be addressed in two ways: through formal psychological intervention and/or by fostering confidence and self-efficacy through engaging the client in interventions to enhance current cognitive function. Many persons with MCI and their caregivers report that quality of life and self-efficacy are the most desirable outcomes for intervention, not improved cognitive performance per se (Barrios et al., 2016). In parallel to their program for healthy older adults, the Rotman–Baycrest Center has created Learning the Ropes for Living with MCI, a manualized intervention protocol that provides psychoeducation to persons with MCI (Anderson, Murphy, & Troyer, 2012). This program provides education about MCI, ways to enhance cognitive reserve, compensatory strategy training for memory, as well as family support for those caring for someone with MCI.

Dementia

Clients with dementia demonstrate pronounced cognitive impairment beyond normal aging, at levels that impair everyday functioning. Depending on the severity of dementia, clients may be experiencing anosognosia, which can interfere with treatment. At some point in their course, they may transition from living in their own home to full-time care (e.g., nursing home). The goal at this stage is to slow the rate of continued decline, while maintaining as much as possible the client's autonomy and dignity and overall engagement with life. As noted earlier, there is limited but promising evidence that cognitive rehabilitation may be productive for persons with dementia, as well as training in task-specific routines using preserved procedural memory (e.g., self-care/hygiene, use of a memory book). Cognitive stimulation may also be beneficial, although the literature does not indicate that one specific activity is more beneficial than another. Given the importance of enjoyment and intrinsic motivation to support experience-dependent plasticity (Kleim & Jones, 2008), we recommend maintaining optimal mental and social stimulation and engagement, congruent with the individual client's previous interests (e.g., music, dance, art, movies). The movie *Alive Inside* (Rossato-Bennett, 2014) provides a vivid illustration of the therapeutic power of personalized music in clients with significant cognitive and communicative impairments. Finally, there is little evidence to suggest that cognitive training is beneficial for persons with dementia, above and beyond any effects of stimulation that may come from particularly engaging computerized platforms. As always, to the degree possible, any intervention program should be grounded in a collaborative process based on identifying the client's most meaningful (yet realistic) goals.

Process-Specific versus Task-Specific Interventions

After taking into consideration a client's current level of cognitive decline, and working with him or her in a collaborative fashion to delineate goals, efforts can then be made to implement a variety of interventions to achieve those goals. There are two broad approaches to cognitive intervention— process-specific versus task-specific intervention (Tuokko & Smart, 2014). First, one can target a specific cognitive process with the notion that this will transfer to real-world activities that require that skill. Within process-specific interventions, one can take a *restitution approach* (i.e., akin to cognitive training) or a *compensation approach* (i.e., a compensatory approach).

As noted in the prior evidence-based reviews, the literature on cognitive training shows best evidence for impact on trained tasks, with diminishing evidence for untrained tasks (near-transfer) and everyday behaviors (far-transfer). If cognitive training is to be used, for example, to keep a healthy older adult mentally engaged and stimulated, then ecological transfer may be less of a concern. However, if transfer to everyday behaviors is the goal, then this is most likely to occur with therapist-guided practice, including metacognitive reflection and explicit connections to real-world situations (Mowzowski et al., 2016). Working memory is known to decline with normal aging (Daselaar & Cabeza, 2013), and training in this area has been the subject of many studies, again with limited evidence of transfer (Melby-Lervåg & Hume, 2013; Melby-Lervåg, Redick, & Hulme, 2016). However, inclusion of metacognitive support as well as explicit connection to everyday scenarios (e.g., recalling phone numbers or grocery lists or following the thread of a conversation) may promote transfer. Some interventions actually blend restitution and compensation. A good example is mindfulness training, which requires participants to engage in daily practice that enhances self-regulation of attention and emotion, with the explicit intent to carry mindful awareness into everyday life. Research has consistently documented the positive impact of mindfulness on the brain and psychological functions in healthy and clinical populations (Chiesa, Calati, & Serretti, 2011; Lutz, Slagter, Dunne, & Davidson, 2008; MacLean et al., 2010), as well as neurologic populations (Azulay, Smart, Mott, & Cicerone, 2013; Cairncross & Miller, 2016; Chen et al., 2011; Novakovic-Agopian et al., 2010). Mindfulness training in older adults is in its relative infancy, but it holds promise in terms of enhanced neural and cognitive function (Gard, Hölzel, & Lazar, 2014; Luders, 2014; Smart et al., 2016; Smart & Segalowitz, 2017; Smoski, McClintock, & Keeling, 2016). Based on the existing literature, process-specific interventions may be beneficial for older adults at all stages of decline.

The second approach is task-specific intervention, where the goal is to train to a specific task such as grooming and hygiene or even more complex, multistep tasks such as preparing simple meals or remembering to take medication (Loewenstein & Acevedo, 2009). The benefit of this type of intervention is that it does not require episodic memory (or explicit memory) or metacognitive abilities. As such, it may be most beneficial in persons with significant cognitive impairment and dementia. After controlling for the effects of processing speed or working memory (Seidler, Bo, & Anguera, 2012), one can train a client on task-specific behaviors using implicit memory systems such as procedural memory that are often relatively preserved in aging (Voelcker-Rehage, 2008). Employing this approach would mean specifying and sequencing a series of steps in which the client would train using errorless learning and behavioral practice to ensure encoding only the accurate steps and not off-task behaviors (Wilson, Baddeley, Evans, & Shiel, 1994). Reinforcement and positive feedback would strengthen the acquisition and subsequent implementation of these steps. One example is implementing a daily habit of writing things down in a memory book and remembering to check the book every day to review that day's activities, as well as look ahead to a subsequent day's events. An evidence-based review of the occupational therapy literature found strong evidence in support of multicomponent interventions to improve and maintain instrumental activities of daily living in older adults (Orellano, Colon, & Arbesman, 2012). The benefit of this type of intervention is that even clients with more severe cognitive impairment can actively engage in cognitive and behavioral intervention in service of promoting their own self-efficacy and autonomy. However, it should be noted that training effects are usually specific to the task and tend not to generalize to other tasks (Lustig, Shah, Seidler, & Reuter-Lorenz, 2009). Nor do they provide the individual with the necessary skills to handle a situation where there is an unanticipated deviation from the routine, such as overdrawing one's bank account unexpectedly (Tuokko & Smart, 2014).

Principles of EDP

While a clinician may choose the appropriate intervention type, if it is not implemented properly, it may fail to produce significant effects. This is where returning to the concept of neuroplasticity becomes useful. If a treatment does not have the sufficient dose (i.e., frequency, intensity, and longevity), then any resultant plasticity is likely to be fragile and subject to decay over time. Kleim and Jones (2008), in their theoretical paper on experience-dependent plasticity, discuss ten core principles that should be considered in the application of interventions to facilitate neuroplasticity. In broad terms, it is important that any intervention consider the following:

- Is the intervention sufficiently engaging and reinforcing?
- Does the client understand the relevance of this intervention to everyday behaviors?
- Is the intervention sufficiently challenging as to encourage new learning?
- Is the intervention occurring at sufficient intensity and frequency to promote change?

In Table 11.2, we summarize these principles, as well as their particular meaning, in the context of interventions for older adults.

TABLE 11.2. Summary of Kleim and Jones (2008) Principles of Experience-Dependent Plasticity, Adapted with Additional Implications for Older Adult Interventions

Principle	Description	Implications
Use it or lose it	Failure to drive specific brain functions can lead to functional degradation.	Stresses the importance of older adults remaining mentally engaged and challenged, regardless of level of cognitive decline.
Use it and improve it	Training that drives a specific brain function can lead to an enhancement of that function.	Improvements in behavioral performance cause changes in underlying brain structure and function. This supports the importance of direct neural measures (e.g., EEG/ERP, fMRI, sMRI) as outcomes of cognitive and behavioral interventions in older adults, not just those focused on cognition.
Specificity	The nature of the training experience dictates the nature of the plasticity.	Learning new material is what drives plasticity, not mere repetition of already-learned skills and abilities. This underscores the importance of novelty and challenge in any training activity.
Repetition matters	Induction of plasticity requires sufficient repetition.	Regular intervention sessions and home practice, over a several-week period, will support neuroplasticity "taking hold" (i.e., long-term potentiation). There is no gold standard available, but some reviews suggest one to three sessions per week.
Intensity matters	Induction of plasticity requires sufficient training intensity.	The individual dose (i.e., length) of any particular session matters, as well as the challenge within that session. There is no gold standard available, but some reviews suggest sessions of at least 30–60 minutes for plasticity to occur.
Time matters	Different forms of plasticity occur at different times during training.	This points to the fact that molecular, cellular, and structural events can occur on different time-orders, including prior to behavioral change, supporting the need for direct neural measures to ascertain intervention effects.
Salience matters	The training experience must be sufficiently salient to induce plasticity.	Sufficient repetition is needed to induce plasticity. To sustain engagement over time, there is a need for motivation and reward due to the "positivity bias," whereby older adults are more likely to orient toward positive experiences. Connecting intervention to stated life goals will further support salience.

(continued)

TABLE 11.2. *(continued)*

Principle	Description	Implications
Age matters	Training-induced plasticity occurs more readily in younger brains.	Plasticity may also occur more readily in more intact brains (i.e., earlier on the trajectory of cognitive decline). This is consistent with available evidence suggesting that restitution following cognitive training is more evident for less impaired individuals.
Transference	Plasticity in response to one training experience can enhance the acquisition of similar behaviors.	The authors discuss evidence that, in animal models, exercise can have a potentiating effect on other forms of training-induced plasticity. This lends support to studies that have combined physical exercise with cognitive training, and also suggests that multimodal programs may have greater effects than those focused on individual domains of function (although this latter claim warrants further investigation).
Interference	Plasticity in response to one experience can interfere with the acquisition of other behaviors.	Allowing individuals to develop compensatory strategies that are easier to perform (i.e., "bad habits") can cause maladaptive forms of plasticity that interfere with recovery of other functions. This suggests a need to teach compensatory strategies early on and supports the use of strategy training in less impaired individuals as a form of primary prevention.

Outcome Measurement

In reviewing published individual intervention studies in the empirical literature, it is clear that there are times when the outcome measurements are not appropriate for the construct under study or lack sufficient sensitivity to detect meaningful change over time. This obscures potential therapeutic effects and may account for some null results. Outcome measurement can occur on a variety of levels; in research studies, outcomes may be more sophisticated and involve one or more types of neuroimaging, such as sMRI and fMRI or cognitive electrophysiology. Such tools provide a complement to behavioral and self-report measurements, and may provide insight into mechanisms of action of the intervention itself (e.g., Campanella, 2013; Suo et al., 2016). However, the average clinician may not have ready access to such tools for individual clients. Nevertheless, it is crucial that the outcome measures chosen be specific to the construct subject to intervention, and include far-transfer to everyday behaviors as well as changes in objective cognitive test scores.

Neuropsychometric tests and self-report measures are considered a standard part of baseline assessment prior to treatment and provide important information about potential targets of intervention and moderating factors (e.g., severe depressive symptoms). Care should be taken to use measures with sufficient reliability, validity, and normative data appropriate to older adults. Ideally, measures have been specifically designed with the older adult population in mind (e.g., the Geriatric Depression Scale and the Adult Manifest Anxiety Scale–Elderly Version). Based on the evidence-based reviews previously discussed, neuropsychometric tests may be most useful in assessing near-transfer for cognitive training interventions, but they may result in false negatives for cognitive rehabilitation or cognitive stimulation interventions. If it is determined that repeat neuropsychometric assessment is an appropriate outcome measurement, it is important to take steps to ensure that any observed changes are clinically meaningful above and beyond mere practice effects. Where possible, it is beneficial to compute RCIs to assess pre/postchange. As there are many different ways to compute RCIs, the reader is referred to Duff (2012) and Frerichs and Tuokko (2005) for an introduction to RCIs and their practical application, as well as Chapter 5 where the assessment of change was discussed in some detail.

For cognitive rehabilitation and stimulation, the goal of intervention may not be improvement of cognitive function per se, but restoration of functional ability and functional adaptation to cognitive decline (Chandler et al., 2016). This renders neuropsychometric tests a less productive metric of improvement postintervention. For those who wish to use standardized tests, more ecologically relevant assessment methods are likely to have greater sensitivity to intervention effects. These are becoming more frequently used as a complement to typical neuropsychometric tests that were initially designed to ascertain levels of brain impairment, but not necessarily represent everyday function (Rabin, Burton, & Barr, 2007). Examples of standardized ecologically oriented instruments include tests such as the Test of Everyday Attention (Robertson, Ward, Ridgeway, & Nimmo-Smith, 1996) or the Memory for Intentions Test (Raskin & Buckheit, 2010). Alternatively, one could use a strictly behavioral approach to measure an increase in desirable behaviors (e.g., prosocial behaviors) and a decrease in maladaptive behaviors (e.g., kicking, swearing). This requires identifying concrete and specific target behaviors that are readily observable and reliably measured. The clinician should specify a baseline period of observation during which the target behavior is observed and frequency counts specified; further frequency counts can be obtained during the intervention and at follow-up, and chi-square statistical tests run to directly test the impact of the intervention.

Special Considerations in Addressing Anosognosia

In the application of any cognitive and behavioral intervention, the clinician should consider the client's current level of awareness. Specifically, the presence of anosognosia is increasingly likely as cognitive decline progresses, particularly from MCI to dementia (Kalbe et al., 2005; Lehrer et al., 2015). Anosognosia is likely to influence a client's ability to identify meaningful and tractable goals, as well as his or her willingness to participate in intervention altogether. The impact of anosognosia should be addressed before pursuing any specific cognitive intervention, and requires its own treatment approach, discussed in Chapter 9.

Creating an Overall Case Conceptualization

The empirical literature on cognitive and behavioral intervention in older adults is mired by inconsistencies in terminology regarding types of intervention. Moreover, failure to match the intervention's purported mechanism of action to the specified target of intervention, with appropriately sensitive and specific outcome measures, may have led to an underestimation of therapeutic effects. The scientist–practitioner approach is to treat each individual client as an $n = 1$ case study, with clear clinical hypotheses, an active intervention, and appropriate outcome measures. Implementing interventions with older adults requires the same case conceptualization skills familiar to clinical psychologists from other domains of practice. In Table 11.3, we provide some examples of how to create a theoretically sound, empirically informed case conceptualization, one that is flexible and responsive to emerging data about client response to intervention. As noted in this table, impaired everyday behavior can be associated with disturbance in more than one specific cognitive function (e.g., failure to recall details of a conversation could be episodic memory retrieval difficulties, or failure to sufficiently attend that impairs initial encoding of information). In part, this question is answered by performance on neuropsychometric tests; however, response to intervention may in and of itself provide information on the underlying impairment. One clinical hypothesis may be addressed initially (e.g., memory compensation strategies), and if the target behavior does not improve, alternate clinical hypotheses are pursued (e.g., attention training). This underscores the iterative nature of theoretically informed clinical practice, as well as the need for continuous assessment at each step of intervention. Appendix 11.1 provides a sampling of different types of intervention strategies that may be beneficial for different clinical problems.

To conclude, we return to the case of Sam, first introduced in Chapter 9, illustrating the first few sessions of how we engaged him in cognitive and behavioral intervention integrated with psychological work.

TABLE 11.3. Creating a Theoretically Informed Case Conceptualization for Cognitive and Behavioral Intervention

Everyday behavior and impact	Clinical hypotheses	Intervention	Outcome assessment
Difficulty recalling information about day-to-day events that impact participation in conversations and create embarrassment and social anxiety	1. Episodic memory retrieval impairment interferes with accessing information that has been previously consolidated 2. Impaired concentration that interferes with initial encoding of information, which means it is not available for later access	1. Compensatory strategy training (e.g., use of a memory book to write down important details as they come up) 2. Mindfulness training to promote self-regulation of attention to the present moment	1. Frequency counts of memory failures pre/postimplementation of a memory book 2. Psychometric assessment of attention pre/postintervention, as well as frequency counts of memory failures pre/posttraining 3. Self-report measures of anxiety and memory self-efficacy included with either intervention
Concerns about occasionally forgetting the names of acquaintances, phone numbers, and items from a shopping list	Symptoms of normal aging or possibly SCD	Provision of psychoeducation that includes: 1. Information on normal cognitive aging 2. Compensatory strategy training (e.g., use of a memory book) 3. Encourage maintenance of physical health	1. Endorsement of strategy use and positive health behaviors 2. Self-report measures of cognitive complaints, metamemory, and memory self-efficacy, as well as depression and anxiety 3. Monitor over time in case individual has SCD
Difficulties in remembering when to take medication and attend doctors' appointments	Failures in prospective memory, either due to: 1. Failure to encode the association between the cue and the target behavior (i.e., episodic remembering), and/or 2. Failure to monitor the environment for the incidence of the cue (i.e., cognitive control/prospective remembering)	1. Errorless learning to ensure accurate encoding of the meaning of cues 2. Use procedural memory to train habit of using and checking an assistive device (e.g., smartphone with calendar with alerts)	1. Frequency counts of memory failures pre/posttraining 2. Self-report measures of metamemory and memory self-efficacy included with either intervention

When we first encountered Sam in Chapter 9, he had recently undergone a neuropsychological evaluation. Results indicated a decline in intellectual functioning, as well as impairments in executive functions (i.e., difficulty with set-shifting, adaptation to novelty, and problem solving, self-monitoring and self-regulation) as well as slowed processing speed. These difficulties were occurring in the context of symptoms of depression and anxiety, some of which were in response to changing life circumstances due to having PD, as well as conflict in his relationship with one of his sons.

After providing Sam with feedback on the neuropsychological evaluation, we presented the possibility of nonpharmacological intervention, for which he was eager. We explained that there were a variety of intervention methods at our disposal, but these would only be useful if we could situate them within his own goals. After thinking about this, Sam identified the following treatment goals:

1. To decrease his social anxiety, so that he could make more friends, and
2. To improve his relationship with his son.

In forming a case conceptualization of Sam, the following key points emerged:

- Sam was a friendly, sociable guy who wanted to meet new people and make new friends, and being sociable was very much part of his culture as someone of Italian heritage. Unfortunately, his efforts to pursue this goal were often unsuccessful. When he tried to initiate small talk with strangers in coffee shops or other social contexts, he was unable to effectively express himself, and he would notice people would get frustrated with him and walk away. Over time, this led to an increase in social anxiety.
- It became evident that, at certain times when he would try to initiate new social contacts, he was feeling sluggish or mentally fatigued and had difficulty organizing his thoughts.
- Because of Sam's difficulties with self-monitoring and self-regulation, he was unaware of the times during which he was feeling less mentally sharp, thereby inadvertently setting himself up for failure.

Reviewing Sam's treatment goals presents another opportunity for us to provide psychoeducation to Sam about the effects of having PD, how it affected not only his cognition but also interfered with his goals of increasing social contact. As clinicians, we identified self-monitoring and self-regulation as domains for cognitive rehabilitation. However, we contextualized this for Sam in the context of helping him achieve his goal of increased socialization. That is, if he learned to self-monitor his cognitive, physiological, and emotional state, he could better plan ahead to make social contact at times when he was feeling his best. This way, we could set him up for success. Along the way, we would also address any self-sabotaging or automatic negative thoughts that were getting in the way of his making progress. The first 6 weeks of treatment consisted of the following steps:

- *Session 1:* For the first week, we asked Sam to track his arousal and attention over the course of each day, as a means of finding times when he was feeling more or less mentally sharp. He was to rate his arousal and energy on a 5-point scale, with 1 being underaroused, 5 being over-aroused, and 3 being optimally aroused. We asked that he minimally rate his arousal three times a day—morning, afternoon, and evening. Because we were concerned that Sam might not have sufficient prospective memory to remember to make these ratings, we asked him if he would be willing to do this activity on his smartphone. This meant that we could program in a recurring alarm three times a day to prompt Sam in the moment about how he was feeling, which he could then record in the notes program of his phone. Not only would this allow him to gather data on his arousal, but it would also serve as an external cue for self-monitoring, which we hoped would begin to generalize over time. In other words, we provided a form of "external mindfulness."

- *Session 2:* After a week of gathering arousal data, we were able to take the data from Sam's smartphone and visually plot them out on a rudimentary graph, so that he could see his arousal and energy fluctuate within and across days. Using these data, we established that he felt at his optimal self around midmorning, after he had had a good breakfast and his first dose of dopaminergic medication. This became the target time to engage in behavioral practice and work on both self-monitoring and social anxiety. We had Sam complete another week of logs, to verify his optimal arousal and energy and also to provide further scaffolding in external mindfulness. We then scheduled the next session during midmorning so that we could engage in an *in vivo* behavioral experiment around self-monitoring and social anxiety.

- *Session 3:* At the next session, Sam felt some trepidation but was willing to try a behavioral experiment. His self-identified goal was to go to a coffee shop and strike up a conversation with a stranger. We created a 10-point hierarchy of potentially anxiety-provoking experiences, with "talking to a beautiful woman" at an 8 of 10, and talking to the barista serving his drink at 4 of 10; thus, the goal of this experiment became to talk to the barista. Next, we had Sam rate his current arousal and energy, which he said was 2 of 5. He also rated his SUDs (subjective units of distress) at a

4 of 10, being mildly anxious. Although this was Sam's self-identified optimal time of day, we wanted to set him up for success. In case he encountered cognitive difficulties in the moment, we had him rehearse some small talk he could say to the barista, which he wrote out on a cue card to keep in his pocket. Then we walked to the coffee shop with Sam and stayed at a safe distance, so that he could engage in the behavioral experiment independently, but also know that a clinician was nearby should he need help. He successfully completed the exercise, and we returned to the office to debrief. Sam rated his arousal at 3 of 5, and his SUDs at 6 of 10—so there was an increase in both arousal and anxiety, but these were tolerable. Sam stated that he was a little disappointed in himself because he got confused about how to make change for his drink, and then he sensed that the barista was getting impatient. We addressed his negative self-talk about his performance, and we helped him reappraise the situation with praise and positive feedback for being willing to try the experiment and moving one step closer to his goal. For homework, we agreed that Sam would try at least one behavioral experiment where he would try to talk to a stranger at his optimal time of day and report back next week.

- *Session 4:* In Session 4, we checked in about the last week's experience. Sam reported being somewhat demoralized by his performance in the in-session experiment, but over the week he was able to tell himself that at least he was trying. At this point, we developed the hypothesis that more direct exposure to mindfulness training could be helpful for Sam. By practicing mindfulness, he could improve his ability to attend to the present moment, help him focus on conversation, and when he did make a "slip-up," learn to be nonjudgmental and accepting of himself. Based on his baseline cognitive function, we were uncertain that Sam would be able to engage in mindfulness training right away. We continued to use his smartphone pre-programmed with alarms throughout the day, encouraging him to attend to his experience and encouraging him to be kind to himself. In subsequent sessions, we were able to transition to guided mindfulness exercises using an audio recording that Sam practiced at home. He reported that he was feeling more mentally alert and yet was also able to be more aware of when he was becoming fatigued or having difficulty thinking clearly. This was then leveraged into further behavioral experiments in and out of session to move him closer to his goal of increased socialization and making new friends.

Summary and Conclusions

There now exist many exciting possibilities for cognitive and behavioral interventions in older adults, bolstered by advancements in basic and applied neuroscience as well as cognitive rehabilitation. Evidence suggests that older adults at every stage of cognitive decline can and should benefit from a variety of skills and training programs, countering the notion that cognitive decline is something to be passively tolerated and unavoidable. Structural and functional neuroplasticity is possible in older adulthood, albeit on potentially longer time-scales than in younger persons; thus, these interventions may not only enhance current cognitive function, but also provide a buffer against future decline (i.e., primary and secondary prevention).

The last decade in particular has seen a rapid expansion in the amount of literature on nonpharmacological interventions for older adults at each level of the trajectory of cognitive decline, with encouraging findings emerging for various cognitive/behavioral and psychological interventions. However, further work needs to be done to solidify the evidence base and move the field forward. For cognitive and behavioral interventions, again there needs to be better characterization of participants, in terms not only of establishing diagnoses but also of identifying possible moderators to intervention such as premorbid function and baseline neuropsychological function. Additionally, more attention needs to be paid to specifying a priori the mechanism of action of a given intervention as well as specifying appropriate outcomes to ascertain response to intervention. To that end, researchers need to consult the literature in other areas such as cognitive rehabilitation to gain an understanding of which cognitive functions are more or less amenable to restitution (e.g., attention) and which would likely benefit more from compensatory approaches (e.g., memory). Neuropsychometric measures may be appropriate for interventions based on restitution, but less appropriate for compensatory approaches that may be better measured by examining ecologically relevant measures and everyday behavior. Moreover, studies such as the ACTIVE trial indicate that intervention effects may not occur for months or even years until after the active intervention phase has ended. This underscores the importance of longitudinal follow-up and also cautions against assuming that a lack of significant findings at immediate postintervention is necessarily a true null result. Finally, much of the existing literature is based on a proof-of-principle model using tightly controlled RCT designs with relatively homogeneous populations. Several systematic reviews and meta-analyses have supported the efficacy of various cognitive and behavioral interventions. Given the rapidly escalating number of older adults who need care, the field needs to move "from the benches to the trenches" and start to focus more on effectiveness designs that test some of these same interventions in more representative clinical samples. For a more detailed discussion of factors to consider in cognitive and behavioral interventions, we refer to the recommendations proposed in Smart et al.'s (2017) systematic review and meta-analysis on nonpharmacological interventions for persons with SCD.

KEY POINTS

✓ In this chapter, we covered the three major modalities of cognitive training, cognitive rehabilitation, and cognitive stimulation, each of which seems to have differential effects based on the stage of cognitive decline.

✓ Cognitive training in general seems to be more efficacious for individuals with minimal manifest cognitive impairment (i.e., healthy older adults and those with SCD), although transfer of training to daily life remains controversial.

✓ Cognitive rehabilitation shows promise in individuals with MCI as well as those with dementia.

✓ Cognitive stimulation is also efficacious in persons with dementia. Although not always empirically tested, cognitive training may actually function as a form of cognitive stimulation in less impaired individuals, providing a means to boost mental engagement and contribute to cognitive reserve.

✓ We recommend grounding any intervention within the context of the client's goals. This will make the intervention more ecologically relevant and promote intrinsic motivation, particularly when tasks become challenging.

✓ Psychoeducation also seems to be effective in healthy older adults, those with SCD, and those with MCI, and, if presented judiciously, can enhance motivation and engagement in other forms of intervention.

✓ Finally, it is critical that the appropriate outcome be used for the type of intervention employed, noting that neuropsychological test scores may not always be the most appropriate outcome measure.

Resources for Cognitive and Behavioral Interventions

For readers unfamiliar with the various types of cognitive and behavioral interventions, we provide a sampling here of those worth further investigation, as well as other sources of information to support engaging in this work.

Overview of Cognitive Rehabilitation

Sohlberg, M. M., & Mateer, C. A. (2001). *Cognitive rehabilitation: An integrative neuropsychological approach* (2nd ed.). New York: Guilford Press.

Although this is an older book, it is a classic scientist–practitioner text that discusses basic and applied neuroscience and neuroplasticity, as well as provides an introduction to various types of intervention for attention, memory, and executive functions. The book is extremely practical and includes various case examples for how to apply these interventions. For the reader new to cognitive rehabilitation, this would be an excellent starting point.

Manualized Interventions for Healthy Aging and MCI

The Rotman–Baycrest Institute has created manualized intervention programs that are available for purchase to qualified individuals. These include:

- *Memory and Aging Program* for healthy older adults, and
- *Learning the Ropes Program* for persons with MCI.

Information on purchasing these programs can be found at www.baycrest. org/care/care-programs/centre-for-memory-and-neurotherapeutics/ neuropsychology-and-cognitive-health/clinical-tools.

Researchers at Rotman–Baycrest have also created an intervention for executive function difficulties entitled goal management training (GMT), which has been investigated in older adults:

Levine, B., Stuss, D. T., Winocur, G., Binns, M. A., Fahy, L., Mandic, M., . . . Robertson, I. H. (2007). Cognitive rehabilitation in the elderly: Effects on strategic behavior in relation to goal management. *Journal of the International Neuropsychological Society, 13*, 143–152.
Stuss, D. T., Robertson, I. H., Craik, F. I., Levine, B., Alexander, M. P., Black, S., . . . Winocur, G. (2007). Cognitive rehabilitation in the elderly: A randomized trial to evaluate a new protocol. *Journal of the International Neuropsychological Society, 13*, 120–131.

(continued)

van Hooren, S. A., Valentijn, S. A., Bosma, H., Ponds, R. W., van Boxtel, M. P., Levine, B., . . . Jolles, J. (2007). Effect of a structured course involving goal management training in older adults: A randomised controlled trial. *Patient Education and Counseling, 65*, 205–213.

Information on training in GMT, as well as how to purchase intervention materials, can be found at *http://shop.baycrest.org/collections/the-goal-management-training-program*.

Rotman–Baycrest also hosts regular "train-the-trainer" workshops for these various programs, information on which can also be found on their website.

Books on MCI

Anderson, N. A., Murphy, K. J., & Troyer, A. K. (2012). *Living with mild cognitive impairment: A guide to maximizing brain health and reducing risk of dementia*. New York: Oxford University Press.

This popular-press book will be useful for clinicians and clients alike, presenting material from the Learning the Ropes for MCIprogram designed at the Rotman–Baycrest Institute.

Organizations

The American Congress of Rehabilitation Medicine (*www.acrm.org*) is one of the most well-respected interdisciplinary organizations for evidence-based practice in rehabilitation. The organization provides information on evidence-based interventions as well as workshop and other training for professionals. They also have special interest groups in brain injury rehabilitation and also geriatric rehabilitation, which would be useful networking opportunities for those seeking to learn more and connect with other professionals using cognitive and behavioral interventions with older adults.

The Alzheimer's Association (*www.alz.org*) hosts one of the world's largest yearly conferences on cutting-edge science and practice in SCD, MCI, and dementia. As a member of the Alzheimer's Association's organization, International Society to Advance Alzheimer's Research and Treatment (ISTA-ART), one can join various Professional Interest Areas (PIAs). Of particular interest for those pursuing cognitive and behavioral interventions would be the PIA on nonpharmacological interventions (*https://act.alz.org/site/SPageServer?pagename=ISTAART_PIA_NPI*). PIAs host a variety of business and research meetings at the yearly conference, again providing an important opportunity to network and collaborate with other clinicians and researchers.

CHAPTER 12

Psychological Interventions

Older adults at various stages of cognitive decline can present with significant psychological difficulties. Understood within the biopsychosocial framework, psychological symptoms can influence cognitive function or, conversely, be an expression of underlying cognitive decline. In addition, psychological symptoms can manifest in adjustment to health difficulties or arise iatrogenically from the pharmacological management of those difficulties. Assessment and management of psychological difficulties should be a routine aspect of care for older adults. In Chapter 10, we discussed pharmacological approaches to the management of psychological and cognitive symptoms. In the current chapter, we present a conceptual framework of how psychological difficulties may manifest in older adulthood, as well as introduce the reader to various psychotherapeutic approaches to address these challenges. Finally, we end with a case example of how psychological intervention might be implemented in clients with cognitive impairment. First, let us return to the case of Sam, to illustrate some of the material presented in this chapter.

> Sam is a 66-year-old, Italian Canadian, right-handed gentleman with PD. He was referred for assessment of current cognitive function due to complaints about perceived cognitive decline particularly over the past 3 years. However, during the assessment, it came to light that Sam had a history of depression, as well as PTSD associated with witnessing many traumatic events as a career police officer. He has had prior treatment for the PTSD, with an improvement in many of his symptoms. However, he presents with ongoing complaints of social anxiety associated with his cognitive difficulties and motor symptoms, which interferes with his ability to make new friends. Some of the social anxiety is also related to a change in self-concept associated

with motor symptoms due to PD, as Sam is no longer able to be as active as he once was. Moreover, Sam reports significant distress over a conflicted relationship with one of his adult sons and desperately wants to find ways improve this relationship. Sam's relationship with his father was very difficult, in part because his father may have been suffering from his own PTSD due to serving in World War II. While Sam has a very loving relationship with his wife and other son, current and historical description of relationships suggests that Sam has an anxious attachment style. This is likely in part due to an unstable relationship with his father, as well as immigrating to Canada as a young child and leaving behind many family members in Italy. Although he has a history of depression, Sam denies current symptoms. He has no history or current report of suicidal ideation, plans, or intent. Rather, he reports a strong awareness of his mortality and a desire to make the best of his retirement. Aside from PD, Sam's medical history is noncontributory, and recent medical work-up was unremarkable. Individuals taking dopamine agonists for PD may be at risk for dopamine dysregulation syndrome, a neurobehavioral syndrome that involves impulse control symptoms such as pathological gambling and hypersexuality. However, Sam denies any such symptoms and has no prior history of addiction, which may be a risk factor for dopamine dysregulation syndrome. He denies any current substance use (including tobacco), and only has one to two drinks on the weekend with his wife.

Consideration of Factors That Contribute to Psychological Functioning

Although Sam has presented for neuropsychological evaluation in the context of (assumed) PD-related cognitive decline, in learning more about him we see that a variety of factors could be contributing to his current psychological functioning beyond the mere presence of PD. Before developing PD, Sam accrued a lifetime of experiences that could be influencing his current presentation, including immigration, early attachment issues, work stress, and family functioning. As we have advocated consistently throughout this text, taking a developmentally informed, biopsychosocial approach is necessary to provide the most comprehensive case formulation of Sam's current function and therefore the required treatment to help him.

A great many factors can affect mood and behavior at any age, including in older adulthood. In order to provide the most effective care, a detailed assessment of these factors is necessary before beginning intervention. *Physiological factors* such as inadequate sleep, blood sugar dysregulation, substance use, and medications can all impact psychological status, with delirium being the most extreme example. To the extent that these factors are modifiable and treatable, a comprehensive medical work-up should always be a foundational step before beginning more psychologically based intervention. Consultation with the client's primary physician can facilitate this goal, who may refer the client to a provider in neurology or psychiatry for more detailed testing, such as a comprehensive medical work-up.

Premorbid psychological functioning is crucial to understand the longevity, course, and evolution of current difficulties, including establishing what interventions, if any, have been useful in the past. Due to cohort effects, the oldest-old (i.e., >80 years) may have had limited exposure to psychological interventions, as well as carrying cultural stigma about mental illness (Faber, 2014). This will necessitate socializing these clients to the idea of psychological intervention in a thoughtful and sensitive manner. Aside from prior diagnoses, premorbid psychological functioning can also include attachment styles and premorbid personality factors (e.g., neuroticism, locus of control, self-efficacy) that may influence engagement in intervention. The broader *psychosocial context* includes factors such as economic stability, current living situation, and interpersonal support. Cultural determinants—including cohort effects—will likely influence a person's response to current circumstances, including ideas about the meaning of mental illness and associated stigma (Gerolimatos, Gregg, & Edelstein, 2014). Likewise, culture can affect an individual's engagement in, and subsequent response to, intervention, which may necessitate culturally appropriate tailoring of standard evidence-based interventions (Flynn, Cooper, & Gary-Webb, 2013). Finally, *legal issues* have a unique place for consideration in working with an older adult clientele, particularly being able to discern suicidal ideation from a desire to pursue medically assisted suicide, which is legal in some jurisdictions (Gerolimatos et al., 2014).

Assessment of Psychological Functioning

It is crucial that any plan for intervention begin with an appropriate assessment of current psychological functioning. Comprehensive assessment of the client's current and premorbid psychological function will help determine the appropriate clinical conceptualization of current difficulties and in turn the most appropriate form of intervention. The phenomenology of mood and anxiety disorders in older adults, and in persons with neurological disorders, can differ from that of psychiatric populations. For example, geriatric depression may include symptoms of perceived or actual cognitive impairment (Steffens & Potter, 2008), as reflected by items on the Geriatric Depression Scale (Yesavage et al., 1983) such as "Do you feel you have more problems with memory than most?" Measures such as the Adult Manifest Anxiety Scale—Elderly Version (AMAS-E; Lowe & Reynolds, 2006) allow for separation of physiological symptoms of anxiety (which are often artificially elevated in certain neurologic diseases such as PD), while also addressing symptoms that may be more developmentally relevant to older adults, such as fear of aging. It also stands to reason that the assessment measure should be relevant to the intervention being used (e.g., the use of a mindfulness-based self-report measure for mindfulness-based cognitive therapy). In Appendix 12.1, we present a checklist of core areas of inquiry for a psychological interview prior to intervention.

Although certain interventions may be more or less relevant depending on the individual's stage of cognitive decline, there is not always a 1:1 association between the two. In the following sections, we present a framework for providing psychological intervention in older adults, organized not by stage of cognitive decline, but rather according to the following four broad areas that warrant clinical attention: (1) adjustment to change in late life, (2) diagnosable psychological conditions, (3) neuropsychiatric and neurobehavioral syndromes, and (4) family and caregiver functioning. This framework is summarized in Table 12.1. Given that therapeutic tailoring may need to occur according to current cognitive function, we discuss this where relevant. Here we focus on psychological interventions, but these comprise only one piece of a holistic intervention plan that may include any or all of pharmacologic intervention, cognitive intervention, and psychological intervention.

Adjustment to Change in Late Life

Developmental Trends in Emotional Experience

Contrary to popular stereotypes, growing older is not "all doom and gloom." Of course, those who have a prior history of mental health issues may bring those same issues into late life, but this is different from the common assumption that aging in and of itself is a cause for major psychological distress. The normative trajectory for most adults is a successful transition into late life, readily navigating the challenges of that developmental period. One reason for this may be the prioritization of emotional goals in later life. For example, a fairly robust body of research has documented the so-called positivity bias, or the tendency for older adults to favor positive states of mind and be more likely to orient their attention to positive information (Reed et al., 2014). In understanding the roots of this positivity bias, Carstensen's socioemotional selectivity theory (Carstensen, Isaacowitz, & Charles, 1999; Mather, 2012) posits that with advancing age comes a heightened awareness of one's mortality and the sense that "time is running out." This thought causes older adults to prioritize the quality of their relationships and make the most of the time that is remaining. Indeed, Carstensen and colleagues (2011) conducted an impressive 10-year longitudinal study that incorporated multiple age cohorts. Using

TABLE 12.1. Summary of Psychological Management Approaches

Clinical issue	Characteristics	Management approach	Intervention strategies	Considerations for consultation
Adjustment to change in late life	Difficulty with adaptation to changes in late life (e.g., age-related cognitive decline, physical health impairments, change in housing). Grief and bereavement. Loss of quality of life and well-being with mild cognitive impairment and dementia	Balancing symptom management with allowing the individual to experience normative feelings of grief or sadness associated with the developmental challenges of late life (e.g., partner loss, retirement)	• Life review therapy for existential concerns or normative grief • Complicated grief therapy or IPT for complicated bereavement • CBT for chronic health impairments, including mood/anxiety symptoms arising in this context • For mood/anxiety disorders, provision of psychotherapy	Regular follow-up with general practitioner, particularly in the context of chronic health impairments
Diagnosable psychological conditions	Ongoing presence or reoccurrence of symptoms of depression, anxiety, bipolar disorder, and so on	Multimodal management of symptoms, including psychotherapy and medication, where appropriate	• Empirically supported psychotherapy (e.g., CBT, IPT, MBSR) that aligns with the client's preferences • Modification, where appropriate, for cognitive decline	Geriatric psychiatrist or neuropsychiatrist for medication consultation

Neuropsychiatric syndromes	Symptoms and syndromes that may be part of an underlying neurological disease process (e.g., depression associated with VaD, hallucinations associated with DLB dementia, Capgras syndrome, and anosognosia)	Minimization of symptoms, particularly those that lead to agitation or cause safety concerns	• For psychotic symptoms (e.g., hallucinations and delusions), providing psychoeducation to the client, family, and caregivers, working to minimize agitation (e.g., avoiding directly challenging delusional beliefs) • Behavioral approaches to minimize agitation • For ICD/DDS, use CBT to decrease antecedent conditions (e.g., anxiety) and/or MI to engage the client in harm reduction around medication overuse	Neuropsychiatrist or behavioral neurologist for medication consultation
Family and caregiver function	Change in relationships with age-related declines. Caregiver burden associated with having a family member with significant cognitive and/or neurobehavioral impairment	Provide caregivers with strategies on how to best engage with client, as well as ways to manage psychological distress associated with caregiving	• Psychoeducation regarding the impact of MCI and dementia • Provision of caregiving resources (websites, support groups, etc.) • Stress management techniques • Making room for the grief process and ambiguous loss	Family therapist, where appropriate; instrumental support resources such as social worker or eldercare attorney

Note. IPT, interpersonal psychotherapy; CBT, cognitive-behavioral therapy; MBSR, mindfulness-based stress reduction; ICD, impulse control disorders; DDS, dopamine dysregulation syndrome; MI, motivational interviewing.

experience sampling methods, they found that emotion regulation abilities enhance with increasing age, with greater experiences of positive emotion and also *poignancy,* or mixed emotions—for example, the bittersweet feeling that comes when spending time with a loved one and realizing that future moments may be limited. Moreover, an accumulation of life experience and concomitant increase in wisdom with age may improve decision making, including a tendency to see the big picture in life and "not sweat the small stuff" (Worthy, Gorlick, Pacheco, Schyner, & Maddox, 2011).

Such research from lifespan developmental science indicates that significant psychological distress is not expected to be the norm for the majority of older adults. That said, there are many stressors and difficulties that older adults face with the passage of time that, if not addressed, can adversely impact psychological functioning, well-being, and quality of life. These include but are not limited to the onset of cognitive decline itself (both age-related and non-normative), chronic health impairments, changes in living arrangements, the loss of loved ones, and the desire to find meaning in one's life. Losses that are unpredicted or "off-time" may be more challenging to deal with as compared to those that are considered "on-time" (Cheek, 2010; Gorman, 2011). Many of these changes may occur with the aging process itself, and it may only be when an individual reaches a critical level of difficulty that he or she seeks intervention. Conversely, an older adult who assumes that stress is simply part and parcel of "getting older" may fail to seek out clinical intervention. Thus, it is important that the clinician consider how an older adult is adjusting to such life changes and whether intervention is indeed warranted.

Chronic Health Issues

As mentioned in Chapter 10, the CDC estimate that approximately 80% of older adults have at least one chronic health impairment and 50% have two or more conditions, which elevates the possibility of clinical depression (CDC, 2015). Cognitive-behavioral therapy (CBT) already has a robust literature of application for a variety of chronic health conditions, including chronic pain, fatigue, and general medical conditions (Hofmann, Asnaan, Vonk, Sawyer, & Fang, 2012). As we have discussed many times, a biopsychosocial understanding of current function is the primary framework for a majority of clinical psychologists. This includes the understanding of chronic illness, which has both biological and psychosocial determinants. In the context of chronic illness, CBT may be helpful in directly reducing symptoms of the disease itself. In addition, CBT may address emotional distress such as depression that may arise from having to deal with a chronic health impairment, distress that may in turn worsen the experience of the medical condition. Braun, Karlin, and Zeiss (2015) provide a fairly comprehensive review of the evidence of the application of CBT to older adults with various medical conditions. They found evidence in support of CBT for insomnia, arthritis, cardiac conditions, diabetes, and other medical issues such as various pain conditions, irritable bowel syndrome, and chronic fatigue syndrome. In certain contexts (e.g., insomnia), CBT was at least as effective as pharmacological interventions, which is encouraging considering the many issues related to polypharmacy and increased risk of adverse drug reactions when older adults are taking multiple medications (see Chapter 10 for more details). In a later section in this chapter, we discuss in more detail the application of CBT to older adults with primary mood and anxiety issues, including tailoring to individuals with cognitive impairment.

Existential Concerns

As older adults move closer to the end of life than the beginning, they may begin to face existential concerns about the meaning and purpose of their life, and how to "gain closure" before their life comes to an end. These concerns may occur in the context of the various transitions or losses that can occur in older adulthood, such as retirement, changes in physical health, and the loss of loved ones. Depending on the life circumstances of the individual, both current and past, such an existential review can create feelings of anxiety or depression. In this context, we do not wish to pathologize what may be part of negotiating a normative life stage. That said, this does not mean that steps cannot be taken to help an older adult navigate this stage effectively.

Reminiscence therapy pertains to a broad category of interventions that involve reflection on autobiographical memories, from more free-form approaches such as simple reminiscence to the more structured approach of life review and life review therapy. Specifically reminiscing about positive events has been shown to engender positive mood states (Bryant, Smart, & King, 2005); unsurprisingly, then, reminiscence therapy has been investigated as an intervention for late-life depression (Scogin, Welsh, Hanson, Stump, & Coates, 2005). Bhar (2014) provided an extensive review of the topic of reminiscence therapy in older adulthood. In his review of empirical literature through 2013, he surveyed fourteen systematic reviews and/or meta-analyses, noting that the findings were quite mixed regarding the efficacy of this intervention approach on improving mental health outcomes. This may be a function of the fact that "reminiscence therapy" is a broad term for a variety of different therapies with different clinical targets.

The findings from the various reviews Bhar (2014) discussed seemed to suggest that the more structured the therapy was (i.e., life review and life review therapy versus simple reminiscence), the greater the benefits on mood and cognitive functioning. Moreover, the benefits of these structured therapies seemed to be most pronounced for depression, with insufficient evidence for other clinical issues such as anxiety, memory problems, or problematic behaviors associated with dementia. Erik Erikson, the developmental psychologist, described older adulthood as a life stage where the main developmental conflict is *ego integrity versus despair* (Erikson, 1963). This conflict can be resolved by reviewing one's past and coming to terms with one's decisions in order to make peace with one's life as a whole and one's resultant identity. Failure to resolve this conflict can result in depression and despair. During the process of life review, the individual is guided through a structured protocol that progresses in chronological order from early childhood to the present time. By reflecting on positive and negative events across time, the intention is to facilitate the individual in developing a meaningful life story that involves the integration of, and coming to terms with, both positive and negative events (Afonso, Bueno, Loureiro, & Pereira, 2011; Westerhof, Bohlmeijer, & Webster, 2010). Not only does structured life review support the development of ego integrity, but when done in conjunction with younger family members (or younger persons such as students in university courses on aging) it can also promote intergenerational dialogue and the transmission of cohort-specific information. This can allow older adults to feel that they are passing along wisdom and understanding to the younger generations, which may be another aspect of cultivating ego integrity.

Therapies for Grief and Bereavement

As we age, we face a variety of "on-time" losses, such as changes in relationships, jobs, physical health status, and of course bereavement over the death of loved ones. Grief in response to those losses is a normal and natural part of life (Malkinson & Bar-Tur, 2014). As such, grief in and of itself is not a disorder that warrants clinical attention but may be an issue to be explored in a supportive psychotherapy context. For clinicians and clients, we find that Francis Weller's (2015) *Wild Edge of Sorrow* could be an excellent resource. Weller, an experienced psychotherapist, discusses grief and loss from a pan-cultural perspective, emphasizing its universality and the importance of doing grief work consciously and mindfully. He also discusses the importance of ritual and ceremony, and provides resources for how this work can be done. As discussed below in the context of family and caregiver interventions, exploring the role of ritual and ceremony may be one way to support a culturally sensitive approach to the discussion of grief.

While most people navigate grief successfully, a significant minority of individuals may have difficulty with processing grief, for a variety of reasons. For example, grief due to the death of a loved one is a relatively common experience for older adults. However, for those who have difficulty transitioning beyond normative grief, they may develop what is referred to as complicated bereavement (Hartz, 1986; Horowitz et al., 1997) or, in the nomenclature of DSM-5, persistent complex bereavement disorder (PCBD). In PCBD, an individual experiences symptoms 12 months after the death of someone, symptoms that involve preoccupation with the deceased, reactive distress related to the death, and social identity disruption, including a desire to die to be reunited with the deceased. There is some evidence that complicated bereavement is more likely to be associated with losses that are "off-time" or traumatic in some way, such as the loss of a child (MacCallum & Bryant, 2013; Shear, 2015). Shear (2015) discusses available evidence supporting the application of complicated grief therapy, suggesting it should be considered a frontline treatment for this condition. In terms of interventions specific to older adults, some RCTs have recently been published examining their efficacy. Shear et al. (2014) compared the efficacy of sixteen weekly sessions of complicated grief therapy (CGT) to grief-focused interpersonal therapy (IPT). They found that, while both groups showed an improvement in complicated grief symptoms, CGT resulted in a significantly larger effect on illness severity, rate of symptom reduction, and rate of improvement in those symptoms. These findings are notable given that grief is one of the core conceptual foci of IPT, suggesting that a specific therapy focused on complicated grief is more efficacious. Similarly, Supiano and Luptak (2014) found that group therapy specifically tailored to complicated grief was more efficacious in reducing symptoms than standard group therapy. We would also direct the reader Stroebe, Schut, and van den Bout (2013), whose edited book provides several chapters on different therapeutic approaches to managing complicated bereavement.

Bereavement would be considered to be a finite loss, meaning it is a discrete event in time with well-defined boundaries. However, older adults may also be faced with nonfinite losses, those that lack such boundaries and may occur in an iterative fashion over a protracted period of time. Ambiguous loss is defined as a loss wherein an individual is either physically absent but still psychologically present in the minds of loved ones (such as in military personnel missing in action), or psychologically absent, yet physically present (such as persons with dementia) (Boss & Yeats, 2014). Ambiguous loss has been reported in caregivers of persons with MCI and dementia (Alzheimer Society of Canada, 2013). In recent work, Ali and Smart (2016) also found that individuals with MCI themselves experienced ambiguous loss associated with the erosion of one's sense of self as well as the uncertain course of decline in MCI. Moreover, their loved ones tended to minimize emotional distress associated with the individual's experience of cognitive loss. While they likely believed that they were being helpful, this contributed to feelings of disenfranchised grief (Corr, 2002). In a later section on family and caregiver interventions, we discuss resources for dealing with ambiguous loss and grief.

Diagnosable Psychological Disorders

Older adults may present with significant psychological symptoms beyond the scope of adjustment to normal aging, symptoms that warrant clinical attention. The most common of these symptoms include mood and anxiety disorders. These may be first-episode, late-life onset, or they could represent a persistence or reoccurrence of long-standing mental health concerns. Luppa and colleagues (2012) conducted a systematic review and meta-analysis of the prevalence of late-life depression. They found that, while prevalence estimates vary significantly based on classification methods (i.e., up to 9.3% for major depression and as high as 37.4% for depressive disorders), late-life depression is relatively common. Anxiety disorders are also relatively common in older adults and highly comorbid with depression, but they tend to be less prevalent in older as compared to younger adults (Wolitzky-Taylor et al., 2010). Psychological disorders can negatively impact quality of life and well-being, and interfere with adjustment to normative changes in late life. Moreover, evidence suggests that depression and anxiety in particular can have secondary effects on cognitive function in late life and in some cases herald a risk for subsequent pathological (i.e., non-normal) cognitive decline. For example, late-life depression has been associated with increased risk of all-cause dementia, including Alzheimer's and vascular dementia (da Silva et al., 2013; Diniz et al., 2013). Recent research suggests that anxiety may moderate the level of cognitive decline in clinically normal older adults who are Aβ positive, a risk factor for AD, whereby greater anxiety predicts accelerated decline (Pietrzak et al., 2015a). Even stress in midlife can herald a risk for future cognitive decline, where stress is taken as a marker for dysfunction of the hypothalamic–pituitary–adrenal axis, which in turn confers risk for the development of AD (Joshi & Pratico, 2013).

A formidable amount of literature is available on empirically supported psychological interventions for older adults; this includes many excellent chapters and entire books written on this topic (e.g., Braun et al., 2015; Cuijpers, Kaylotaki, Pot, Park, & Reynolds, 2014; Holland & Gallagher-Thompson, 2014; Laidlaw, 2014), several of which we reference in our review. The overarching consensus is that many or most empirically supported therapies used in younger age groups can be effectively applied in older adults, either with or without specific developmental tailoring. As such, the focus of this section is to introduce the reader to some of the more prominent empirically supported treatments and how these may be applied or modified for use with older adults. We provide additional information on modifications that may be needed to support the delivery of these interventions in persons with cognitive decline. We remind the reader that, while a client may present with a primary psychological disorder, this does not preclude the presence of some of the adjustment or existential issues discussed in the prior section, and these may need to be woven into the overall psychotherapeutic approach. Finally, as noted, many psychotherapies seem to be effective for older adults. Choosing a particular psychotherapeutic approach for a given client will depend on client-specific factors (e.g., world-view, values), as well as so-called common factors such as the ability to build a collaborative and supportive relationship between client and therapist. As such, we believe that to effectively provide psychotherapy to older adults, it is worthwhile for clinicians to be trained in a variety of modalities in order to best serve their clients' needs.

Cognitive-Behavioral Therapy

CBT is one of the most popular evidence-based treatments for adults, widely applied for a variety of psychological disorders and diagnoses. CBT has been shown to be efficacious for a wide variety of psychological disorders, and there are many disorder-specific manuals for the application of CBT. For those relatively new to CBT, Judith Beck's (2011) book, *Cognitive Behavior Therapy: Basics and Beyond,* is a classic scientist–practitioner text that introduces the core principles of this therapy as well as practical guidance for its implementation in a variety of contexts. Laidlaw (2014) and Braun et al. (2015) have both written excellent reviews of the evidence for and application of CBT specific to older adult populations. We draw on their work here and direct the reader to these citations for a more in-depth discussion of this topic.

Laidlaw (2014) has provided a comprehensive overview of the evidence for CBT in older adults, as well as its application for depression and anxiety. Based on available evidence, CBT does appear to be efficacious for late-life depression, although there is insufficient evidence to say that it is unequivocally more effective than other forms of psychotherapy. Individual CBT is more efficacious than group CBT and is comparable in efficacy to medication, although data on this topic are limited. One limitation of this literature is that a majority of studies are conducted on youngest-old participants, and data are lacking on the oldest-old cohort. We direct the interested reader to Thompson, Dick-Siskin, Coon, Powers, and Gallagher-Thompson (2010), who have created a specific protocol for applying CBT to late-life depression. In terms of anxiety, there is some evidence to support the efficacy of CBT, but it is far less robust than that for depression. For example, CBT for anxiety seems to be substantially more efficacious for working-age adults as compared to older adults. Laidlaw (2014) does not discuss why, but one could speculate that the reason for this discrepancy could be due to some of the sources of anxiety in older adulthood, which may be more existential in nature. For example, if an older adult's concerns are associated with death anxiety (Fortner & Neimeyer, 1999; Hoelterhoff & Chung, 2013), it may be inappropriate to conceptualize these concerns as based on dysfunctional or irrational thought patterns. Rather, existential or acceptance-based therapies (discussed below) may be more appropriate. In addition, Laidlaw (2014) notes several methodological issues with the literature on CBT for anxiety, including a tendency to use younger-old participants as well as those of higher socioeconomic status who have better physical health. This raises questions about the generalizability of any positive findings. Given that anxiety disorders are a heterogeneous class of disorders, it is notable that most clinical trials focus on generalized anxiety disorder, with comparatively less evidence on phobias, obsessive–compulsive disorder, and PTSD.

Tailoring of CBT

Much of the evidence on CBT for older adults is likely based on cognitively intact participants. As such, one might wonder whether CBT could be used for older adults showing significant cognitive decline. Laidlaw (2014) notes that the current evidence base is limited and consists primarily of case studies or studies with small sample sizes and mixed findings. The author reports on one promising study by Paukert and colleagues (2010, 2013) that showed positive results following a modified CBT, where family members were trained to act as collateral therapists for clients with anxiety in dementia. Greater emphasis was placed on behaviorally oriented techniques versus cognitive techniques, as well as the inclusion of cues and other specific strategies to facilitate memory retrieval. While the current evidence is limited, this does not preclude clinicians from attempting this work with individual clients. Below we provide several strategies to tailor CBT and other evidence-based therapies to older adults with cognitive impairment, evaluating the impact of such tailored therapy in an $n = 1$ case study manner.

There is some preliminary evidence that such tailoring may be beneficial. For example, Mohlman (2008) found that older adults who received CBT for generalized anxiety disorder plus concurrent executive skills training benefited more than those who received CBT alone. One caveat we would mention is the application of CBT to clients with *perseveration,* a specific aspect of executive dysfunction. Rumination is a common symptom in various psychological disorders, and asking clients to focus on attending to and tracking their thoughts may become counterproductive to the extent to which they perseverate on these thoughts and are unable to effectively disengage with them. As such, thought work should be used judiciously in clients with this symptom. In such cases, mindfulness-based approaches such as mindfulness-based cognitive therapy may be more effective as there is less emphasis on restructuring thoughts as opposed to simply noticing and de-identifying with difficult thoughts. Modified CBT has also been developed specifically to target behavioral problems in dementia (James,

2014), which we discuss in the section on agitation and challenging behaviors.

Interpersonal Psychotherapy

Although a variety of therapies have an interpersonal focus, IPT as a specific approach conceptualizes depression as arising from interpersonal distress that has one of three main foci: role transition, role dispute, and complicated grief (Klerman, Weissman, Rounsaville, & Chevron, 1984). It is a short-term, problem-focused treatment that takes a medical model approach to depression and connects current life situations to the triggering of depression. The main goals of treatment are to resolve disturbing life events, build social skills, and organize one's life (Markowitz & Weissman, 2004). IPT is one of the most well-validated interventions for depression.

Although there is a fairly substantial evidence base for IPT in youth and adult samples (Cuijpers et al., 2011), the number of recent studies documenting its application to older adults is limited, although some older studies report that it can be beneficial in conjunction with pharmacotherapy (e.g., Lenze et al., 2002; Reynolds et al., 1999, 2006). This relative dearth of literature is surprising, given that the theoretical model of IPT would seem to translate well to the presenting concerns of older adults. For example, retirement as a normative late-life event could give rise to changing roles and emotional challenges in adjusting to those new roles. Moreover, as previously discussed, grief and bereavement are issues that most older adults are likely to encounter at some point in their lives, whether it be normative grief or complicated bereavement.

In terms of recent studies, Heisel, Talbot, King, Tu, and Duberstein (2015) adapted IPT for older adults at risk for suicide. In this small, uncontrolled pilot trial, seventeen older adults received a sixteen-session course of IPT that focused on discussions of suicide risk, enhancing meaning in life (MIL), and psychological well-being. In terms of MIL, they further focused on participants' existential concerns, helping them to find meaning and cultivate meaningful relationships. At posttest, participants showed enhanced psychological well-being, as well as reduced symptoms of depression and suicidal ideation. While further replications are needed with control comparisons, the findings suggest that tailored IPT for older adults may be worth pursuing. The aforementioned study by Shear et al. (2014) found that IPT was beneficial in helping older adults with complicated bereavement, although not as effective as specific complicated grief therapy. Given the robust evidence base for IPT for depression at other developmental stages, it would seem that further trials are worth pursuing on IPT for older adults. For the interested reader, Hinrichsen and Clougherty (2006) have devoted an entire book to the specific application of IPT to depressed older adults.

Mindfulness-Based Interventions

Mindfulness-based interventions (MBIs) are included in what are considered "third-wave" psychotherapies, a heterogeneous group of psychotherapy interventions that have proven effectiveness, particularly in clinical populations that have been seen as difficult to treat (Kahl, Winter, & Schweiger, 2012). Examples of third-wave psychotherapies include mindfulness-based cognitive therapy (MBCT; Segal, Williams, & Teasdale, 2012), mindfulness-based stress reduction (MBSR; Kabat-Zinn, 1990), dialectical behavior therapy (DBT; Linehan, 2015), and acceptance and commitment therapy (ACT; Hayes, Strosahl, & Wilson, 2012), a common ingredient of which is some component of mindfulness. There has been an explosion of research on various MBIs over the past decade, with evidence that it is effective for a variety of mental health issues, both those with primary psychiatric disorders (Hofmann, Sawyer, Witt, & Oh, 2010) and those with psychological disorders in the context of chronic illness (Bohlmeijer, Prenger, Taal, & Cuijpers, 2010). MBIs may be particularly relevant to older adults. Although CBT has been shown to be effective in older adults, there are ways in which it may be less beneficial or relevant. For example, challenging the validity of "negative thoughts" about losses and challenges in late life may be less productive because the thoughts themselves, while perhaps excessive, may not be unrealistic per se (Petkus & Wetherell, 2013). Conversely, MBIs focus more on de-identifying with thoughts rather than trying to change them, such that thoughts do not define who we are or our value in the world. This is one of the various rationales Gillanders and Laidlaw (2014) use in their conceptual framework supporting the application of ACT to older adults. ACT has much fewer empirical studies available than CBT or even other MBIs, but does show promise in this population. An additional benefit of MBIs for older adults may come in the form of cognitive enhancement, given the evidence that certain types of MBI such as MBSR can improve different aspects of cognitive function in both healthy and clinical populations (Chiesa et al., 2011; Gotink, Meijboom, Vernooij, Smits, & Hunink, 2016), including older adults (Gard et al., 2014; Luders, 2014; Smart et al., 2016; Smart & Segalowitz, 2017). We discuss just two of the recent reviews examining the potential benefit of MBI in older adults. This is likely to become an area of increasing focus given the proliferation of research on mindfulness in general, as well as the growing recognition that the aging population is growing rapidly and is in need of care.

Kishita, Takei, and Stewart (2016) conducted a meta-analysis of MBCT and ACT for anxiety and depression in older adults with a variety of physical and psychological conditions. Ten studies were included, five each of MBCT and ACT, with most delivered in a group format and most ($n = 7$) focused on community versus residential samples. Of these, seven reported significant reductions in anxiety, and nine reported significant reductions in depression, both with moderate effect sizes (Hedges's $g = 0.58$ and 0.55, respectively). However, the authors noted several methodological issues in the included trials, including a general lack of active control conditions (only found in one trial), significant methodological heterogeneity, and possible publication bias that may have led to an overestimate of the anxiety effect size specifically.

Geiger and colleagues (2016) also conducted a review to examine the impact of MBI trials on physical and emotional well-being in older adults. Fifteen studies were included in their review, seven of which used standard MBSR or MBCT, with the remaining studies using modified versions of these interventions tailored according to the particular sample (e.g., introduction of elements of age-related psychoeducation, shortening of practice sessions). Results across studies indicated generally positive effects on a variety of psychological variables such as depression, anxiety, stress, sleep problems, and rumination, although some studies found null results. Substantially more inconsistency was found in physical health outcomes, including immune response, blood pressure, and self-reported physical symptoms. Interestingly, the few studies that included a self-report measure of mindfulness consistently showed null effects. Geiger et al. noted that this could be because of high baseline scores resulting in a ceiling effect. That is, older adults in general may report higher levels of dispositional mindfulness due to increased attention to emotional goals and positive emotion as previously discussed within the context of Carstensen et al.'s (1999) socioemotional selectivity theory. As such, while the intervention may show positive impact in other areas, the self-report of mindfulness per se may show limited change as older adults already report high levels of this as an individual difference characteristic.

Similar to the Kishita et al.'s (2016) review, Geiger et al. (2016) noted methodological flaws and inconsistencies across studies that may account for some of the mixed findings, including inconsistent modification of protocols in some of the studies. However, rather than seeing this as a weakness, it may be the individual study authors' attempt to ascertain *effectiveness* rather than *efficacy*. That is, once a standard protocol has been shown to be effective using the most tightly controlled RCT design, the next step is to ascertain how that treatment performs in a typical clinical sample that is more complex and heterogeneous in presentation. Efficacy studies are easier to evaluate in a meta-analysis due to homogeneous application of the intervention, but this does not make effectiveness studies any less valid. Moreover, the lack of consistent findings in physical health outcomes is perhaps not surprising, given that older adults are likely to vary in the level of medical comorbidities, medication usage, and so on. If studies were able to stratify samples to tightly control for such variables, it is questionable how generalizable the resultant studies would be to the typical older adult.

Finally, neither the Kishita et al. (2016) nor the Geiger et al. (2016) review discussed the influence of cognitive status of participants in the various studies. Participants at different levels of cognitive decline may have unique psychological concerns (e.g., persons with MCI having specific fears about an uncertain future), as well as unique cognitive needs in terms of how the material is made accessible. This is the topic of our next section, as we provide suggestions on how to appropriately tailor psychological interventions for persons at different levels of cognitive decline.

Appropriate Tailoring of Interventions for Cognitive Decline

The interventions discussed in this section are evidence-based treatments that have documented efficacy in an older adult population. For clinicians and researchers familiar with the application of these protocols in other age groups and populations, it is important to note that specific modifications and adaptations are likely warranted when using these protocols with older adults. This is the process referred to as *tailoring* (Kreuter & Skinner, 2000). Tailoring can occur along many dimensions, but perhaps the one most salient to the current context is tailoring as a function of the individual's current level of cognitive decline. Mood and anxiety disorders could theoretically occur at any stage of the trajectory of cognitive decline. However, the manner in which the intervention is delivered needs to account for the client's current cognitive ability and include modifications, where necessary, to maximize the likelihood of positive impact.

The term *neuropsychotherapy* has been coined to refer to the process of tailoring psychotherapy for individuals with cognitive impairment, where psychotherapy is implemented as part of a holistic neurorehabilitation treatment plan (Judd, 1999). Neuropsychotherapy considers that the goals of therapy for persons with neurological disorders and cognitive impairment may differ from those clients with primary psychiatric disorders. Likewise, therapy needs to be adapted and made accessible for clients with cognitive challenges. For example, many types of intervention involve the client engaging in activities between session (e.g., practicing mindfulness of breathing in MBSR, thought work in CBT). Before assigning these activities, one must consider whether the client has cognitive difficulties that will interfere with the implementation of such homework. In addition, cognitive difficulties may contraindicate certain interventions entirely (e.g., severely impaired abstract reasoning likely precludes cognitive restructuring in CBT). The interventions discussed in Chapter 10 can be used not only for the primary purpose of improving current cognitive function, but also for providing effective psychotherapy. Below we present some examples of neuropsychotherapy tailoring. These can be applied to the evidence-based treatments discussed in this section, but they would apply equally to other types of interventions discussed in this chapter (e.g., life review therapy, grief therapy).

Episodic Memory Difficulties

Clients with episodic memory difficulties may benefit from having a therapy journal that is used to record information from each session, as well as keeping track of any homework exercises (e.g., tracking negative automatic thoughts, remembering positive reframing of negative thoughts). The journal can be referred to each day to promote consolidation of information. Of course, if the client has difficulties with memory, he or she may forget to check the journal. Thus, before the formal psychological homework tasks can be implemented, several sessions may be needed to implement use of the therapy journal. Procedural memory is one form of memory comparatively robust to late-life cognitive decline, even as other forms of memory are declining (Seidler et al., 2012; Voelcker-Rehage, 2008). Procedural memory can be harnessed to develop a habit of keeping the therapy journal in the same place and checking it at the same time every day (e.g., placing it by the nightstand and checking it before bed). In implementing this habit, the client could be cued by an alarm or by a prompt from a partner or family member. After the implicit memory of checking the journal has been established, then the journal can be used for more traditional psychological homework exercises. Family involvement at this stage could be particularly productive if it facilitates episodic memory retrieval of important events to be recorded in the journal. Aside from structured therapy exercises, a therapy journal could be a way to record personal narratives in life review therapy, as discussed in the previous section. A therapy journal can also be a place for clients to write out, in their own words, the purpose of discrete therapy exercises and how these can move them closer to their own goals. This tool can be used to build intrinsic motivation, which is an essential part of any cognitive or psychological intervention.

Prospective Memory Difficulties

Various forms of therapy utilize behavioral practice. Considering the work on neuroplasticity, clients are likely to benefit to the extent that they regularly engage in such practice. However, difficulties with prospective memory may mean forgetting to engage in such practice on a regular basis. External cueing can be employed to remind the client to engage in practice. This could be accomplished through a smartphone or other device with an auditory alarm. Of course, if the client has episodic memory difficulties as well, the cue in and of itself may not remind the client what is to be done. Many smartphones have alarms that can be programmed with a label (e.g., "time for thought record"), or a written sign could be placed next to any other form of alarm being used.

Language Difficulties

Language difficulties do not necessarily preclude an individual's engagement with psychotherapy, but it requires the clinician to be more creative in being able to harness the client's experience in a meaningful way to bring into session. Art therapy is often employed in individuals with dementia as a means of cognitive stimulation (Chancellor, Duncan, & Chatterjee, 2013; Cowl & Gaugler, 2014; Young, Camic, & Tischler, 2016), but artistic formats could also be used to facilitate engagement in higher functioning clients. For example, instead of completing a thought record, a client may wish to draw or paint his or her responses. Likewise, instead of keeping a written therapy journal, a client may wish to photograph salient events across the day. Wearable cameras such as SenseCam have been investigated in individuals with various forms of anterograde amnesia as a means to investigate and remediate memory impairment (Allé et al., 2017). An additional benefit of photographs or video is that they may be more emotionally evocative than written material, which in turn benefits memory, given that affectively salient material has been shown to be subject to deeper levels of encoding (Kensinger, Allard, & Krendl, 2014; LaBar & Cabeza, 2006). Finally, clients may have issues with comprehension (or concept formation) that interfere with understanding therapy tasks. At the end of each session, it is important to take time to review the session material and have the client report back in his or her own words the main "take-home points," as well as his or her understanding of the purpose and benefits of any homework exercises. Clients should be encouraged to record such understanding in their therapy journal.

Executive Dysfunction

Issues with executive dysfunction could impact psychotherapy in a variety of ways. In particular, there is some evidence to suggest that older adults with executive dysfunction show less benefit from CBT (Mohlman & Gorman, 2005). Executive dysfunction is a broad term that applies to several different discrete processes, each of which may impact psychotherapy participation in unique ways and requires its own strategy for management. For clients who have difficulty with planning and organization, the aforementioned therapy journal could serve an additional benefit beyond memory, if the journal is organized into different sections pertaining to different aspects of the client's life. Ensuring that the client only ever uses the one book is also likely to be more productive for a client who may otherwise take notes in many different journals that could be lost or misplaced. For clients with difficulty in conceptual thinking, the use of visual imagery or analogy can prove helpful to convey abstract concepts. For example, in MBSR, one useful analogy is to describe the mind as being like the sky, open and clear, while the negative or difficult thoughts are merely clouds passing by. For clients with difficulties in emergent awareness (Crosson et al., 1989), they may intellectually grasp that they have a problem (e.g., negative thinking, emotional reactivity) but be unable to track in the moment when it is occurring. Having a smartphone or other alarm that sounds multiple times a day can act as an external aid to cue the clients to attend to their present moment experience as a way to cultivate this ability. While various types of executive difficulties can be accommodated, as we noted earlier, perseveration and inability to engage in abstract reasoning may be contraindications for CBT, and so in these cases it may be fruitful to explore other therapeutic approaches instead.

In sum, many evidence-based treatments for younger and middle-aged populations can be effectively used with older adults. For those who are showing significant cognitive decline, modifications can be made to support full participation and benefit from those treatments. However, cognitive or neurobehavioral impairment may be so significant as to preclude these approaches. In the next section we discuss some therapeutic approaches that may be beneficial for clients at this level of impairment.

Neuropsychiatric and Neurobehavioral Syndromes

The prior two sections describe circumstances under which an older adult may develop psychological distress associated with situational factors or a long-standing, premorbid history of such issues. In complement to these contexts, older adults may present with symptoms and syndromes that are neurogenic in origin (i.e., endogenous to an underlying neurological disease process). Some examples include hallucinations associated with DLB, delusional misidentification syndromes such as Capgras syndrome, and dopamine dysregulation syndrome associated with dopamine agonist overuse in movement disorders. Some of these neuropsychiatric symptoms and syndromes may be associated with cognitive impairment that improves with treatment (e.g., delirium associated with a urinary tract infection). Conversely, symptoms can appear iatrogenically in relation to medication prescribed for another condition, such as impulse control disorders. Accordingly, it is crucial that a comprehensive medical work-up be completed on any older adult presenting with neuropsychiatric symptoms, as treating any underlying conditions may likewise attenuate these symptoms. Pharmacological management of an underlying neurodegenerative disease process may also attenuate symptoms, such as PD. Conversely, treating physicians may wish to explore psychotropic medications to manage neuropsychiatric symptoms (Kales, Gitlin, & Lysekos, 2015), although medications cannot be relied on, given the many challenges associated with use of pharmacological agents in the elderly. Even though symptoms may be neurogenic in origin, this presents a unique opportunity for psychologists to bring their skills and expertise in psychological interventions to help manage some of these difficult symptoms.

Psychosis in Late Life

There are a variety of causes for psychosis in older adulthood, including long-standing, premorbid conditions such as schizophrenia and bipolar disorder. If the disorder is long-standing, the individual may already be maintained on an effective treatment regimen. However, much more common in older adulthood is psychosis associated with both delirium and dementia. Jeste and Finkel (2000) compared the features of psychosis due to AD as compared with schizophrenia, suggesting that the phenomenology of these disorders is quite distinct, sufficiently different to be considered separate syndromes. For example, while auditory hallucinations are common in schizophrenia, visual hallucinations are much more common in AD (and also DLB). Another feature more common to dementia-related psychosis is the presence of delusional misidentification syndromes (DMS). The most well-known DMS is Capgras syndrome, in which the affected individual believes that another person, usually someone with whom he or she is close, has been replaced by an imposter. Paranoia often co-occurs with Capgras syndrome, whereby the imposter or "evil twin" is associated with malevolent intentions toward the individual. Other reduplications can occur, for example, for places such as one's home (i.e., reduplicative paramnesia) and for strangers who are misidentified as friends or family members (i.e., Fregoli syndrome) (Cipriani et al., 2013). Despite the striking nature of these symptoms, we have found that often clients will not disclose them unless a specific inquiry about them is made. Thus, it is crucial that screening questions about psychosis and DMS be included in any psychological intake; they may include the following:

- "Have you ever had the feeling that someone close to you had a twin or a double? Did that ever make you uncomfortable or afraid?"
- "Have you ever had the feeling that there were two versions of the same place, like two versions of your home or your hometown?"
- "Do you ever have the feeling that people are out to hurt you or harm you in some way?"
- "Do you ever have the experience of seeing things that other people can't see or hearing things that other people can't hear?"

Ceglowski, de Dios, and Depp (2014) reviewed the available literature on psychosis in older adults, noting that, despite its common occurrence, there is still a limited understanding of how to manage it effectively. This is particularly concerning, given the high caregiver burden associated with neuropsychiatric symptoms such as psychosis. As noted in Chapter 9, while pharmacological agents are a first-line treatment for earlier-onset psychotic presentations such as schizophrenia, there are serious cautions about using antipsychotic medications in older adults due to the elevated risks of morbidity and mortality. This puts a heavy emphasis on the need for psychological interventions to manage these symptoms. Fortunately, there is an accumulating evidence base in support of cognitive behavioral social skills training (CBSST), a form of cognitive-behavioral therapy combined with social skills training to improve everyday function in individuals with psychotic disorders (Granholm, McQuaid, & Holden, 2016). A meta-analysis of thirty-five CBT trials indicated improvement not only for positive symptoms, but also for negative symptoms and everyday functioning (Wykes, Steel, Everitt, & Tarrier, 2008).

Granholm, Holden, Link, McQuaid, and Jeste (2013) have evaluated the application of CBSST specifically to middle-aged and older participants with schizophrenia and schizoaffective disorder. Sixty-four participants were randomized to either CBSST or supportive group contact. The active treatment consisted of thirty-six weekly group sessions over a course of 9 months. A thought-challenging module was used to address defeatist and ageist beliefs (e.g., "I'm too old to change"), as well as frank delusional beliefs (e.g., "Spirits will harm me"). Two other modules focused on social skills training and problem-solving skills, respectively. Results indicated that, compared to the control condition, CBSST led to significant post-treatment improvements in functioning and skills acquisition. Both groups improved on measures of negative symptoms (e.g., motivation), anxiety, depression, life satisfaction, and positive self-esteem. Interestingly, in an earlier study by this same group, Granholm and colleagues (2008) examined the influence of baseline neuropsychological function on response to CBSST versus treatment-as-usual (TAU) in older persons with schizophrenia. They found that although poorer neuropsychological performance was associated with poorer functional outcome for both treatment groups, the effect sizes for the active intervention were the same regardless of whether neuropsychological impairment was rated mild or severe. As such, CBSST improved functioning relative to TAU, even for persons with substantial neuropsychological impairment. Taken together, these findings suggest that CBSST for DMS or dementia-related psychosis may be worth pursuing. For the reader interested in learning more about CBSST, a clinician's treatment manual by Granholm et al. (2016) is available.

One of the biggest challenges with DMS and psychosis is that they can lead to agitation and escalate the possibility of harm to self or other.

Clinically we have observed that, despite their best intentions, family and caregivers often inadvertently escalate agitation by arguing with the client's delusions. In general, we have found that it is beneficial to provide psychoeducation to both family and health care providers (e.g., physicians, nurses, home health care aides) on the nature of DMS as well as how to minimize agitation. One area of future investigation (and clinical application) could be to involve family as co-therapists, teaching them rudimentary CBT skills such as those incorporated in CBSST, as a way to engage with the client's delusions without escalating the agitation. The studies by Paukert et al. (2010, 2013) indicated that modified CBT for anxiety in dementia was helpful when family members were trained to act as collateral therapists. While outside the realm of older adults, Landa and colleagues (2016) obtained promising results in response to a group and family-based CBT program for adolescents and young adults at risk for psychosis where family were taught how to apply basic CBT skills. In addition, recovery-oriented CBT for psychosis recommends placing the client's recovery and goals at the center of treatment, rather than reducing symptoms such as delusions. Symptoms are directly addressed when they interfere with the achievement of the client's goals (Grant, Huh, Perivoliotis, Stolar, & Beck, 2012). This goal-oriented approach is very much in line with the approach we advocated in Chapter 11 on cognitive and behavioral interventions. In a later section, we provide a case example of an older adult we worked with who had DMS following a traumatic brain injury.

Agitation and Challenging Behaviors

In the context of both delirium and dementia, an older adult can present not only with cognitive disturbance but also agitation and challenging behaviors. These behaviors can manifest themselves in a variety of ways, including hitting, punching, kicking, swearing, and spitting, to name just a few examples. The source of such behaviors is likely multifactorial and can include physical difficulties, perceptual difficulties, metabolic changes, drug effects, current and premorbid emotional state, and current cognitive function (James, 2014; McGrath, 2008). In persons with dementia, agitation also seems to increase during the transition from day to night, a phenomenon referred to as sundowning (Alzheimer's Association, 2017). While anxiolytics and antipsychotics can be prescribed to calm these symptoms, many physicians are understandably reticent to prescribe these medications, and if they do, certainly for only a brief period of time. As we have emphasized, the use of pharmacological agents in older adults, particularly antipsychotic medication, should come with extreme caution, owing to the increased risk of morbidity and mortality associated with these agents. This makes it more imperative that clinicians seek out nonpharmacological approaches to manage agitation and challenging behaviors.

James (2014) has provided a comprehensive review of nonpharmacological intervention approaches in treating dementia, including behavioral approaches, reality orientation therapy (nowadays subsumed under cognitive stimulation), multisensory stimulation, environmental manipulation, and music therapy, to name just a few. In most cases, James found that the available evidence was either very limited or of questionable quality to permit broad statements about the efficacy of any one approach on its own or in comparison to other approaches. However, this may be a function of how the quality of evidence is adjudicated. The field tends to favor the conduct and publishing of RCTs as the primary form of robust evidence for an intervention. While RCTs do have the most internally valid design, in many situations the application of an RCT model does not make sense. For example, being able to run an RCT usually means having a critical mass of participants who are randomized en masse to one versus another treatment and participants who are relatively homogeneous or present with one primary diagnosis. One can quickly see why this model might not work well in any evaluation of the efficacy of interventions for agitation and challenging behaviors. Instead, contributions to the evidence base could be made in this area by placing greater focus on rigorously controlled $n = 1$ case studies, only nine of which are required to meet the Chambless criteria for efficacious treatments (Chambless et al., 1998).

James (2014) has provided a model for how to apply CBT to older adults with challenging behaviors, but this approach requires that the client have some requisite level of cognitive function. This approach requires that the client have a grasp of the basics of the CBT model such as abstract reasoning, be able to link his or her own thoughts and behaviors to consequences, and so on. For many older adults with challenging behaviors in the context of dementia, this approach may not be tractable owing to the scope of cognitive impairment. From a practical clinical standpoint, principles of behaviorism and behavioral therapy may be effective in older adults with greater levels of cognitive impairment. The benefit of a behaviorist approach is that it places minimal cognitive demands on the individual, which makes its use particularly appealing in individuals with severe cognitive impairment and even anosognosia. Moniz-Cook et al. (2012) conducted a *Cochrane Review* of eighteen multicomponent programs that included a behavioral component. The available evidence was inconclusive but promising, noting positive postintervention effects for the frequency of challenging behavior (but not incidence or severity), and also for caregiver reactions to such behavior (but not burden or depression).

In creating a case formulation for dealing with agitation and challenging behaviors, it is crucial to create a biopsychosocial analysis of the context of these behaviors, given that their causes and contributors are likely multifactorial (James, 2014). Moreover, a solid grasp of principles of reinforcement learning and conditioning will inform how the maladaptive behavior can be extinguished in favor of more adaptive behaviors. For the clinician who is relatively inexperienced in behavioral approaches, we recommend Karen Pryor's (2006) *Don't Shoot the Dog!* Although this book discusses behavior modification in a canine context, it deftly illustrates the way that behavioral therapy can work in clients who cannot communicate the sources of their distress or lack the cognitive capacity to engage in other types of therapies. Another useful, practical resource is McGrath (2008)'s work on individuals with severe brain injury in an inpatient context, where many of the same types of challenging behaviors may be observed as in older adults with dementia or severe cognitive impairment. In our case example of a client with DMS, we discuss the application of behavioral principles in decreasing agitation and challenging behaviors, including the use of McGrath's (2008) behavioral analysis decision tree.

Impulse Control Disorders

PD is a neurodegenerative disease associated with progressive loss of dopaminergic neurons in the nigrostriatal pathways. Motor impairment associated with PD is typically treated by medications that increase dopaminergic availability, including L-dopa (a dopamine precursor) and dopamine agonists. These medications can be quite effective in improving motor function, although individuals with PD typically need to take them in the long term to maintain functionality. Unfortunately, the last decade has revealed that long-term usage can result in significant neurobehavioral side effects for a significant minority of persons. Impulse control disorders (ICD) pertain to a class of disorders that involve maladaptive behaviors associated with a loss of impulse control, including disinhibition and repetitive, purposeless behaviors. For example, persons with PD have been observed to develop ICD such as pathological gambling, hypersexuality, and compulsive eating and shopping.

Dopamine dysregulation syndrome (DDS) refers to a specific form of ICD that is associated with overuse of dopamine agonists. Often, DDS may start as a response to severe anxiety about "off" periods (i.e., fluctuations in motor function as a particular medication dose wears off), whereby individuals hoard their medication and then take in higher-than-usual quantities. However, over time, affected individuals experience positive hedonic states associated with this overuse in a manner similar to addiction, a symptom referred to as hedonic homeostatic dysregulation. Additional symptoms of DDS including *punding* (i.e., purposeless, stereotyped motor behaviors such as compulsively checking or manipulating objects, writing and rewriting emails) and *walkabouts* (i.e., where clients will literally go walking for hours at a time, often when large amounts of dopamine agonists have been ingested).

Similar to DMS, we have found that, unless clients are specifically asked, they may not spontaneously disclose symptoms of ICD. Although advanced PD can be associated with cognitive impairment such as executive dysfunction, persons with ICD and DDS often retain intellectual awareness about their maladaptive behavior, yet feel powerless to stop engaging in such behavior. This can cause additional psychological distress, embarrassment, and shame. Thus, it is crucial to ask sensitively, yet directly, about ICD and DDS in persons with PD, particularly those taking dopamine agonists. For those unfamiliar with ICD and DDS in PD, we refer the reader to Katzenschlager and Evans (2014) for a comprehensive overview of these syndromes.

Tanwani and colleagues (2015) conducted a systematic review of treatments for ICDs and related behaviors in PD. Seven studies met the criteria for inclusion. Although each study showed a positive effect on ICD symptoms, most of the studies were of lower quality (i.e., class IV evidence), suggesting a great need for a more robust evidence base. Six of the seven trials involved pharmacological intervention. The single psychological intervention reported was an RCT comparing CBT plus standard medical care versus medical care alone for forty-five individuals with ICD (Okai et al., 2013). The active intervention consisted of twelve nurse-led sessions that consisted of psychoeducation pertaining to treatment and potential adverse effects. Compared to the control condition, the active intervention was associated with a statistically significant reduction in impulse control behaviors ($p = .002$) and a decrease in overall severity of symptoms ($p = .004$).

There is a paucity of intervention research in this area, and this is not simply due to ICD and DDS being low base-rate disorders. In their review, Katzenschlager and Evans (2014) cite lifetime prevalence estimates as high as 13.7% for ICD. The behaviors associated with these conditions often cause embarrassment and shame to the sufferer, and clients may be reluctant to disclose these behaviors unless specifically asked about them. Thus, available figures may actually underestimate the true incidence and prevalence of these disorders. Nevertheless, given the potential for significant suffering caused by these conditions, it behooves professionals working with individuals with PD or those taking dopaminergic medications to inquire about the symptoms of these conditions. DDS in particular can be particularly challenging to manage. Although affected individuals may use their medications in a manner similar to other drugs of abuse, unlike many addictions, persons with PD truly need these medications to function motorically. Thus, abstinence may not be an option. Clearly, more research is required in this area.

In the interim, for clinicians working with individuals with ICD and DDS, existing empirically supported interventions can be used to target the symptoms of these disorders. For example, DDS often develops within a context of anxiety about "on"/"off" fluctuations, and hedonic homeostatic dysregulation is often associated with a belief that to be "on" is equivalent to feeling "high." If the client has the requisite cognitive capacity, CBT for anxiety may be useful to challenge erroneous thoughts such as catastrophizing about the impact of going "off" as well as misattributions about the experience of being "on." Psychoeducation about the therapeutic use of medication (versus seeking of hedonic states) may also be helpful. Conversely, motivational interviewing (MI) has been shown to be successful in addictions such as gambling (Yakovenko, Quigley, Hemmelgarn, Hodgins, & Ronksley, 2015), which is a common manifestation of ICD in PD. We have found clinically that persons with ICD often retain intellectual awareness of the maladaptive nature of their behavior, which suggests they could engage in some of the self-reflection and weighing of pros and cons involved in MI. Finally, family and caregiver involvement may also be useful, for example, to monitor access to medication, although this must be done in a sensitive manner so as not to remove the client's autonomy.

Family and Caregiver Functioning

Involving family and caregivers is often an integral part of the care of older adults all along the trajectory of cognitive decline. For example, cognitively normal older adults may experience changes in relational status associated with major life events such as retirement, relocation, and physical illness. Conversely, for those older adults with significant cognitive impairment such as MCI and dementia, caregiving can take a significant toll that is multifactorial, including the social, emotional, physical, and financial aspects of life (Beinart, Weiman, Wade, & Brady, 2012; Kales et al., 2015; Richardson, Lee, Berg-Weger, & Grossberg, 2013). Early work in the field of psychoneuroimmunology noted that caregivers of persons with AD continued to show suppressed immune function even after their loved one was deceased (Graham et al., 2006). Although caring for someone with cognitive impairment can be challenging, often it is the presence of neurobehavioral symptoms that creates the most distress for caregivers. Late-life psychosis is associated with significant caregiver burden (Ceglowski et al., 2014). Moreover, while greater levels of anosognosia are often found to be correlated to better psychological function in the affected individual, this lack of insight is associated with higher levels of distress in their caregivers (Kelleher, Tolea, & Galvin, 2015; Maki, Amari, Yamaguchi, Nakaaki, & Yamaguchi, 2012). In this section, we discuss the available evidence for psychological interventions specifically targeted to families and caregivers of older adults with cognitive and neurobehavioral impairments.

Review of Available Literature

In the last 5 years alone, a considerable number of evidence-based reviews and chapters have been written on the topic of family and caregiver interventions for persons with dementia, respecting the fact that this is an area of prominent interest for those serving the older adult population. Here we summarize and comment on just a selection of those recent empirical and theoretical reviews.

Providing information about dementia, how it may affect the client, and how the family can prepare for anticipated changes are important factors in supporting caregivers. Beinart and colleagues (2012) reviewed the literature on psychoeducation and caregiver burden in AD. They found that a lack of accurate information on AD, as well as a sense of moral obligation to provide complete care for their loved one, led families to withdraw from their social milieu, and in turn experience hopelessness and depression. Their review indicated that multicomponent interventions (e.g., including education and psychosocial support), as well as individually tailored interventions, were particularly effective in reducing caregiver burden. This finding echoes the observation of other reviews (e.g., Qualls, 2014) that families and caregivers have unique needs and challenges and must be supported accordingly.

Caregiving for a family member with dementia represents a chronic stressor over which the family may have limited perceived control, as well as facing chronic feelings of grief and ambiguous loss (Boss & Yeats, 2014). Earlier, we discussed the application of ACT to older adults in general (Gillanders & Laidlaw, 2014). Márquez-González, Losada, and Romero-Moreno (2014) recently explored the application of ACT for dementia caregivers. ACT acknowledges individuals' tendency to deploy experiential avoidance as a way of dealing with negative emotion, which may provide short-term relief from distress but is ultimately maladaptive. As such, ACT encourages clients to make contact with their present moment experience in a way that decreases the need for experiential avoidance. The appeal of ACT in this population is learning to tolerate what may be chronic emotional distress, as well as cultivate psychological flexibility and the ability to act in accordance with one's own values. While ACT holds theoretical promise for the alleviation of suffering in dementia caregivers, Márquez-González and colleagues note that, again, a limited amount of work has been pursued in this area, including only three pilot studies examining ACT or mindfulness-based interventions in this population. For readers interested in pursuing this work with caregivers, Márquez-González and colleagues (2014) provide a comprehensive theoretical explanation of how this therapy could be applied to dementia caregivers.

Many caregiver interventions may not be accessible for family members if they require that they have to leave their loved one at home while they come to a clinic for treatment. At best, such interventions may impose an extra financial burden on the family, who must now find a temporary caregiver to be with the client while the family attends therapy. With the advent of telehealth, researchers and clinicians are becoming more creative about how interventions are delivered, including across the Internet. Boots et al. (2014) have conducted a systematic review of Internet-based supportive interventions for caregivers of persons with dementia. They included twelve studies in the review, which represented one of four types of intervention: a website with information and support on caregiving; a website with additional caregiving strategies; a website with email support; and a website with a combination of individual work and exchange with other caregivers online. There was significant variation in the methods employed across studies (e.g., dosage, use of a control group), and the evidence overall was adjudicated as low quality. Fifty percent of studies showed a small but statistically significant effect on measures of caregiver well-being, including depression, sense of competence, self-efficacy, and decision-making confidence; yet no significant effects were found for caregiver burden. The interventions that seemed to create the most positive effects were multicomponent in nature (i.e., combining information, contact with other caregivers) and tailored to individual caregiving needs. These findings suggest that Internet-based interventions hold promise, and, with higher quality studies, more robust evidence may be found.

Practical Strategies for Supporting Families and Caregivers

As has been described, the literature on providing support to families and caregivers is mixed. However, one should not therefore assume that working with families does not provide some comfort or is not effective. The lack of consistent evidence is more likely a reflection of the fact that the needs of these individuals are very diverse and unique to the person and that a "one-size-fits-all" approach may not be appropriate. In her discussion of the application of family therapy for caregivers of persons with dementia, Qualls (2014) notes that the type of supports that families need is very individualized; such an idiographic application of family support is difficult to evaluate in RCTs, where the intention is to provide the same types of supports and strategies to all participants. Each family system is different and has different levels of function before a family member experiences cognitive decline. Moreover, different types of dementia will take a different toll on loved ones, from the prominent memory impairment in AD to the executive and neurobehavioral disturbances in FTLD and PD (Nunnemann, Kurz, Leucht, & Diehl-Schmid, 2012). Reviews such as those by Boots et al. (2014) support the contention that personalized intervention programs tend to be more effective than programs that are generic to all participants. Finally, family systems will differ in their relational style, understanding of dementia, and approach to caregiving as a function of cultural heritage (Pharr, Francis, Terry, & Clark, 2014), and this may be a dimension along which tailoring needs to occur (Napoles, Chadila, Eversley, & Moreno-John, 2010). In this context, culture may interface with religious or spiritual practices and coping styles, and room should be made for the diverse ways in which families cope with stress and make meaning of adversity. In this next section, we provide practical suggestions for how to support families and caregivers.

Psychoeducation

Psychoeducation is a standard intervention approach used both for persons with cognitive impairment and for their families and caregivers. We believe that families who are well informed will be more empowered to make choices that support their own goals and the goals of their loved one. As has been noted, Beinart and colleagues (2012) found evidence that psychoeducation, particularly when tailored to the individual caregivers, is beneficial. Psychoeducation often begins during the neuropsychological feedback session, but it can continue over the course of repeated visits occurring with treatment or repeat assessment. In terms of the content of psychoeducation, the first way to start is to provide education about the specific type of dementia or cognitive decline the individual is experiencing. Considering that "dementia" is not a global term, the specific effects on families may vary substantially according to the type of dementia involved. For example, in caring for a person with AD, family stress may come from the individual's eroding memory and associated lack of continuity in their relationships. For someone with DLB, stress may be associated with the presence of prominent visual hallucinations and paranoia. Finally, significant neurobehavioral impairment and features such as apathy and diminishing empathy can be particularly challenging for caregivers of individuals with FTLD and may relate to higher caregiving burden than AD (Nunnemann et al., 2012). For families who have some prior knowledge of dementia, it may be based primarily on AD, given its status as the most well-known and commonly diagnosed form of dementia. Thus, it may be surprising and confusing to have a loved one experiencing symptoms that are quite different from those expected if their loved one had AD. Being able to connect an individual's symptoms to a certain type of dementia can be validating, as well as signalling recognition and empathy for the family's difficulty in relating to these symptoms.

The content of psychoeducation will likely change over the course of a client's decline as a function of family and caregiver needs; thus:

- Initial phase—providing information about the diagnosis; linking observed behaviors to the particular diagnosis; providing strategies to families to help compensate for difficulties (e.g., using reminders/cueing) or avoid escalating agitation (e.g., refrain from arguing with delusional beliefs).
- While the client retains capacity, supporting the family and the

client in discussing choices about the future and preferences for care (e.g., health care proxy, living will).
- As decline continues, providing emotional validation and support for stress as well as possible grief reactions as their family member declines.

Ideally, the clinician will be monitoring a client over time with repeat assessment, thereby allowing the establishment of a relationship not only with the client but also the client's family and caregivers. Psychologists often have a luxury that physicians do not: they have much more face-to-face time to spend with their clients than physicians do. We have found that clients and their families are often extremely appreciative of this extra time, where a simple word or two of recognition or validation goes a long way. This developing relationship allows the clinician to unfold psychoeducation at a pace and in a manner that families can effectively integrate. Families will be going through their own emotional journey as their loved one declines, and this emotional toll will likely impact their information-processing capacity. In-person feedback meetings with the psychologist can be helpful and provide caring and reassurance, but one cannot assume that all of the factual information provided in those meetings will be retained. We find it helpful to provide additional resources that reinforce the information being given; that way, the family can review these resources at their leisure and follow up with questions at a later date. It is also important to strike a balance between being factual and not being overly pessimistic. In this technological age, the average client or family will often go to the Internet seeking information, and unfortunately much of the information available on dementia can foster a very depressing outlook. Fortunately, there are some excellent resources that clinicians can recommend to families and caregivers. For example, the University of California, San Francisco Memory and Aging Center has a comprehensive and very accessible set of resources and YouTube videos for caregivers (*http://memory. ucsf.edu/caregiving*). Specific resources for AD, FTLD, and PD can also be found through the Alzheimer's Association (*www.alz.org/care/overview. asp*), the Association for Frontotemporal Dementia (*www.theaftd.org*), and the Parkinson's Disease Foundation, respectively (*www.pdf.org/en/ caregiving_fam_issues*). Providing psychoeducation and neuropsychological feedback is, in and of itself, a nuanced and important skill to master. As noted elsewhere, an excellent resource to which we would refer the clinician is Armstrong and Postal's (2013) *Feedback That Sticks*.

Stress Management Techniques

The chronic stress associated with caregiving can take an emotional and physical toll, as discussed earlier on the research on psychoneuroimmunology.

Psychologists have a variety of techniques at their disposal that can support families in managing their stress, such as relaxation exercises, guided imagery, and deep breathing. Mindfulness-based psychotherapies may be particularly useful in this context; not only does mindfulness practice provide relief from stress and support emotional well-being, but it may also attend to some of the existential issues that arise from watching one's loved one experience cognitive decline. As noted earlier, ACT may be one such promising approach (Márquez-González et al., 2014). In engaging with caregivers, it is also important to emphasize their strengths as well as their challenges. In their review of the psychobiology of dementia caregiving, Harmell, Chattillion, Roepke, and Mausbach (2011) identified three broad resilience domains that may support caregiver health—personal mastery, self-efficacy, and coping style. These are useful domains to bear in mind when helping caregivers find sources of resilience.

Acknowledging the Grieving Process

As mentioned earlier, it is not uncommon for caregivers to experience ambiguous loss in the face of caring for a loved one with significant cognitive decline and dementia. While it is important to minimize the acute stressors associated with caregiving, there is an aspect of emotional experience that must be considered: the very real, and understandable, chronic grieving process that can occur in this context. For those interested in learning more about ambiguous loss, we direct the reader to Pauline Boss, the researcher and clinician who has become most synonymous with this topic. In particular, her book *Loving Someone Who Has Dementia* (Boss, 2011) is written for caregivers but would be a useful introduction to clinicians as well. In addition, the Alzheimer Society of Canada (2013) has created an excellent fact sheet for caregivers that explains the experience of ambiguous loss and includes many helpful strategies for self-care as well as other resources for support. As noted previously, it is imperative to take a culturally sensitive approach in this area, as norms for grieving are likely to differ significantly across cultural groups (Rosenblatt, 2012). Clinicians need to have some working knowledge of different cultural, religious, and spiritual practices involved in attending to matters of death and dying. Ultimately, however, clinicians should take the family as their own expert in this area, inquiring in an open-ended manner about how the family could use ritual and ceremony and finding ways to support them in this endeavor. As previously discussed, in this regard, Francis Weller's (2015) *Wild Edge of Sorrow* is an excellent resource for both clinicians and families. Weller discusses the normative aspects of grief and the necessity to do grief work in one's community. Encouraging families to grieve together and with other caregivers, in community, could go a long way to addressing the disenfranchisement that caregivers may feel.

Referrals to Other Providers

Families and caregivers will need different types of support at different times along the trajectory of their loved one's decline. While psychologists have a broad and diverse skill set, part of their role may be to triage families to other providers who can best fulfill those needs. For example, a need for emotional support may include referral to individual, couples, or family psychotherapy. In her chapter on family therapy with aging families, Qualls (2014) discusses caregiver family therapy—a specific family therapy model that may be beneficial in supporting families of persons with cognitive decline and dementia. Conversely, a need for instrumental support may involve referral to a social worker who can help with accessing financial and practical assistance or referral to an eldercare lawyer who can assist in advanced care planning decisions.

We conclude this chapter with a case presentation of Kate, a client with DMS; this case involved provision of care for the client, her family, and formal care staff. For additional case examples, we refer the reader to Chapter 11, where we discussed treating Sam through an approach that integrated cognitive/behavioral and psychological intervention.

> Kate is an 82-year-old, right-handed Canadian woman of European descent. She has spinal stenosis and osteoarthritis, but otherwise is relatively healthy with no major signs of cognitive decline or dementia. She copes with her pain quite well with over-the-counter medication and does not currently suffer from depression or anxiety. Two months ago, Kate was walking home from the grocery store when she was struck by a motor vehicle as she was crossing the street. As a result of this accident, she suffered a traumatic brain injury. Acute neuroimaging indicated frontoparietal contusions, which were greater on the right side, as well as mild diffuse axonal injury. Before the accident, Kate was living in her own apartment and was relatively independent. Unfortunately, since the accident, Kate has evidenced such severe behavioral disturbance that her children have had to procure full-time nursing care for her. They bring Kate in to our clinic for neuropsychological evaluation to understand her current problems and determine if any type of treatment could be beneficial.
>
> On interview, we discover that Kate seems to have developed Capgras syndrome since her accident. She is convinced that her daughter, Maria, has been replaced by multiple imposters, each of whom is trying to kill her. This is extremely distressing for Maria, as they previously had a very good relationship. More recently, Kate's Capgras syndrome seems to have extended to the nurses and aides in the care facility. She exhibits intense paranoia and believes that her room has been bugged with microphones and cameras. At times she becomes agitated to the point of requiring sedation. Most of the historical information is provided by Kate's daughter and son-in-law, as Kate seems

to have <u>anosognosia</u> and believes that everything is fine, other than the imposters trying to hurt her. Neuropsychometric testing indicates that Kate has an amnestic memory profile (i.e., impaired encoding, consolidation, and retrieval), visuospatial impairment, and executive dysfunction.

Working effectively with Kate involves trying to understand her behavior, its antecedents and consequences, as well as providing psychoeducation to the family and formal care staff so as to avoid escalating her agitation. To begin with, we took the following steps to derive a functional analysis of challenging behavior:

- We precisely defined the challenging behaviors (i.e., swearing and punching).
- We tracked the frequency and occurrence of those behaviors for a set period of time (i.e., over a 3-day period, at various points during the day).
- Next, we used a chi-square analysis to ascertain the time or contexts in which the maladaptive behaviors were most prevalent, determining that these behaviors were most prevalent under three conditions: (1) when her daughter came to visit, (2) at lunchtime, and (3) prior to dinnertime.
- Next, we examined the *antecedents* and *consequences* of acting out in the different contexts: (1) visits from her daughter triggered the experience of Capgras; (2) lunchtime was determined to be a period during the day when there was a lot of activity on the unit, and Kate's room was close to the nurses' station; and (3) changes in behavior prior to dinnertime were speculated to be a manifestation of sundowning. In each case, the other person would try to logically debate or argue with Kate about her delusions, which led to an escalation of the agitation until finally the other person left.

Next, we applied McGrath's (2008) behavioral analysis decision tree to further understand the context of Kate's challenging behaviors. This involved considering the following issues:

- *Is the behavior a response to an internal physiological state?* There was some concern that Kate's chronic pain was not adequately being managed and that her pain may have been worsening at the end of the day, increasing her irritability and tendency to act out. To address this possibility, her pain medication dose was increased and her response was monitored over subsequent days.
- *Is the level of stimulation appropriate?* Kate recently suffered a brain injury, and it is common for affected individuals to experience

sensitivity to sensory stimulation, which can lead to emotional dys-regulation. Kate's room was next to the nurses' station because the staff wanted to keep a close eye on her. However, lunchtime can be a quite chaotic and noisy time, and it was speculated that Kate would get overstimulated, further triggering her paranoia and challenging behaviors. To address this problem, we suggested to the staff that they move her to a room that was further from the nurses' station, but make more frequent check-ins to ensure she was doing okay. The staff was also encouraged to check in with Kate about the level of lighting and noise in her room; given her anosognosia, we could not assume that Kate would make the connection between overstimula-tion and becoming agitated.

- *Is the person confused or amnestic?* Formal assessment data revealed that Kate did have an amnestic memory profile, which likely con-tributed to her anosognosia. That is, Kate could not remember that she had suffered a brain injury and could not retain awareness that she was impaired, which further exacerbated her persecutory ide-ation and paranoia.

- *Is the behavior a response to a specific trigger in the environment?* As discussed, environmental stimulation was already identified as a possible trigger. A further trigger was the fact that Kate's daughter and the nursing staff would try to debate and argue with Kate in a logical way when she became paranoid. Given Kate's lack of aware-ness as well as her other cognitive impairments, this argumentation only served to escalate her agitation.

Kate's family had never heard of Capgras syndrome. Likewise, the staff in the care facility was more accustomed to working with clients with AD and other types of dementias, and were unfamiliar with how to work skillfully with individuals with DMS. Thus, it was necessary to provide some psychoeducation to both Kate's family and the formal caregivers, both to support Kate and to reduce stress and the burden stemming from having to navigate Kate's challenging behaviors. Following is an excerpt from a handout we created:

Kate is suffering from Capgras syndrome. Because of her injury, there has been a disconnect between her "emotional brain" and her "logical brain." She might look at her daughter Maria and visually recognize her, but something "feels off" to her. Because she has experienced a decline in logical reasoning (executive functions), she cannot make sense of the fact that things feel off. So her only other option is to assume that Maria and others are trying to hurt her. This process is not rational; trying to explain or debate with Kate does not work. In fact, this seems to make her more agitated. Our main goal in supporting Kate is to keep her calm and avoid letting her escalate into agitation. We have identified some environmental triggers, such as inadequate pain management and too much sensory stimulation. Another thing we can do is avoid arguing with Kate when she reports persecutory delusions. We can be empathic with Kate and reflect how distressing it might be to feel what she's feeling. We can also acknowledge what she is feeling and then redirect her attention to something else such as another topic of conversation (reflect-and-redirect). For example, Kate identified her grandchildren as a source of joy and happiness, so when Kate's delusions intensify, we could engage Kate in a conversation about them or have her knit something for them, as we know she likes to knit. If her acting out becomes extreme, we can engage in a "time-out on the spot" (TOOTS)—we let Kate know we are taking a time-out and walk to the other side of the room for a moment or two until she calms down. By employing TOOTS, we are removing positive reinforcement for her agitated behavior. In other words, if her agitated behavior gets no response, she is less likely to continue engaging in it. This approach will be most effective if we all agree to use it as consistently as possible.

After a month, Kate's family and care staff observed some reduction in her challenging behaviors. Kate continued to exhibit paranoia and persecutory delusions, but family and staff were able to deescalate her in these situations before things reached a level of agitation. Kate was still only 4 months postinjury at this point. Given that individuals with traumatic brain injury continue to show spontaneous recovery over the first year postinjury, we were hopeful that, over time, she might show some remittance of these symptoms, particularly if there was concurrent improvement in her cognitive function that could be used to build awareness of her difficulties. Kate's daughter, Maria, was able to have some interactions with her mother without triggering the Capgras delusions, but the delusions would still occur with some frequency. Maria was understandably very sad about this abrupt change in her relationship with her mother and had to remind herself that this was "not personal," but rather directly attributable to the brain injury. With therapeutic support, she was able to learn to notice and appreciate the positive moments with her mother when they did occur.

Summary and Conclusions

Provision of psychological care for older adults is a rich and engaging process, requiring the clinician to draw on a variety of skill sets and resources to provide such care. It is our hope that this chapter has introduced the reader to some of the major issues that might bring an older adult to clinical attention.

In addition to improving psychological well-being, boosting current psychological function can also provide the requisite stability and self-efficacy to facilitate an older adult's engagement in cognitive and behavioral interventions. At the same time, knowing the individual's current stage of cognitive decline is necessary in considering the most appropriate goals of psychotherapy for that individual, including where tailoring may be necessary to accommodate concurrent cognitive deficits. Relatedly, it is important to consider that some of the concerns an older adult presents with may be developmentally appropriate, such as grief associated with change in roles and activities as well as bereavement. While provision of support is appropriate in these cases, it is important not to pathologize what may be normative reactions to developmentally relevant life experiences.

The literature on psychological interventions is promising, containing evidence suggesting that many or most of the major empirically supported interventions for younger or working-age adults are effective with older adults. In certain areas of practice, such as anxiety disorders and psychosis, these interventions may carry even greater weight, given that medications for these conditions come with significant risks, if they are not contraindicated entirely. However, greater efforts need to be directed to establishing the effectiveness of these interventions in routine clinical practice, as well as the impact of tailoring (e.g., for level of cognitive decline). Particularly in the area of family and caregiver interventions, while there has been a proliferation of research in the last 5 to 10 years, the findings remain mixed owing to the observation that personalized, multicomponent interventions may be more impactful than many of the interventions that are more tightly controlled or disseminated in a homogeneous way. The single-case experimental design (Tate et al., 2016) that we have referred to previously provides one concrete avenue through which practitioners could begin to test and document the effectiveness of a variety of interventions in routine clinical practice with individual clients.

KEY POINTS

✓ Contrary to popular stereotypes, a majority of older adults approach aging with positive emotions and psychological well-being. At the same time, psychological interventions can benefit older adults by enhancing psychological health and secondarily improving cognitive function.

✓ Broad classes of clinical concerns include (1) those that are developmentally relevant, such as adjustment to change in late life, (2) diagnosable psychological conditions, (3) neuropsychiatric and neurobehavioral syndromes, and (4) family and caregiver functioning. Empirically supported approaches are available for each of these classes of clinical issue.

✓ Any intervention plan should begin with a comprehensive assessment of current and premorbid psychological functioning, as well as a consideration of factors that could negatively impact mental health (e.g., chronic illness, social support).

✓ Psychotherapy may need to be tailored to accommodate the older adult's current cognitive function, including difficulties with memory, language, and executive functions.

✓ Family and caregivers often require their own emotional support, and clinicians and researchers are encouraged to be innovative in how they make such supports accessible.

Core Questions Regarding Psychological Function to Be Asked during Assessment or Prior to Intervention

Premorbid Psychological History

_____ Prior psychiatric diagnoses (e.g., depression, anxiety, bipolar disorder, schizophrenia)

_____ Prior history of treatment (psychological or pharmacological)

_____ Premorbid personality factors (e.g., locus of control, self-efficacy, coping style)

_____ Developmental history

_____ Early family relationships

_____ Attachment style

_____ Developmental trauma

_____ Family mental health history

Psychosocial Context

_____ Attitudes toward mental health and treatment

_____ Cultural factors (e.g., language, acculturation, attitudes toward intervention)

_____ Socioeconomic factors that may influence treatment accessibility

_____ Social support

Current Psychological Function

_____ Symptoms of mood and anxiety disorders

_____ Suicidal ideation, plans, or intent; differentiate from desire to pursue medically assisted suicide

_____ Symptoms of psychosis (e.g., hallucinations, delusions such as Capgras syndrome, reduplicative paramnesia)

(continued)

For clients with movement disorders:

_____ Symptoms of ICD (e.g., pathological gambling, hypersexuality, compulsive shopping or eating)

_____ Symptoms of DDS (e.g., hoarding of medication, walkabouts, punding, hedonic homeostatic dysregulation)

Medical/Physiological Factors

_____ Sleep quality/presence of sleep disturbance

_____ Quality of nutrition/dietary habits/blood sugar management

_____ Current and past alcohol and substance use

_____ Comorbid medical conditions

_____ Current medications

_____ Reversible dementia work-up

Readiness for Intervention

_____ Stage of change; motivation for change

_____ Awareness/insight into current difficulties

_____ Clearly identifiable goals

_____ Family/caregiver support to engage in intervention

References

Aarts, S., van den Akker, M., Tan, F. E., Verhey, F. R., Metsemakers, J. F., & van Boxtel, M. P. (2011). Influence of multimorbidity on cognition in a normal aging population: A 12-year follow-up in the Maastricht Aging Study. *International Journal of Geriatric Psychiatry, 26*(10), 1046–1053.

Abbott, R. D., White, L. R., Ross, G. W., Masaki, K. H., Curb, J. D., & Petrovitch, H. (2004). Walking and dementia in physically capable elderly men. *JAMA, 292*(12), 1447–1453.

Abdulrab, K., & Heun, R. (2008). Subjective memory impairment: A review of its definitions indicates the need for a comprehensive set of standardized and validated criteria. *European Psychiatry, 23,* 321–330.

Adamis, D., Devaney, A., Shanahan, E., McCarthy, G., & Meagher, D. (2015). Defining "recovery" for delirium research: A systematic review. *Age and Ageing, 44*(2), 318–321.

Afonso, R. M., Bueno, B., Loureiro, M. J., & Pereira, H. (2011). Reminiscence, psychological well-being, and ego integrity in Portuguese elderly people. *Educational Gerontology, 37,* 1063–1080.

Ahmed, S., de Jager, C., & Wilcock, G. (2012). A comparison of screening tools for the assessment of mild cognitive impairment: Preliminary findings. *Neurocase, 18*(4), 336–351.

Alaszewski, A., Alaszewski, H., & Potter, J. (2004). The bereavement model, stroke and rehabilitation: A critical analysis of the use of a psychological model in professional practice. *Disability and Rehabilitation: An International, Multidisciplinary Journal, 26,* 1067–1078.

Albert, M., & Cohen, C. (1992). The Test for Severe Impairment: An instrument for the assessment of patients with severe cognitive dysfunction. *Journal of the American Geriatrics Society, 40*(5), 449–453.

Albert, M. S., DeKosky, S. T., Dickson, D., Dubois, B., Feldman, H. H., Fox, N. C., . . . Phelps, C. H. (2011). The diagnosis of mild cognitive impairment due to Alzheimer's disease: Recommendations from the National Institute on Aging-Alzheimer's Association workgroups on diagnostic guidelines for Alzheimer's disease. *Alzheimer's and Dementia, 7*(3), 270–279.

311

Albrecht, M. A., Masters, C. L., Ames, D., & Foster, J. K. (2016). Impact of mild head injury on neuropsychological performance in healthy older adults: Longitudinal assessment in the AIBL Cohort. *Frontiers in Aging Neuroscience, 8,* 105.

Ali, J. I., & Smart, C. M. (2016). Mourning me: An interpretive description of grief and identity loss in older adults with mild cognitive impairment. *Alzheimer's and Dementia, 12*(7, Suppl.), 302.

Alladi, S., Bak, T. H., Duggirala, V., Surampudi, B., Shailaja, M., Shukla, A. K., . . . Kaul, S. (2013). Bilingualism delays age at onset of dementia, independent of education and immigration status. *Neurology, 81*(22), 1938–1944.

Allan, C. L., Sexton, C. E., Filippini, N., Topiwala, A., Mahmood, A., Zsoldos, E., . . . Ebmeier, K. P. (2016). Sub-threshold depressive symptoms and brain structure: A magnetic resonance imaging study within the Whitehall II cohort. *Journal of Affective Disorders, 204,* 219–225.

Allaz, A.-F., & Cedraschi, C. (2015). Emotional aspects of chronic pain. In G. Pickering & S. Gibson (Eds.), *Pain, emotion and cognition: A complex nexus* (pp. 21–34). New York: Springer.

Allé, M. C., Manning, L., Potheegadoo, J., Coutelle, R., Danion, J.-M., & Berna, F. (2017). Wearable cameras are useful tools to investigate and remediate autobiographical memory impairment: A systematic PRISMA review. *Neuropsychology Review, 27*(1), 81–99.

Almeida, O. P., Hulse, G. K., Lawrence, D., & Flicker, L. (2002). Smoking as a risk factor for Alzheimer's disease: Contrasting evidence from a systematic review of case–control and cohort studies. *Addiction, 97*(1), 15–28.

Alzheimer Society of Canada. (2013). Ambiguous loss and grief in dementia: A resource for individuals and families. Retrieved February 18, 2017, from *www.alzheimer.ca/~/media/Files/national/Core-lit brochures/ambiguous_loss_family_e.pdf.*

Alzheimer's Association. (2017). Sleep issues and sundowning. Retrieved February 16, 2017, from *www.alz.org/care/alzheimers-dementia-sleep-issues-sundowning.asp.*

Alzheimer's Association. (n.d.). Vascular dementia. Retrieved January 23, 2017, from *www.alz.org/dementia/vascular-dementia-symptoms.asp.*

Alzheimer's Disease Neuroimaging Initiative. (2011). ADNI 2 defining Alzheimer's disease procedures manual. Retrieved February 4, 2017, from *http://adni.loni.usc.edu/wp content/uploads/2008/07/adni2-procedures-manual.pdf.*

Alzheimer's Disease Neuroimaging Initiative. (n.d.). About. Retrieved February 4, 2017, from *http://adni.loni.usc.edu/about.*

Amariglio, R. E., Becker, J. A., Carmasin, J., Wadsworth, L. P., Lorius, N., Sullivan, C., . . . Rentz, D. M. (2012). Subjective cognitive complaints and amyloid burden in cognitively normal older individuals. *Neuropsychologia, 50,* 2880–2886.

Amariglio, R. E., Townsend, M. K., Grodstein, F., Sperling, R. A., & Rentz, D. M. (2011). Specific subjective memory complaints in older persons may indicate poor cognitive function. *Journal of the American Geriatric Society, 59,* 1612–1617.

Amato, M. P., Zipoli, V., & Portaccio, E. (2006). Multiple sclerosis-related cognitive changes: A review of cross-sectional and longitudinal studies. *Journal of the Neurolgical Sciences, 245*(1–2), 41–46.

American Academy of Neurology. (n.d.). AAN guideline summary for clinicians: Detection, diagnosis and management of dementia. Retrieved January 23, 2017, from *http://tools.aan.com/professionals/practice/pdfs/dementia_guideline.pdf.*

American Bar Association Commission on Law and Aging & American Psychological Association. (2008). Assessment of older adults with diminished capacity: A handbook for psychologists. Retrieved from *www.apa.org/pi/aging/programs/assessment/capacity-psychologist-handbook.pdf*.

American Educational Research Association, American Psychological Association, National Council on Measurement in Education. (2014). *Standards for educational and psychological testing*. Washington, DC: Author.

American Geriatrics Society, Beers Criteria Update Expert Panel. (2015). American Geriatrics Society updated Beers criteria for potentially inappropriate medication use in older adults. *Journal of the American Geriatrics Society, 63*, 2227–2246.

American Psychiatric Association. (1994). *Diagnostic and statistical manual of mental disorders* (4th ed.). Washington, DC: Author.

American Psychiatric Association. (2013). *Diagnostic and statistical manual of mental disorders* (5th ed.). Arlington, VA: Author.

American Psychological Association. (2002). Ethical principles of psychologists and code of conduct. *American Psychologist, 57*(12), 1060–1073. Retrieved January 23, 2017, from *www.apa.org/ethics/code*.

American Psychological Association. (2010). 2010 amendments to the 2002 "Ethical principles of psychologists and code of conduct." *American Psychologist, 65*(5), 493.

American Psychological Association. (2012). Guidelines for the evaluation of dementia and age-related cognitive change. *American Psychologist, 67*(1), 1–9.

American Psychological Association. (2014). Guidelines for psychological practice with older adults. *American Psychologist, 69*(1), 34–65.

American Society for Pharmacology and Experimental Therapeutics. (n.d.). Explore pharmacology. Retrieved October 15, 2016, from *www.aspet.org/uploadedfiles/knowledge_center/pharmacology_resources/explorephm.pdf?n=7741*.

Amieva, H., Le Goff, M., Millet, X., Orgogozo, J. M., Peres, M., Barberger-Gateau, P., . . . Dartigues, J. F. (2008). Prodromal Alzheimer's disease: Successive emergence of the clinical symptoms. *Annals of Neurology, 64*, 492–498.

Amieva, H., Stoykova, R., Matharan, F., Helmer, C., Antonucci, T. C., & Dartigues, J.-F. (2010). What aspects of social network are protective for dementia?: Not the quantity but the quality of social interactions is protective up to 15 years later. *Psychosomatic Medicine, 72*(9), 905–911.

Andel, R., Crowe, M., Pedersen, N. L., Mortimer, J., Crimmins, E., Johansson, B., & Gatz, M. (2005). Complexity of work and risk of Alzheimer's disease: A population-based study of Swedish twins. *Journals of Gerontology: Series B: Psychological Sciences and Social Sciences, 60B*(5), P251–P258.

Andel, R., Kåreholt, I., Parker, M. G., Thorslund, M., & Gatz, M. (2007). Complexity of primary lifetime occupation and cognition in advanced old age. *Journal of Aging and Health, 19*(3), 397–415.

Andel, R., Vigen, C., Mack, W. J., Clark, L. J., & Gatz, M. (2006). The effect of education and occupational complexity on rate of cognitive decline in Alzheimer's patients. *Journal of the International Neuropsycholgical Society, 12*(1), 147–152.

Anderson, N. A., Murphy, K. J., & Troyer, A. K. (2012). *Living with mild cognitive impairment: A guide to maximizing brain health and reducing risk of dementia*. New York: Oxford University Press.

Anderson-Mooney, A. J., Schmitt, F. A., Head, E., Lott, I. T., & Heilman, K. M. (2016). Gait dyspraxia as a clinical marker of cognitive decline in Down syndrome: A review of theory and proposed mechanisms. *Brain and Cognition, 104*, 48–57.

Anstey, K. J., Cherbuin, N., & Herath, P. M. (2013). Development of a new method for assessing global risk of Alzheimer's disease for use in population health approaches to prevention. *Prevention Science, 14*(4), 411–421.

Anstey, K. J., Lipnicki, D. M., & Low, L.-F. (2008). Cholesterol as a risk factor for dementia and cognitive decline: A systematic review of prospective studies with meta-analysis. *American Journal of Geriatric Psychiatry, 16*(5), 343–354.

Antonell, A., Fortea, J., Rami, L., Bosch, B., Balasa, M., Sánchez-Valle, R., . . . Lladó, A. (2011). Different profiles of Alzheimer's disease cerebrospinal fluid biomarkers in controls and subjects with subjective memory complaints. *Journal of Neural Transmission (Vienna), 118,* 259–262.

Appollonio, I., Gori, C., Riva, G. P., Spiga, D., Ferrari, A., Ferrarese, C., & Frattola, L. (2001). Cognitive assessment of severe dementia: The test of severe impairment (TSI). *Archives of Gerontology and Geriatrics, 7*(Suppl.), 25–31.

Araujo, J. R., Martel, F., Borges, N., Araujo, J. M., & Keating, E. (2015). Folates and aging: Role in mild cognitive impairment, dementia and depression. *Ageing Research Review, 22,* 9–19.

Ardila, A. (2003). Culture in our brains: Cross-cultural differences in the brain-behavior relationships. In A. Toomela (Ed.), *Cultural guidance in the development of the human mind* (pp. 63–78). Westport, CT: Ablex.

Ardila, A. (2005). Cultural values underlying psychometric cognitive testing. *Neuropsychology Review, 15*(4), 185–195.

Ardila, A. (2007). The impact of culture on neuropsychological test performance. In B. P. Uzzell, M. Ponton, & A. Ardila (Eds.), *International handbook of cross-cultural neuropsychology* (pp. 23–44). Mahwah, NJ: Erlbaum.

Armstrong, C. L., & Morrow, L. (Eds.). (2010). *Handbook of medical neuropsychology: Applications of cognitive neuroscience.* New York: Springer Science + Business Media.

Armstrong, K., & Postal K. (2013). *Feedback that sticks: The art of effectively communicating neuropsychological assessment results.* New York: Oxford University Press.

Attems, J., & Jellinger, K. A. (2014). The overlap between vascular disease and Alzheimer's disease—lessons from pathology. *BMC Medicine, 12,* 206.

Attix, D. K., & Welsh-Bohmer, K. A. (Eds.). (2006). *Geriatric neuropsychology: Assessment and intervention.* New York: Guilford Press.

Auer, S. R., Sclan, S. G., Yaffee, R. A., & Reisberg, B. (1994). The neglected half of Alzheimer disease: Cognitive and functional concomitants of severe dementia. *Journal of the American Geriatrics Society, 42*(12), 1266–1272.

Australian and New Zealand Society for Geriatric Medicine. (2016). Position statement—Delirium in older people. *Australasian Journal on Ageing, 35*(4), 292.

Azulay, J., Smart, C. M., Mott, T., & Cicerone, K. D. (2013). A pilot study examining the effect of mindfulness-based stress reduction on symptoms of chronic mild traumatic brain injury/post-concussive syndrome. *Journal of Head Trauma Rehabilitation, 28,* 323–331.

Bahar-Fuchs, A., Clare, L., & Woods, B. (2013). Cognitive training and cognitive rehabilitation for mild to moderate Alzheimer's disease and vascular dementia [Review]. *Cochrane Database of Systematic Reviews, 6,* CD003260

Bak, T. H., Nissan, J. J., Allerhand, M. M., & Deary, I. J. (2014). Does bilingualism influence cognitive aging? *Annals of Neurology, 75*(6), 959–963.

Ball, K., Berch, D. B., Helmers, K. F., Jobe, J. B., Leveck, M. D., Marsiske, M., . . . the Advanced Cognitive Training for Independent and Vital Elderly Study Group.

(2002). Effects of cognitive training interventions with older adults: A randomized controlled trial. *Journal of the American Medical Association, 288,* 2271–2281.

Baltes, P. B. (1987). Theoretical propositions of life-span developmental psychology: On the dynamics between growth and decline. *Developmental Psychology, 23*(5), 611–626.

Baltes, P. B., & Baltes, M. M. (1990). Psychological perspectives on successful aging: The model of selective optimization with compensation. In P. B. Baltes & M. M. Baltes (Eds.), *Successful aging: Perspectives from the behavioral sciences* (pp. 1–34). New York: Cambridge University Press.

Bandura, A. (1994). Self-efficacy. In V. S. Ramachandran (Ed.), *Encyclopedia of human behavior* (Vol. 4, pp. 71–81). New York: Academic Press.

Barnes, D. E., Cenzer, I. S., Yaffe, K., Ritchie, C. S., & Lee, S. J. (2014). A point-based tool to predict conversion from mild cognitive impairment to probable Alzheimer's disease. *Alzheimer's and Dementia, 10*(6), 646–655.

Barnes, D. E., Covinsky, K. E., Whitmer, R. A., Kuller, L. H., Lopez, O. L., & Yaffe, K. (2009). Predicting risk of dementia in older adults: The late-life dementia risk index. *Neurology, 73*(3), 173–179.

Barnes, D. E., & Yaffe, K. (2011). The projected effect of risk factor reduction on Alzheimer's disease prevalence. *The Lancet Neurology, 10*(9), 819–828.

Barrios, P. G., Pabon, R. G., Hanna, S. M., Lunde, A. M., Fields, J. A., Locke, D. E. C., & Smith, G. E. (2016). Priority of treatment outcomes for caregivers and patients with mild cognitive impairment: Preliminary analyses. *Neurology and Therapy,* 1–10.

Baskys, A. (2004). Lewy body dementia: The litmus test for neuroleptic sensitivity and extrapyramidal symptoms. *Journal of Clinical Psychiatry, 65*(Suppl. 1), 16–22.

Bassuk, S. S., Glass, T. A., & Berkman, L. F. (1999). Social disengagement and incident cognitive decline in community-dwelling elderly persons. *Annals of Internal Medicine, 131*(3), 165–173.

Beard, R. L., & Neary, T. M. (2013). Making sense of nonsense: Experiences of mild cognitive impairment. *Sociology of Health and Illness, 35,* 130–146.

Beauchamp, T. L., & Childress, J. F. (2009). *Principles of biomedical ethics* (6th ed.). New York: Oxford University Press.

Beaudoin, M., & Desrichards, O. (2011). Are memory self-efficacy and memory performance related?: A meta-analysis. *Psychological Bulletin, 137,* 211–241.

Bechara, A. (2007). *Iowa gambling task.* Lutz, FL: Psychological Assessment Resources.

Bechara, A., Damasio, A. R., Damasio, H., & Anderson, S. W. (1994). Insensitivity to future consequences following damage to human prefrontal cortex. *Cognition, 50,* 7–15.

Beck, J. S. (2011). *Cognitive behavior therapy: Basics and beyond* (2nd ed.). New York: Guilford Press.

Beinart, N., Weinman, J., Wade, D., & Brady, R. (2012). Caregiver burden and psychoeducational interventions in Alzheimer's disease: A review. *Dementia and Geriatric Cognitive Disorders Extra, 2,* 638–648.

Beland, F., Zunzunegui, M. V., Alvarado, B., Otero, A., & Del Ser, T. (2005). Trajectories of cognitive decline and social relations. *Journals of Gerontology: Series B: Psychological Sciences Social Sciences, 60*(6), 320–330.

Ben-Porath, Y., & Tellegen, A. (2008). *Minnesota Multiphasic Personality Inventory-2—Restructured Format.* San Antonio, TX: Pearson Assessments.

Ben-Yishay, Y., & Gold, J. (1990). Therapeutic milieu approach to neuropsychological rehabilitation. In R. L. Wood (Ed.), *Neurobehavioural sequelae of traumatic brain injury* (pp. 194–218). London: Taylor & Francis.

Bergman, I., & Almkvist, O. (2015). Neuropsychological test norms controlled for physical health: Does it matter? *Scandinavian Journal of Psychology, 56*(2), 140–150.

Berkman, L. F., Glass, T., Brissette, I., & Seeman, T. E. (2000). From social integration to health: Durkheim in the new millennium. *Social Sciences and Medicine, 51*(6), 843–857.

Bhar, S. S. (2014). Reminiscence therapy: A review. In N. A. Pachana & K. Laidlaw (Eds.), *The Oxford handbook of clinical geropsychology* (pp. 675–690). New York: Oxford University Press.

Bialystok, E., Craik, F. I., Binns, M. A., Ossher, L., & Freedman, M. (2014). Effects of bilingualism on the age of onset and progression of MCI and AD: Evidence from executive function tests. *Neuropsychology, 28*(2), 290–304.

Bialystok, E., Craik, F. I., & Freedman, M. (2007). Bilingualism as a protection against the onset of symptoms of dementia. *Neuropsychologia, 45*(2), 459–464.

Bielak, A. A. M., Hultsch, D. F., Strauss, E., MacDonald, S. W. S., & Hunter, M. A. (2010). Intraindividual variability in reaction time predicts cognitive outcomes 5 years later. *Neuropsychology, 24*(6), 731–741.

Billioti de Gage, S., Moride, Y., Ducruet, T., Kurth, T., Verdoux, H., Tournier, M., . . . Begaud, B. (2014). Benzodiazepine use and risk of Alzheimer's disease: Case–control study. *British Medical Journal, 349,* g5205.

Birks, J. (2006, January 25). Cholinesterase inhibitors for Alzheimer's disease. *Cochrane Database of Systematic Reviews, 1,* CD005593.

Birks, J., McGuinness, B., & Craig, D. (2013). Rivastigmine for vascular cognitive impairment. *Database of Systematic Reviews, 5,* CD004744.

Bittles, A. H., Petterson, B. A., Sullivan, S. G., Hussain, R., Glasson, E. J., & Montgomery, P. D. (2002). The influence of intellectual disability on life expectancy. *Journals of Gerontology: Series A: Biological Sciences and Medical Sciences, 57*(7), M470–M472.

Blacker, D., Lee, H., Muzikansky, A., Martin, E. C., Tanzi, R., McArdle, J. J., . . . Albert, M. (2007). Neuropsychological measures in normal individuals that predict subsequent cognitive decline. *Archives of Neurology, 64,* 862–871.

Blackford, R. C., & La Rue, A. (1989). Criteria for diagnosing age-associated memory impairment: Proposed improvements for the field. *Developmental Neuropsychology, 5,* 295–306.

Blom, K., Emmelot-Vonk, M. H., & Koek, H. L. (2013). The influence of vascular risk factors on cognitive decline in patients with dementia: A systematic review. *Maturitas, 76*(2), 113–117.

Bohlmeijer, E., Prenger, R., Taal, E., & Cuijpers, P. (2010). The effects of mindfulness-based stress reduction therapy on mental health of adults with a chronic medical disease: A meta-analysis. *Journal of Psychosomatic Research, 68,* 539–544.

Boller, F., Verny, M., Hugonot-Diener, L., & Saxton, J. (2002). Clinical features and assessment of severe dementia: A review. *European Journal of Neurology, 9*(2), 125–136.

Bond, M., Rogers, G., Peters, J., Anderson, R., Hoyle, M., Miners, A., . . . & Hyde, C. (2012). The effectiveness and cost-effectiveness of donepezil, galantamine, rivastigmine and memantine for the treatment of Alzheimer's disease (review of Technology Appraisal No. 111): A systematic review and economic model. *Health Technology Assessment, 16,* 1–470.

Bondi, M. W., Edmonds, E. C., Jak, A. J., Clark, L. R., Delano-Wood, L., McDonald, C. R., . . . the Alzheimer's Disease Neuroimaging Initiative. (2014). Neuropsychological criteria for mild cognitive impairment improves diagnostic precision, biomarker associations, and progression rates. *Journal of Alzheimer's Disease, 42,* 275–289.

Bondi, M. W., & Smith, G. E. (2014). Mild cognitive impairment: A concept and diagnostic entity in need of input from neuropsychology. *Journal of the International Neuropsychological Society, 20,* 129–134.

Bookheimer, S. Y., Strojwas, M. H., Cohen, M. S., Saunders, A. M., Pericak-Vance, M. A., Mazziotta, J. C., & Small, G. W. (2000). Patterns of brain activation in people at risk for Alzheimer's disease. *New England Journal of Medicine, 343*(7), 450–456.

Boone, K. B. (2009). Fixed belief in cognitive dysfunction despite normal neuropsychological scores: Neurocognitive hypochondriasis? *The Clinical Neuropsychologist, 23,* 1016–1036.

Boots, L. M. M., Vugt, M. E., Knippenberg, R. J. M., Kempen, G. I. J. M., & Verhey, F. R. J. (2014). A systematic review of Internet-based supportive interventions for caregivers of patients with dementia. *International Journal of Geriatric Psychiatry, 29,* 331–344.

Borghesani, P. R., Weaver, K. E., Aylward, E. H., Richards, A. L., Madhyastha, T. M., Kahn, A. R., . . . Willis, S. L. (2012). Midlife memory improvement predicts preservation of hippocampal volume in old age. *Neurobiology of Aging, 33*(7), 1148–1155.

Bosma, H., van Boxtel, M. P. J., Ponds, R. W. H. M., Houx, P. J., Burdorf, A., & Jolles, J. (2003). Mental work demands protect against cognitive impairment: MAAS prospective cohort study. *Experimental Aging Research, 29*(1), 33–45.

Bosma, H., van Boxtel, M. P., Ponds, R. W., Jelicic, M., Houx, P., Metsemakers, J., & Jolles, J. (2002). Engaged lifestyle and cognitive function in middle and old-aged, non-demented persons: A reciprocal association? *Zeitschrift für Gerontologie und Geriatrie, 35*(6), 575–581.

Boss, P. (2011). *Loving someone who has dementia: How to find hope while coping with stress and grief.* San Francisco: Jossey-Bass.

Boss, P., & Yeats, J. R. (2014). Ambiguous loss: A complicated type of grief when loved ones disappear. *Bereavement Care, 33,* 63–69.

Bouazzaoui, B., Angel, L., Fay, S., Taconnat, L., Charlotte, F., & Isingrini, M. (2013). Does the greater involvement of executive control in memory with age act as a compensatory mechanism? *Canadian Journal of Experimental Psychology, 68,* 59–66.

Bowers, M. E., & Yehuda, R. (2016). Intergenerational effects of PTSD on offspring glucocorticoid receptor methylation. In D. Spengler & E. Binder (Eds.), *Epigenetics and neuroendocrinology: Clinical focus on psychiatry* (Vol. 2, pp. 141–155). New York: Springer.

Braak, H., & Braak, E. (1998). Evolution of neuronal changes in the course of Alzheimer's disease. *Journal of Neural Transmission Supplementum, 53,* 127–140.

Brandt, J., Spencer, M., & Folstein, M. (1988). The Telephone Interview for Cognitive Status. *Neuropsychiatry, Neuropsychology, and Behavioral Neurology, 1*(2), 111–117.

Braun, M. M., Karlin, B. E., & Zeiss, A. M. (2015). Cognitive-behavioral therapies in older adult populations. In C. M. Nezu & A. Nezu (Eds.), *The Oxford handbook of cognitive and behavioral therapies* (pp. 349–362). New York: Oxford University Press.

Bravo, G., Dubois, M.-F., Wildeman, S. M., Graham, J. E., Cohen, C. A., Painter, K., & Bellemare, S. (2010). Research with decisionally incapacitated older adults: Practices of Canadian research ethics boards. *IRB: Ethics and Human Research, 32*(6), 1–8.

Brink, T. L., Yesavage, J. A., Lum, O., Heersema, P. H., Adey, M., & Rose, T. L. (1982). Screening tests for geriatric depression. *The Clinical Gerontologist, 1*(1), 37–43.

Broadway, J., & Mintzer, J. (2007). The many faces of psychosis in the elderly. *Current Opinion in Psychiatry, 20,* 551–558.

Brown, G. G., Lazar, R. M., & Delano-Wood, L. (2009). Cerebrovascular disease. In I. Grant & K. Adams (Eds.), *Neuropsychological assessment of neuropsychiatric and neuromedical disorders* (3rd ed., pp. 306–335). New York: Oxford University Press.

Bruscoli, M., & Lovestone, S. (2004). Is MCI really just early dementia?: A systematic review of conversion studies. *International Psychogeriatrics, 16,* 129–140.

Bryant, F. B., Smart, C. M., & King, S. P. (2005). Using the past to enhance the present: Boosting happiness through positive reminiscence. *Journal of Happiness Studies, 6,* 227–260.

Buckley, R. F., Maruff, P., Ames, D., Bourgeat, P., Martins, R. N., Masters, C. L., . . . the AIBL Study. (2016a). Subjective memory decline predicts greater rates of clinical progression in preclinical Alzheimer's disease. *Alzheimer's and Dementia, 12,* 796–804.

Buckley, R., Saling, M. M., Ames, D., Rowe, C. C., Lautenschlager, N. T., Macaulay, S. L., . . . the Australian Imaging Biomarkers and Lifestyle Study of Aging (AIBL) Research Group. (2013). Factors affecting subjective memory complaints in the AIBL aging study: Biomarkers, memory, affect, and age. *International Psychogeriatrics, 25,* 1307–1315.

Buckley, R. F., Saling, M. M., Fromann, I., Wolfsgruber, S., & Wagner, M. (2015). Subjective cognitive decline from a phenomenological perspective: A review of the qualitative literature. *Journal of Alzheimer's Disease, 48,* S125–S140.

Buckley, R. F., Villemagne, V. L., Masters, C. L., Ellis, K. A., Rowe, C. C., Johnson, K., . . . Amariglio, R. (2016b). A conceptualization of the utility of subjective cognitive decline in clinical trials of preclinical Alzheimer's disease. *Journal of Molecular Neuroscience, 60,* 354–361.

Bugnicourt, J. M., Godefroy, O., Chillon, J. M., Choukroun, G., & Massy, Z. A. (2013). Cognitive disorders and dementia in CKD: The neglected kidney–brain axis. *Journal of American Society of Nephrology, 24*(3), 353–363.

Burt, D. B., & Aylward, E. H. (1998). *Test battery for the diagnosis of dementia in individuals with intellectual disability.* Washington, DC: American Association on Mental Retardation.

Burt, D. B., & Aylward, E. H. (2000). Test battery for the diagnosis of dementia in individuals with intellectual disability. *Journal of Intellectual Disability Research, 44*(2), 175–180.

Buschke, H. (1973). Selective reminding for analysis of memory and learning. *Journal of Verbal Learning and Verbal Behavior, 12,* 543–550.

Bush, S. S. (2007). *Ethical decision making in clinical neuropsychology.* New York: Oxford University Press.

Bush, S. S. (2009). *Geriatric mental health ethics: A casebook.* New York: Springer.

Bush, S. S., & Drexler, M. L. (2002). *Ethical issues in clinical neuropsychology.* Lisse, The Netherlands: Swets & Zeitlinger.

Busse, A., Bischkopf, J., Riedel-Heller, S. G., & Angermeyer, M. C. (2003). Mild cognitive impairment: Prevalence and incidence according to different diagnostic criteria: Results of the Leipzig Longitudinal Study of the Aged (LEILA75+). *British Journal of Psychiatry, 182,* 449–454.

Butt, Z. (2008). Sensitivity of the Informant Questionnaire on cognitive decline: An application of item response theory. *Aging, Neuropsychology, and Cognition, 15*(5), 642–655.

Butters, M. A., Young, J. B., Lopez, O., Aizenstein, H. J., Mulsant, B. H., Reynolds, C. F., 3rd, . . . Becker, J. T. (2008). Pathways linking late-life depression to persistent cognitive impairment and dementia. *Dialogues in Clinical Neuroscience, 10*(3), 345–357.

Caamano-Isorna, F., Corral, M., Montes-Martinez, A., & Takkouche, B. (2006). Education and dementia: A meta-analytic study. *Neuroepidemiology, 26*(4), 226–232.

Caddell, L. S., & Clare, L. (2013). How does identity relate to cognition and functional abilities in early-stage dementia? *Aging, Neuropsychology, and Cognition, 20*(1), 1–21.

Cairncross, M., & Miller, C. J. (2016). The effectiveness of mindfulness-based therapies for ADHD: A meta-analytic review. *Journal of Attention Disorders.*

Calamia, M., Markon, K., & Tranel, D. (2012). Scoring higher the second time around: Meta-analyses of practice effects in neuropsychological assessment. *The Clinical Neuropsychologist, 26,* 543–570.

Campanella, S. (2013). Why it is time to develop the use of cognitive event-related potentials in the treatment of psychiatric diseases. *Neuropsychiatric Disease and Treatment, 9,* 1835–1845.

Campbell, D. T., & Stanley, J. C. (1963). *Experimental and quasi-experimental designs for research.* Chicago: Rand McNally.

Canadian Institutes of Health Research, Natural Sciences and Engineering Research Council of Canada, & Social Sciences and Humanities Research Council of Canada. (2010). Tri-council Policy Statement: Ethical Conduct for Research Involving Humans. Retrieved from *www.pre.ethics.gc.ca/eng/policy-politique/initiatives/tcps2-eptc2/Default.*

Canadian Psychological Association. (2017). Canadian code of ethics for psychologists (4th ed.). Retrieved from *www.cpa.ca/aboutcpa/committees/ethics/codeofethics.*

Canadian Study of Health and Aging Working Group. (1994). Canadian Study of Health and Aging: Study methods and prevalence of dementia. *Canadian Medical Association Journal, 150,* 899–913.

Canevelli, M., Adali, N., Tainturier, C., Bruno, G., Cesari, M., & Vellas, B. (2013). Cognitive interventions targeting subjective cognitive complaints. *American Journal of Alzheimer's Disease and Other Dementias, 28,* 560–567.

Carcaillon, L., Brailly-Tabard, S., Ancelin, M. L., Tzourio, C., Foubert-Samier, A., Dartigues, J. F., . . . Scarabin, P. Y. (2014). Low testosterone and the risk of dementia in elderly men: Impact of age and education. *Alzheimer's and Dementia, 10*(5, Suppl.), S306–S314.

Carpenter, B. D., Strauss, M. E., & Ball, A. M. (1995). Telephone assessment of memory in the elderly. *Journal of Clinical Geropsychology, 1*(2), 107–117.

Carroll, E., & Coetzer, R. (2011). Identity, grief and self-awareness after traumatic brain injury. *Neuropsychological Rehabilitation, 21,* 289–305.

Carstensen, L. (1993). Perspective on research with older families: Contributions of older adults to families and to family theory. In P. A. Cowan, D. Field, D. A. Hansen, A. Skolnick, & G. E. Swanson (Eds.), *Family, self, and society: Toward a new agenda for family research* (pp. 353–360). Hillsdale, NJ: Erlbaum.

Carstensen, L., Isaacowitz, D., & Charles, S. T. (1999). Taking time seriously: A theory of socioemotional selectivity. *The American Psychologist, 54,* 165–181.

Carstensen, L. L., Turan, B., Scheibe, S., Ram, N., Ersner-Hershfield, H., Samanez-Larkin, G. R., . . . Nesselroade, J. R. (2011). Emotional experience improves with age: Evidence based on over 10 years of experience sampling. *Psychology and Aging, 26,* 21–33.

Carvalho, J. P., de Almeida, A. R., & Gusmao-Flores, D. (2013). Delirium rating scales in critically ill patients: A systematic literature review. *Revista Brasileira de Terapia Intensiva, 25*(2), 148–154.

Castanho, T. C., Amorim, L., Zihl, J., Palha, J. A., Sousa, N., & Santos, N. C. (2014). Telephone-based screening tools for mild cognitive impairment and dementia in aging studies: A review of validated instruments. *Frontiers in Aging Neuroscience, 6,* 16.

Cato, M. A., & Crosson, B. A. (2006). Stable and slowly progressive dementias. In D. K. Attix & K. A. Welsh-Bohmer (Eds.), *Geriatric neuropsychology: Assessment and intervention* (pp. 89–102). New York: Guilford Press.

Ceglowski, J., de Dios, L. V., & Depp, C. A. (2014). Psychosis in older adults. In N. A. Pachana & K. Laidlaw (Eds.), *The Oxford handbook of clinical geropsychology* (pp. 490–503). New York: Oxford University Press.

Centers for Disease Control and Prevention. (2015). Depression is not a normal part of growing older. Retrieved October 16, 2016, from *www.cdc.gov/aging/mental-health/depression.htm.*

Chambless, D. L., Baker, M. J., Baucom, D. H., Beutler, L. E., Calhoun, K. S., Crits-Christoph, P., . . . Woody, S. R. (1998). Update on empirically validated therapies: II. *The Clinical Psychologist, 51,* 3–16.

Chambless, D., & Hollon, S. D. (1998). Defining empirically supported therapies. *Journal of Consulting and Clinical Psychology, 66,* 7–18.

Chan, R. C. K., Shum, D., Toulopoulou, T., & Chen, E. Y. H. (2008). Assessment of executive functions: Review of instruments and identification of critical issues. *Archives of Clinical Neuropsychology, 23*(2), 201–216.

Chancellor, B., Duncan, A., & Chatterjee, A. (2013). Art therapy for Alzheimer's disease and other dementias. *Journal of Alzheimer's Disease, 39,* 1–11.

Chandler, M. J., Parks, A. C., Marsiske, M., Rotblatt, L. J., & Smith, G. E. (2016). Everyday impact of cognitive interventions in mild cognitive impairment: A systematic review and meta-analysis. *Neuropsychology Review, 26,* 225–251.

Charles, R. F., & Hillis, A. E. (2005). Posterior cortical atrophy: Clinical presentation and cognitive deficits compared to Alzheimer's disease. *Behavioural Neurology, 16*(1), 15–23.

Chatterjee, A., & Farah, M. J. (2013). *Neuroethics in practice: Medicine, mind, and society.* New York: Oxford University Press.

Chatterjee, S., Peters, S. A., Woodward, M., Mejia Arango, S., Batty, G. D., Beckett, N., . . . Huxley, R. R. (2016). Type 2 diabetes as a risk factor for dementia in women compared with men: A pooled analysis of 2.3 million people comprising more than 100,000 cases of dementia. *Diabetes Care, 39*(2), 300–307.

Cheek, C. (2010). Passing over: Identity transition in widows. *International Journal of Aging and Human Development, 70,* 345–364.

Chelune, G. J., Naugle, R. I., Lüders, H., Sedlak, J., & Awad, I. A. (1993). Individual change after epilepsy surgery: Practice effects and base-rate information. *Neuropsychology, 7*(1), 41–52.

Chen, A. J.-W., Novakovic-Agopian, T., Nycum, T., Song, S., Turner, G. R., Hills,

N. K., . . . D'Esposito, M. (2011). Training of goal-directed attention regulation enhances control over neural processing for individuals with brain injury. *Brain, 134,* 1541–1554.

Chen, Y. D., Zhang, J., Wang, Y., Yuan, J. L., & Hu, W. L. (2016). Efficacy of cholinesterase inhibitors in vascular dementia: An updated meta-analysis. *European Neurology, 75,* 132–141.

Cherbuin, N., & Jorm, A. F. (2013). The IQCODE: Using informant reports to assess cognitive change in the clinic and in older individuals living in the community. In A. J. Larner (Ed.), *Cognitive screening instruments: A practical approach* (pp. 165–182). New York: Springer-Verlag.

Chertkow, H., Whitehead, V., Phillips, N., Wolfson, C., Atherton, J., & Bergman, H. (2010). Multilingualism (but not always bilingualism) delays the onset of Alzheimer disease: Evidence from a bilingual community. *Alzheimer Disease and Associated Disorder, 24*(2), 118–125.

Chételat, G., Villemagne, V. L., Bourgeat, P., Pike, K. E., Jones, G., Ames, D., . . . the Australian Imaging Biomarkers and Lifestyle Research Group. (2010). Relationship between atrophy and beta-amyloid deposition in Alzheimer disease. *Annals of Neurology, 67,* 317–324.

Chiesa, A., Calati, R., & Serretti, A. (2011). Does mindfulness improve cognitive abilities?: A systematic review of neuropsychological findings. *Clinical Psychology Review, 31,* 449–464.

Cho, A., Sugimura, M., Nakano, S., & Yamada, T. (2008). The Japanese MCI screen for early detection of Alzheimer's disease and related disorders. *American Journal of Alzheimer's Disease and Other Dementias, 23*(2), 162–166.

Choe, J. Y., Youn, J. C., Park, J. H., Park, I. S., Jeong, J. W., Lee, W. H., . . . Kim, K. W. (2008). The Severe Cognitive Impairment Rating Scale—An instrument for the assessment of cognition in moderate to severe dementia patients. *Dementia and Geriatric Cognitive Disorders, 25*(4), 321–328.

Choi, J., & Twamley, E. W. (2013). Cognitive rehabilitation therapies for Alzheimer's disease: A review of methods to improve treatment engagement and self-efficacy. *Neuropsychology Review, 23,* 48–62.

Christensen, H., Hofer, S. M., Mackinnon, A. J., Korten, A. E., Jorm, A. F., & Henderson, A. S. (2001). Age is no kinder to the better educated: Absence of an association investigated using latent growth techniques in a community sample. *Psychological Medicine, 31*(1), 15–28.

Christensen, H., Mackinnon, A., Jorm, A. F., Henderson, A. S., Scott, L. R., & Korten, A. E. (1994). Age differences and interindividual variation in cognition in community-dwelling elderly. *Psychology and Aging, 9*(3), 381–390.

Cicerone, K. D., & Azulay, J. (2007). Perceived self-efficacy and life satisfaction after traumatic brain injury. *Journal of Head Trauma Rehabilitation, 22,* 257–266.

Cicerone, K. D., Langenbahn, D. M., Braden, C., Malec, J. F., Kalmar, K., Fraas, M., . . . Ashman, T. (2011). Evidence-based cognitive rehabilitation: Updated review of the literature from 2003 through 2008. *Archives of Physical Medicine and Rehabilitation, 92,* 519–530.

Cicerone, K. D., Mott, T., Azulay, J., Sharlow-Galella, M. A., Ellmo, W. J., Paradise, S., & Friel, J. C. (2008). A randomized controlled trial of holistic neuropsychologic rehabilitation after traumatic brain injury. *Archives of Physical Medicine and Rehabilitation, 89,* 2239–2249.

Cipriani, G., Vedovello, M., Ulivi, M., Lucetti, C., Di Fiorino, A., & Nuti, A. (2013). Delusional misidentification syndromes and dementia: A border zone between neurology and psychiatry. *American Journal of Alzheimer's Disease and Other Dementias, 28,* 671–678.

Clare, L. (2003). Managing threats to self: Awareness in early stage Alzheimer's disease. *Social Science and Medicine, 57*(6), 1017–1029.

Clare, L., Linden, D. E. J., Woods, R., Whitaker, R., Evans, S. J., Parkinson, C. H., . . . Rugg, M. D. (2010). Goal-oriented cognitive rehabilitation for people with early-stage Alzheimer disease: A single-blind randomized controlled trial of clinical efficacy. *American Journal of Geriatric Psychiatry, 18,* 928–939.

Clare, L., Whitaker, C. J., Craik, F. I., Bialystok, E., Martyr, A., Martin-Forbes, P. A., . . . Hindle, J. V. (2014). Bilingualism, executive control, and age at diagnosis among people with early-stage Alzheimer's disease in Wales. *Journal of Neuropsychology, 10*(2), 163–185.

Clare, L., & Woods, R. T. (2004). Cognitive training and cognitive rehabilitation for people with early-stage Alzheimer's disease: A review. *Neuropsychological Rehabilitation, 14*(4), 385–401.

Clark, L. R., Delano-Wood, L., Libon, D. J., McDonald, C. R., Nation, D. A., Bangen, K. J., . . . Bondi, M. W. (2013). Are empirically-derived subtypes of mild cognitive impairment consistent with conventional subtypes? *Journal of the International Neuropsychological Society, 19,* 635–645.

Clegg, A., & Young, J. B. (2011). Which medications to avoid in people at risk of delirium: A systematic review. *Age Ageing, 40,* 23–29.

Cohen, J. E. (2003). Human population: The next half century. *Science, 302*(5648), 1172–1175.

Colcombe, S., & Kramer, A. (2003). Fitness effects on the cognitive function of older adults: A meta-analytic study. *Psychological Science, 14,* 125–130.

Cole, M. G., & Dastoor, D. P. (1987). A new hierarchic approach to the measurement of dementia. *Psychosomatics: Journal of Consultation and Liaison Psychiatry, 28*(6), 298–304.

Coley, N., Ousset, P. J., Andrieu, S., Matheix Fortunet, H., Vellas, B., & The GuidAge Study Group. (2008). Memory complaints to the general practitioner: Data from the GuidAge study. *Journal of Nutrition, Health and Aging, 12,* 66S–72S.

Collins, O., & Kenny, R. A. (2007). Is neurocardiovascular instability a risk factor for cognitive decline and/or dementia?: The science to date. *Reviews in Clinical Gerontology, 17*(3), 153–160.

Colsher, P. L., & Wallace, R. B. (1991). Longitudinal application of cognitive function measures in a defined population of community-dwelling elders. *Annals of Epidemiology, 1*(3), 215–230.

Cooper, C., Bebbington, P., Lindesay, J., Meltzer, H., McManus, S., Jenkins, R., & Livingston, G. (2011). The meaning of reporting forgetfulness: A cross-sectional study of adults in the English 2007 Adult Psychiatric Morbidity Survey. *Age and Ageing, 40,* 711–717.

Cooper, C., Sommerlad, A., Lyketsos, C. G., & Livingston, G. (2015). Modifiable predictors of dementia in mild cognitive impairment: A systematic review and meta-analysis. *American Journal of Psychiatry, 172*(4), 323–334.

Corner, L., & Bond, J. (2004). Being at risk of dementia: Fears and anxieties of older adults. *Journal of Aging Studies, 18,* 143–155.

Corr, C. A. (2002). Revisiting the concept of disenfranchised grief. In K. J. Doka (Ed.), *Disenfranchised grief* (pp. 39–60). Champaign, IL: Research Press.

Coval, M., Crockett, D., Holliday, S., & Koch, W. (1985). A multi-focus assessment scale for use with frail elderly populations. *Canadian Journal on Aging, 4*(2), 101–109.

Cowl, A. L., & Gaugler, J. E. (2014). Efficacy of creative arts therapy in treatment of Alzheimer's disease and dementia: A systematic literature review. *Activities, Adaptation, and Aging, 38,* 281–330.

Craik, F. I., Bialystok, E., & Freedman, M. (2010). Delaying the onset of Alzheimer disease: Bilingualism as a form of cognitive reserve. *Neurology, 75*(19), 1726–1729.

Craik, F. I. M., & Salthouse, T. A. (2008). *The handbook of aging and cognition* (3rd ed.). New York: Psychology Press.

Crawford, J. (2004). Psychometric foundations of neuropsychological assessment. In L. H. Goldstein & J. E. Mcneil (Eds.), *Clinical neuropsychology: A practical guide to assessment and management for clinicians* (pp. 121–140). West Sussex, UK: Wiley.

Crawford, J. R., & Garthwaite, P. H. (2004). Statistical methods for single-case studies in neuropsychology: Comparing the slope of a patient's regression line with those of a control sample. *Cortex: A Journal Devoted to the Study of the Nervous System and Behavior, 40*(3), 533–548.

Crawford, J. R., Garthwaite, P. H., Azzalini, A., Howell, D. C., & Laws, K. R. (2006). Testing for a deficit in single-case studies: Effects of departures from normality. *Neuropsychologia, 44*(4), 666–677.

Crawford, J. R., Garthwaite, P. H., & Howell, D. C. (2009). On comparing a single case with a control sample: An alternative perspective. *Neuropsychologia, 47*(13), 2690–2695.

Crawford, J. R., Garthwaite, P. H., & Slick, D. J. (2009). On percentile norms in neuropsychology: Proposed reporting standards and methods for quantifying the uncertainty over the percentile ranks of test scores. *The Clinical Neuropsychologist, 23*(7), 1173–1195.

Crawford, J. R., & Howell, D. C. (1998). Comparing an individual's test score against norms derived from small samples. *The Clinical Neuropsychologist, 12*(4), 482–486.

Crayton, L., Oliver, C., Holland, A., Bradbury, J., & Hall, S. (1998). The neuropsychological assessment of age related cognitive deficits in adults with Down's syndrome. *Journal of Applied Research in Intellectual Disabilities, 11*(3), 255–272.

Crooks, V. C., Lubben, J., Petitti, D. B., Little, D., & Chiu, V. (2008). Social network, cognitive function, and dementia incidence among elderly women. *American Journal of Public Health, 98*(7), 1221–1227.

Crooks, V. C., Parsons, T. D., & Buckwalter, J. G. (2007). Validation of the Cognitive Assessment of Later Life Status (CALLS) instrument: A computerized telephonic measure. *BioMed Central Neurology, 7,* 10.

Crosson, B., Barco, P., Velozo, C., Bolesta, M., Cooper, P., Werts, D., & Brobeck, T. (1989). Awareness and compensation in postacute head injury rehabilitation. *Journal of Head Trauma Rehabilitation, 4,* 46–54.

Crumley, J. J., Stetler, C. A., & Horhota, M. (2014). Examining the relationship between subjective and objective memory performance in older adults: A meta-analysis. *Psychology and Aging, 29,* 250–263.

Crutch, S. J., Lehmann, M., Schott, J. M., Rabinovici, G. D., Rossor, M. N., & Fox, N. C. (2012). Posterior cortical atrophy. *The Lancet Neurology, 11*(2), 170–178.

Cuijpers, P., Geraedts, A. S., van Oppen, P., Andersson, G., Markowitz, J. C., & van Straten, A. (2011). Interpersonal psychotherapy for depression: A meta-analysis. *American Journal of Psychiatry, 168,* 581–592.

Cuijpers, P., Karyotaki, E., Pot, A. M., Park, M., & Reynolds, C. F. (2014). Managing depression in old age: Psychological interventions. *Maturitas, 79,* 160–169.

Cullum, C. M., Hynan, L. S., Grosch, M., Parikh, M., & Weiner, M. F. (2014). Tele-neuropsychology: Evidence for video teleconference-based neuropsychological assessment. *Journal of the International Neuropsychological Society, 20*(10), 1028–1033.

Cullum, C. M., Saine, K., Chan, L. D., Martin-Cook, K., Gray, K. F., & Weiner, M. F. (2001). Performance-based instrument to assess functional capacity in dementia: The Texas Functional Living Scale. *Neuropsychiatry, Neuropsychology, and Behavioral Neurology, 14*(2), 103–108.

Cummings, J., Mega, M., Gray, K., Rosenberg-Thompson, S., Carusi, D. A., & Gornbein, J. (1994). The Neuropsychiatric Inventory: Comprehensive assessment of psychopathology in dementia. *Neurology, 44,* 2308–2314.

Cutler, N. R., Shrotriya, R. C., Sramek, J. J., Veroff, A. E., Seifert, R. D., Reich, L. A., & Hironaka, D. Y. (1993). The use of the Computerized Neuropsychological Test Battery (CNTB) in an efficacy and safety trial of BMY 21,502 in Alzheimer's disease. *Annals of the New York Academy of Science, 695,* 332–336.

da Silva, J., Gonçalves-Pereira, M., Xavier, M., & Mukaetova-Ladinska, E. B. (2013). Affective disorders and risk of developing dementia: Systematic review. *British Journal of Psychiatry, 202*(3), 177–186.

Darby, D. G., Pietrzak, R. H., Fredrickson, J., Woodward, M., Moore, L., Fredrickson, A., . . . Maruff, P. (2012). Intraindividual cognitive decline using a brief computerized cognitive screening test. *Alzheimer's and Dementia, 8*(2), 95–104.

Daselaar, S., & Cabeza, R. (2013). Age-related decline in working memory and episodic memory. In K. N. Ochsner & S. Kosslyn (Eds.), *The Oxford handbook of cognitive neuroscience: Vol. 1. Core topics.* New York: Oxford University Press.

Davies, E. A., & O'Mahony, M. S. (2015). Adverse drug reactions in special populations—the elderly. *British Journal of Clinical Pharmacology, 80,* 796–807.

Davis, J. C., Bryan, S., Marra, C. A., Hsiung, G.-Y. R., & Liu-Ambrose, T. (2015). Challenges with cost-utility analyses of behavioral interventions among older adults at risk for dementia. *British Journal of Sport Medicine, 49,* 1343–1347.

Davis, S. W., Dennis, N. A., Daselaar, S. M., Fleck, M. S., & Cabeza, R. (2008). Qué pasa?: The posterior-anterior shift in aging. *Cerebral Cortex, 18,* 1201–1209.

de Jonghe, J. F. M., Wetzels, R. B., Mulders, A., Zuidema, S. U., & Koopmans, R. T. C. M. (2009). Validity of the Severe Impairment Battery Short Version. *Journal of Neurology, Neurosurgery and Psychiatry, 80*(9), 954–959.

de la Torre, J. C. (2004). Is Alzheimer's disease a neurodegenerative or a vascular disorder?: Data, dogma, and dialectics. *The Lancet Neurology, 3*(3), 184–190.

De Lepeleire, J., Heyrman, J., Baro, F., & Buntinx, F. (2005). A combination of tests for the diagnosis of dementia had a significant diagnostic value. *Journal of Clinical Epidemiology, 58*(3), 217–225.

De Santi, S., Pirraglia, E., Barr, W., Babb, J., Williams, S., Rogers, K., . . . de Leon, M. J. (2008). Robust and conventional neuropsychological norms: Diagnosis and prediction of age-related cognitive decline. *Neuropsychology, 22*(4, Suppl.), 469–484.

Deary, I. J., Gow, A. J., Taylor, M. D., Corley, J., Brett, C., Wilson, V., . . . Starr, J. M. (2007). The Lothian Birth Cohort 1936: A study to examine influences on cognitive ageing from age 11 to age 70 and beyond. *BioMed Cetral Geriatrics, 7,* 28.

Deb, S., Hare, M., Prior, L., & Bhaumik, S. (2007). Dementia Screening Questionnaire for Individuals with Intellectual Disabilities. *British Journal of Psychiatry, 190,* 440–444.

Debanne, S. M., Patterson, M. B., Dick, R., Riedel, T. M., Schnell, A., & Rowland, D. Y. (1997). Validation of a Telephone Cognitive Assessment Battery. *Journal of the American Geriatrics Society, 45*(11), 1352–1359.

DeCarlo, C. A., Tuokko, H. A., Williams, D., Dixon, R. A., & MacDonald, S. W. (2014). BioAge: Toward a multi-determined, mechanistic account of cognitive aging. *Ageing Research Reviews, 18,* 95–105.

Deckers, K., van Boxtel, M. P., Schiepers, O. J., de Vugt, M., Munoz Sanchez, J. L., Anstey, K. J., . . . Kohler, S. (2015). Target risk factors for dementia prevention: A systematic review and Delphi consensus study on the evidence from observational studies. *International Journal of Geriatric Psychiatry, 30*(3), 234–246.

Delis, D. C., Kramer, J. H., Kaplan, E., & Ober, B. A. (2000). *California Verbal Learning Test* (2nd ed.). San Antonio, TX: Pearson Assessments.

Dempster, F. N. (1992). The rise and fall of the inhibitory mechanism: Toward a unified theory of cognitive development and aging. *Developmental Review, 12*(1), 45–75.

Denkinger, M. D., Nikolaus, T., Denkinger, C., & Lukas, A. (2012). Physical activity for the prevention of cognitive decline: Current evidence from observational and controlled studies. *Zeitschrift für Gerontologie und Geriatrie, 45*(1), 11–16.

Detre, J., & Bockow, T. B. (2013). Incidental findings in magnetic resonance imaging research. In A. Chatterjee & M. J. Farah (Eds.), *Neuroethics in practice: Medicine, mind, and society* (pp. 120–127). New York: Oxford University Press.

Di Santo, S. G., Prinelli, F., Adorni, F., Caltagirone, C., & Musicco, M. (2013). A meta-analysis of the efficacy of donepezil, rivastigmine, galantamine, and memantine in relation to severity of Alzheimer's disease. *Journal of Alzheimer's Disease, 35,* 349–361.

Diehl, M., Willis, S. L., & Schaie, K. W. (1995). Everyday problem solving in older adults: Observational assessment and cognitive correlates. *Psychology and Aging, 10*(3), 478–491.

Dik, M., Deeg, D. J., Visser, M., & Jonker, C. (2003). Early life physical activity and cognition at old age. *Journal of Clinical Experimental Neuropsychology, 25*(5), 643–653.

Dik, M. G., Jonker, C., Comijs, H. C., Bouter, L. M., Twisk, J. W., van Kamp, G. J., & Deeg, D. J. H. (2001). Memory complaints and APOE-epsilon4 accelerate cognitive decline in cognitively normal elderly. *Neurology, 57,* 2217–2222.

Diniz, B. S., Butters, M. A., Albert, S. M., Dew, M. A., & Reynolds, C. F., 3rd. (2013). Late-life depression and risk of vascular dementia and Alzheimer's disease: Systematic review and meta-analysis of community-based cohort studies. *British Journal of Psychiatry, 202*(5), 329–335.

Diniz, B. S., Nunes, P. V., Machado-Vieira, R., & Forlenza, O. V. (2011). Current pharmacological approaches and perspectives in the treatment of geriatric mood disorders. *Current Opinion in Psychiatry, 24,* 473–477.

Doniger, G. M., Dwolatzky, T., Zucker, D. M., Chertkow, H., Crystal, H., Schweiger, A., & Simon, E. S. (2006). Computerized cognitive testing battery identifies mild cognitive impairment and mild dementia even in the presence of depressive symptoms. *American Journal of Alzheimer's Disease and Other Dementias, 21*(1), 28–36.

Doody, R. S., Strehlow, S. L., Massman, P. J., Feher, E. P., Clark, C., & Roy, J. R. (1999). Baylor Profound Mental Status Examination: A brief staging measure for profoundly demented Alzheimer disease patients. *Alzheimer Disease and Associated Disorders, 13*(1), 53–59.

Dosa, D., Intrator, O., McNicoll, L., Cang, Y., & Teno, J. (2007). Preliminary derivation of a Nursing Home Confusion Assessment Method based on data from the Minimum Data Set. *Journal of the American Geriatric Society, 55*(7), 1099–1105.

Dougherty, J. H., Jr., Cannon, R. L., Nicholas, C. R., Hall, L., Hare, F., Carr, E., . . . Arunthamakun, J. (2010). The computerized self test (CST): An interactive, Internet accessible cognitive screening test for dementia. *Journal of Alzheimers Disease, 20*(1), 185–195.

Downs, S. H., & Black, N. (1998). The feasibility of creating a checklist for the assessment of the methodological quality of both randomised and non-randomised studies of health care interventions. *Journal of Epidemiology and Community Health, 52,* 377–384.

Draper, B., Peisah, C., Snowdon, J., & Brodaty, H. (2010). Early dementia diagnosis and the risk of suicide and euthanasia. *Alzheimer's and Dementia, 6,* 75–82.

Duberstein, P. R., Chapman, B. P., Tindle, H. A., Sink, K. M., Bamonti, P., Robbins, J., . . . the Ginkgo Evaluation of Memory (GEM) Study Investigators. (2011). Personality and risk for Alzheimer's disease in adults 72 years of age and older: A six-year follow-up. *Psychology and Aging, 26,* 351–362.

Duff, K. (2012). Evidence-based indicators of neuropsychological change in the individual patient: Relevant concepts and methods. *Archives of Clinical Neuropsychology, 27,* 248–261.

Duff, K., Beglinger, L. J., Moser, D. J., & Paulsen, J. S. (2010). Predicting cognitive change within domains. *The Clinical Neuropsychologist, 24*(5), 779–792.

Dwolatzky, T., Dimant, L., Simon, E. S., & Doniger, G. M. (2010). Validity of a short computerized assessment battery for moderate cognitive impairment and dementia. *International Psychogeriatrics, 22*(5), 795–803.

Dwolatzky, T., Whitehead, V., Doniger, G. M., Simon, E. S., Schweiger, A., Jaffe, D., & Chertkow, H. (2003). Validity of a novel computerized cognitive battery for mild cognitive impairment. *BioMed Central Geriatrics, 3,* 4.

Edmonds, E. C., Delano-Wood, L., Clark, L. R., Jak, A. J., Nation, D. A., McDonald, C. R., . . . Bondi, M. W. for the Alzheimer's Disease Neuroimaging Initiative. (2015a). Susceptibility of the conventional criteria for MCI to false positive diagnostic errors. *Alzheimer's and Dementia, 11,* 415–424.

Edmonds, E. C., Delano-Wood, L., Galasko, D. R., Salmon, D. P., Bondi, M. W., & the Alzheimer's Disease Neuroimaging Initiative. (2014). Subjective cognitive complaints contribute to misdiagnosis of mild cognitive impairment. *Journal of the International Neuropsychological Society, 20,* 836–847.

Edmonds, E. C., Delano-Wood, L., Galasko, D. R., Salmon, D. P., & Bondi, M. W., & the Alzheimer's Disease Neuroimaging Initiative. (2015b). Subtle cognitive decline and biomarker staging in preclinical Alzheimer's disease. *Journal of Alzheimer's Disease, 47,* 231–242.

Edwards, E. R., Spira, A. P., Barnes, D. E., & Yaffe, K. (2009). Neuropsychiatric symptoms in mild cognitive impairment: Differences by subtype and progression to dementia. *International Journal of Geriatric Psychiatry, 24*(7), 716–722.

Egerhazi, A., Berecz, R., Bartok, E., & Degrell, I. (2007). Automated Neuropsychological Test Battery (CANTAB) in mild cognitive impairment and in Alzheimer's disease. *Progress in Neuropsychopharmacology and Biology Psychiatry, 31*(3), 746–751.

Einstein, G. O., & McDaniel, M. A. (1990). Normal aging and prospective memory. *Journal of Experimental Psychology: Learning, Memory, and Cognition, 16,* 717–726.

Elliott, R. (2003). Executive functions and their disorders. *British Medical Bulletin, 65,* 49–59.

Elliott-King, J., Shaw, S., Bandelow, S., Devshi, R., Kassam, S., & Hogervorst, E. (2016). A critical literature review of the effectiveness of various instruments in the diagnosis of dementia in adults with intellectual disabilities. *Alzheimers Dement (Amsterdam), 4,* 126–148.

Elwood, R. W. (2001). MicroCog: Assessment of cognitive functioning. *Neuropsychology Review, 11*(2), 89–100.

Engel, G. L. (2012). The need for a new medical model: A challenge for biomedicine. *Psychodynamic Psychiatry, 40*(3), 377–396.

Ericsson, I., Malmberg, B., Langworth, S., Haglund, A., & Almborg, A. H. (2011). KUD—A scale for clinical evaluation of moderate-to-severe dementia. *Journal of Clinical Nursing, 20*(11–12), 1542–1552.

Erikson, E. H. (1963). *Childhood and society.* New York: Norton.

Erlanger, D. M., Kaushik, T., Broshek, D., Freeman, J., Feldman, D., & Festa, J. (2002). Development and validation of a web-based screening tool for monitoring cognitive status. *Journal of Head Trauma Rehabilitation, 17*(5), 458–476.

Ernst, A., Moulin, C. J. A., Souchay, C., Mograbi, D. C., & Morris, R. (2016). Anosognosia and metacognition in Alzheimer's disease: Insights from experimental psychology. In J. Dunlosky & S. Tauber (Eds.), *The Oxford handbook of metamemory* (pp. 451–472). New York: Oxford University Press.

Etgen, T., Chonchol, M., Forstl, H., & Sander, D. (2012). Chronic kidney disease and cognitive impairment: A systematic review and meta-analysis. *American Journal of Nephrology, 35*(5), 474–482.

Evidently Cochrane. (2016, November). What are *Cochrane Reviews?* Retrieved November 20, 2016, from *www.evidentlycochrane.net/what-are-cochrane-reviews.*

Faber, M. A. (2014). The realities of growing older. In J. A. Sugar, R. J. Rieske, H. Holstege, & M. A. Faber (Eds.), *Introduction to aging: A positive, interdisciplinary approach* (pp. 37–112). New York: Springer.

Fagundes, C. P., Glaser, R., & Kiecolt-Glaser, J. K. (2013). Stressful early life experiences and immune dysregulation across the lifespan. *Brain, Behavior, and Immunity, 27C,* 8–12.

Falleti, M. G., Maruff, P., Collie, A., & Darby, D. G. (2006). Practice effects associated with the repeated assessment of cognitive function using the CogState Battery at 10-minute, one week and one month test–retest intervals. *Journal of Clinical and Experimental Neuropsychology, 28*(7), 1095–1112.

Farias, S. T., Mungas, D., Harvey, D. J., Simmons, A., Reed, B. R., & DeCarli, C. (2011). The measurement of everyday cognition: Development and validation of a short form of the Everyday Cognition scales. *Alzheimer's and Dementia, 7*(6), 593–601.

Farias, S. T., Mungas, D., Reed, B. R., Cahn-Weiner, D., Jagust, W., Baynes, K., & DeCarli, C. (2008). The measurement of everyday cognition (ECog): Scale development and psychometric properties. *Neuropsychology, 22,* 531–544.

Farmer, M. E., Kittner, S. J., Rae, D. S., Bartko, J. J., & Regier, D. A. (1995). Education and change in cognitive function: The Epidemiologic Catchment Area Study. *Annal of Epidemiology, 5*(1), 1–7.

Feart, C., Samieri, C., & Barberger-Gateau, P. (2015). Mediterranean diet and cognitive health: An update of available knowledge. *Current Opinion in Clinical Nutrition and Metabolic Care, 18*(1), 51–62.

Federal Trade Commission. (2016, January 5). Lumosity to pay $2 million to settle FTC deceptive advertising charges for its "brain training" program. Retrieved December 27, 2016, from *www.ftc.gov/news-events/press-releases/2016/01/lumosity-pay-2 million-settle-ftc-deceptive-advertising-charges.*

Ferraro, F. R. (Ed.). (2016). *Minority and cross-cultural aspects of neuropsychological assessment: Enduring and emerging trends* (2nd ed.). New York: Taylor & Francis.

Fillenbaum, G. G. (1988). *Multidimensional functional assessment of older adults: The Duke older Americans resources and services procedures.* Hillsdale, NJ: Erlbaum.

Fillit, H. M., Simon, E. S., Doniger, G. M., & Cummings, J. L. (2008). Practicality of a computerized system for cognitive assessment in the elderly. *Alzheimer's and Dementia, 4*(1), 14–21.

Fink, H. A., Hemmy, L. S., MacDonald, R., Carlyle, M. H., Olson, C. M., Dysken, M. W., . . . Wilt, T. J. (2015). Intermediate and long-term cognitive outcomes after cardiovascular procedures in older adults: A systematic review. *Annals of Internal Medicine, 163,* 107–117.

Fitzpatrick-Lewis, D., Warren, R., Ali, M. U., Sherifali, D., & Raina, P. (2015). Treatment for mild cognitive impairment: A systematic review and meta-analysis. *Canadian Medical America Journal Open, 3,* E419–E427.

Fliser, D., Zeier, M., Nowack, R., & Ritz, E. (1993). Renal functional reserve in healthy elderly subjects. *Journal of the American Society of Nephrology, 3,* 1371–1377.

Flynn, S. J., Cooper, L. A., & Gary-Webb, T. L. (2013). The role of culture in promoting effective clinical communication, behavior change, and treatment adherence. In L. R. Martin & M. R. DiMatteo (Eds.), *The Oxford handbook of health communication, behavior change, and treatment adherence* (pp. 267–285). New York: Oxford University Press.

Folstein, M. F., Folstein, S. E., & McHugh, P. R. (1975). "Mini-mental state": A practical method for grading the cognitive state of patients for the clinician. *Journal of Psychiatric Research, 12,* 189–198.

Fong, T. G., Jones, R. N., Shi, P., Marcantonio, E. R., Yap, L., Rudolph, J. L., . . . Inouye, S. K. (2009). Delirium accelerates cognitive decline in Alzheimer disease. *Neurology, 72*(18), 1570–1575.

Fortin, A., & Caza, N. (2014). A validation study of memory and executive functions indexes in French-speaking healthy young and older adults. *Canadian Journal on Aging, 33*(1), 60–71.

Fortner, B. V., & Neimeyer, R. A. (1999). Death anxiety in older adults: A quantitative review. *Death Studies, 23,* 387–411.

Foster, P. P., Rosenblatt, K. P., & Kuljiš, R. O. (2011). Exercise-induced cognitive plasticity, implications for mild cognitive impairment and Alzheimer's disease. *Frontiers in Neurology, 2,* 28.

Fox, C., Lafortune, L., Boustani, M., & Brayne, C. (2013). Debate and analysis: The pros and cons of early diagnosis in dementia. *British Journal of General Practice, 63,* 612.

Franceschi, C., & Campisi, J. (2014). Chronic inflammation (inflammaging) and its potential contribution to age-associated diseases. *Journals of Gerontology Series A: Biological Sciences and Medical Sciences, 69*(1, Suppl.), S4–S9.

Franco, A., Malhotra, N., & Simonovits, G. (2014). Publication bias in the social sciences: Unlocking the file drawer. *Science, 345,* 1502–1505.

Frank, L., Lloyd, A., Flynn, J. A., Kleinman, L., Matza, L. S., Margolis, M. K., . . . Bullock, R. (2006). Impact of cognitive impairment on mild dementia patients and mild cognitive impairment patients and their informants. *International Psychoge-riatrics, 18*, 151–162.

Fratiglioni, L. (1993). Epidemiology of Alzheimer's disease: Issues of etiology and valid-ity. *Acta Neurologica Scandinavica, 145*(Suppl.), 1–70.

Fratiglioni, L., Wang, H. X., Ericsson, K., Maytan, M., & Winblad, B. (2000). Influ-ence of social network on occurrence of dementia: A community-based longitudi-nal study. *The Lancet, 355*(9212), 1315–1319.

Freedman, M., Alladi, S., Chertkow, H., Bialystok, E., Craik, F. I., Phillips, N. A., . . . Bak, T. H. (2014). Delaying onset of dementia: Are two languages enough? *Behav-ioral Neurology, 2014*, 808137.

Frerichs, R. J., & Tuokko, H. A. (2005). A comparison of methods for measuring cogni-tive change in older adults. *Archives of Clinical Neuropsychology, 20*(3), 321–333.

Frerichs, R. J., & Tuokko, H. A. (2006). Reliable change scores and their relation to perceived change in memory: Implications for the diagnosis of mild cognitive impairment. *Archives of Clinical Neuropsychology, 21*(1), 109–115.

Frisardi, V., Panza, F., Seripa, D., Imbimbo, B. P., Vendemiale, G., Pilotto, A., & Sol-frizzi, V. (2010). Nutraceutical properties of Mediterranean diet and cognitive decline: Possible underlying mechanisms. *Journal of Alzheimer's Disease, 22*(3), 715–740.

Fritsch, T., Smyth, K. A., McClendon, M. J., Ogrocki, P. K., Santillan, C., Larsen, J. D., & Strauss, M. E. (2005). Associations between dementia/mild cognitive impair-ment and cognitive performance and activity levels in youth. *Journal of the Ameri-can Geriatrics Society, 53*(7), 1191–1196.

Fujii, D. (2017). *Conducting a culturally informed neuropsychological evaluation.* Washington, DC: American Psychological Association.

Ganguli, M., Lee, C.-W., Snitz, B. E., Hughes, T. F., McDade, E., & Chang, C.-C. H. (2015). Rates and risk factors for progression to incident dementia vary by age in a population cohort. *Neurology, 84*(1), 72–80.

Ganguli, M., Snitz, B. E., Lee, C.-W., Vanderbilt, J., Saxton, J. A., & Chang, C.-C. H. (2010). Age and education effects and norms on a cognitive test battery from a population-based cohort: The Monongahela–Youghiogheny Healthy Aging Team. *Aging and Mental Health, 14*(1), 100–107.

García-Casal, J. A., Loizeau, A., Csipke, E., Franco-Martín, M., Perea-Bartolomé, M. V., & Orrell, M. (2017). Computer-based cognitive interventions for people living with dementia: A systematic review and meta-analysis. *Aging and Mental Health, 21*(5), 454–467.

Gard, T., Hölzel, B. K., & Lazar, S. W. (2014). The potential effects of meditation on age-related cognitive decline: A systematic review. *Annals of the New York Acad-emy of Sciences, 1307*, 89–103.

Gardner, R. C., Burke, J. F., Nettiksimmons, J., Kaup, A., Barnes, D. E., & Yaffe, K. (2014). Dementia risk after traumatic brain injury vs nonbrain trauma: The role of age and severity. *JAMA Neurology, 71*(12), 1490–1497.

Gates, N., & Sachdev, P. (2014). Is cognitive training an effective treatment for preclini-cal and early Alzheimer's disease? *Journal of Alzheimer's Disease, 42*, S551–S559.

Gatz, M., Jang, J. Y., Karlsson, I. K., & Pedersen, N. L. (2014). Dementia: Genes, environments, interactions. In D. Finkel & C. A. Reynolds (Eds.), *Behavior genet-ics of cognition across the lifespan* (pp. 201–231). New York: Springer Science + Business Media.

Gatz, M., Reynolds, C. A., John, R., Johansson, B., Mortimer, J. A., & Pedersen, N. L.

(2002). Telephone screening to identify potential dementia cases in a population-based sample of older adults. *International Psychogeriatrics, 14*(3), 273–289.

Gatz, M., Reynolds, C., Nikolic, J., Lowe, B., Karel, M., & Pedersen, N. (1995). An empirical test of telephone screening to identify potential dementia cases. *International Psychogeriatrics, 7*(3), 429–438.

Geda, Y. E., Roberts, R. O., Knopman, D. S., Christianson, T. J., Pankratz, V. S., Ivnik, R. J., . . . Rocca, W. A. (2010). Physical exercise, aging, and mild cognitive impairment: A population-based study. *Archives Neurology, 67*(1), 80–86.

Geiger, P. J., Boggero, I. A., Brake, C. A., Caldera, C. A., Combs, H. L., Peters, J. R., & Baer, R. A. (2016). Mindfulness-based interventions for older adults: A review of the effects on physical and emotional well-being. *Mindfulness, 7,* 296–307.

Geldmacher, D. S., Levin, B. E., & Wright, C. B. (2012). Characterizing healthy samples for studies of human cognitive aging. *Frontiers in Aging Neuroscience, 4,* 23.

Gerolimatos, L. A., Gregg, J. J., & Edelstein, B. A. (2014). Interviewing older adults. In N. A. Pachana & K. Laidlaw (Eds.), *The Oxford handbook of clinical geropsychology* (pp. 163–183). New York: Oxford University Press.

Ghisletta, P., Bickel, J. F., & Lovden, M. (2006). Does activity engagement protect against cognitive decline in old age?: Methodological and analytical considerations. *Journal of Gerontology Series B: Psychological Sciences and Social Sciences, 61*(5), 253–261.

Gibson, S. J. (2015). The pain, emotion, and cognition nexus in older persons and in dementia. In G. S. Pickering & S. Gibson (Eds.), *Pain, emotion and cognition: A complex nexus* (pp. 231–247). New York: Springer.

Gifford, K. A., Liu, D., Lu, Z., Tripodis, Y., Cantwell, N., Palmisano, J., . . . Jefferson, A. L. (2014). The source of cognitive complaints differentially predicts diagnostic conversion in non-demented older adults. *Alzheimer's and Dementia, 10,* 319–327.

Gillanders, D., & Laidlaw, K. (2014). ACT and CBT in older age: Towards a wise synthesis. In N. A. Pachana & K. Laidlaw (Eds.), *The Oxford handbook of clinical geropsychology* (pp. 637–657). New York: Oxford University Press.

Go, R. C. P., Duke, L. W., Harrell, L. E., Cody, H., Bassett, S. S., Folstein, M. F., . . . Blacker, D. (1997). Development and validation of a Structured Telephone Interview for Dementia Assessment (STIDA): The NIMH Genetics Initiative. *Journal of Geriatric Psychiatry and Neurology, 10*(4), 161–167.

Goesling, J., Clauw, D. J., & Hassett, A. L. (2013). Pain and depression: An integrative review of neurobiological and psychological factors. *Current Psychiatry Reports, 15,* 421.

Gold, B. T., Johnson, N. F., & Powell, D. K. (2013). Lifelong bilingualism contributes to cognitive reserve against white matter integrity declines in aging. *Neuropsychologia, 51*(13), 2841–2846.

Gold, B. T., Kim, C., Johnson, N. F., Kryscio, R. J., & Smith, C. D. (2013). Lifelong bilingualism maintains neural efficiency for cognitive control in aging. *Journal of Neuroscience, 33*(2), 387–396.

Gold, D. A. (2012). An examination of instrumental activities of daily living assessment in older adults and mild cognitive impairment. *Journal of Clinical and Experimental Neuropsychology, 34,* 11–34.

Goldberg, T. E., Harvey, P. D., Wesnes, K. A., Snyder, P. J., & Schneider, L. S. (2015). Practice effects due to serial cognitive assessment: Implications for preclinical Alzheimer's disease randomized controlled trials. *Alzheimer's and Dementia, 1,* 103–111.

Goldstein, F. C., & Levin, H. S. (2001). Cognitive outcomes after mild and moderate traumatic brain injury in older adults. *Journal of Clinical and Experimental Neuropsychology, 23,* 739–752.

Gonçalves, D. C., & Byrne, G. J. (2012). Interventions for generalized anxiety disorder in older adults: Systematic review and meta-analysis. *Journal of Anxiety Disorders, 26,* 1–11.

Gorelick, P. B., Scuteri, A., Black, S. E., Decarli, C., Greenberg, S. M., Iadecola, C., . . . Seshadri, S. (2011). Vascular contributions to cognitive impairment and dementia: A statement for healthcare professionals from the American Heart Association/American Stroke Association. *Stroke, 42,* 2672–2713.

Gorman, E. (2011). Chronic degenerative conditions, disability, and loss. In D. L. Harris (Ed.), *Counting our losses: Reflecting on change, loss, and transition in everyday life* (pp. 195–208). New York: Routledge/Taylor & Francis Group.

Gotink, R. A., Meijboom, R., Vernooij, M. W., Smits, M., & Hunink, M. G. M. (2016). 8-week Mindfulness Based Stress Reduction induces brain changes similar to traditional long term meditation practice: A systematic review. *Brain and Cognition, 108,* 32–41.

Grace, J., & Malloy, P. (2001). *Frontal Systems Behavior Scale: Professional manual.* Lutz, FL: Psychological Assessment Resources.

Grady, C. (2012). The cognitive neuroscience of ageing. *Nature Reviews Neuroscience, 13,* 491–505.

Grady, C. L., McIntosh, A. R., Rajah, M. N., Beig, S., & Craik, F. I. M. (1999). The effects of age on the neural correlates of episodic encoding. *Cerebral Cortex, 9*(8), 805–814.

Graham, J. E., Christian, L. M., & Kiecolt-Glaser, J. K. (2006). Stress, age, and immune function: Toward a lifespan approach. *Journal of Behavioral Medicine, 29*(4), 389–400.

Graham, J. E., Rockwood, K., Beattie, B. L., Eastwood, R., Gauthier, S., Tuokko, H., & McDowell, I. (1997). Prevalence and severity of cognitive impairment with and without dementia in an elderly population. *The Lancet, 349,* 1793–1796.

Granholm, E., Holden, J., Link, P. C., McQuaid, J. R., & Jeste, D. V. (2013). Randomized controlled trial of cognitive behavioral social skills training for older consumers with schizophrenia: Defeatist performance attitudes and functional outcome. *American Journal of Geriatric Psychiatry, 21,* 251–262.

Granholm, E. L., McQuaid, J. R., & Holden, J. L. (2016). *Cognitive-behavioral social skills training for schizophrenia: A practical treatment guide.* New York: Guilford Press.

Granholm, E. L., McQuaid, J. R., Link, P. C., Fish, S., Patterson, T., & Jeste, D. V. (2008). Neuropsychological predictors of functional outcome in Cognitive Behavioral Social Skills Training for older people with schizophrenia. *Schizophrenia Research, 100,* 133–143.

Grant, P. M., Huh, G. A., Perivoliotis, D., Stolar, N. M., & Beck, A. T. (2012). Randomized trial to evaluate the efficacy of cognitive therapy for low-functioning patients with schizophrenia. *Archives of General Psychiatry, 69,* 121–127.

Green, R. C., Green, J., Harrison, J. M., & Kutner, M. H. (1994). Screening for cognitive impairment in older individuals: Validation study of a computer-based test. *Archives Neurology, 51*(8), 779–786.

Greenblatt, H. K., & Greenblatt, D. J. (2016). Use of antipsychotics for the treatment of behavioral symptoms of dementia. *Journal of Clinical Pharmacology, 56,* 1048–1057.

Greenwood, P., & Parasuraman, R. (2010). Neuronal and cognitive plasticity: A neurocognitive framework for ameliorating cognitive aging. *Frontiers in Aging Neuroscience, 2,* 150.

Grosch, M. C., Weiner, M. F., Hynan, L. S., Shore, J., & Cullum, C. M. (2015). Video teleconference-based neurocognitive screening in geropsychiatry. *Psychiatry Research, 225*(3), 734–735.

Gualtieri, C. T. (2004). Computerized neurocognitive testing and its potential for modern psychiatry. *Psychiatry (Edgmont), 1*(2), 29–36.

Gualtieri, C. T., & Johnson, L. G. (2005). Neurocognitive testing supports a broader concept of mild cognitive impairment. *American Journal of Alzheimer's Disease and Other Dementias, 20*(6), 359–366.

Gualtieri, C. T., & Johnson, L. G. (2006). Reliability and validity of a computerized neurocognitive test battery, CNS Vital Signs. *Archives of Clinical Neuropsychology, 21*(7), 623–643.

Gurland, B. J., Dean, L. L., Copeland, J., Gurland, R., & Golden, R. (1982). Criteria for the diagnosis of dementia in the community elderly. *The Gerontologist, 22,* 180–186.

Haag, M. D., Hofman, A., Koudstaal, P. J., Stricker, B. H., & Breteler, M. M. (2009). Statins are associated with a reduced risk of Alzheimer disease regardless of lipophilicity: The Rotterdam Study. *Journal of Neurology, Neurosurgery and Psychiatry, 80*(1), 13–17.

Hageman, W. J., & Arrindell, W. A. (1993). A further refinement of the Reliable Change (RC) Index by improving the pre–post difference score: Introducing RCID. *Behaviour Research and Therapy, 31*(7), 693–700.

Hageman, W. J., & Arrindell, W. A. (1999a). Clinically significant and practical!: Enhancing precision does make a difference: Reply to McGlinchey and Jacobson, Hsu, and Speer. *Behaviour Research and Therapy, 37*(12), 1219–1233.

Hageman, W. J., & Arrindell, W. A. (1999b). Establishing clinically significant change: Increment of precision and the distinction between individual and group level of analysis. *Behaviour Research and Therapy, 37*(12), 1169–1193.

Hamer, M., & Chida, Y. (2009). Physical activity and risk of neurodegenerative disease: A systematic review of prospective evidence. *Psychological Medicine, 39*(1), 3–11.

Hamid, A. A., Pettibone, J. R., Mabrouk, O. S., Hetrick, V. L., Schmidt, R., Vander Weele, C. M., . . . Berke, J. D. (2016). Mesolimbic dopamine signals the value of work. *Nature Neuroscience, 19,* 117–126.

Hammers, D., Spurgeon, E., Ryan, K., Persad, C., Barbas, N., Heidebrink, J., . . . Giordani, B. (2012). Validity of a brief computerized cognitive screening test in dementia. *Journal of Geriatric Psychiatry and Neurology, 25*(2), 89–99.

Hammers, D., Spurgeon, E., Ryan, K., Persad, C., Heidebrink, J., Barbas, N., . . . Giordani, B. (2011). Reliability of repeated cognitive assessment of dementia using a brief computerized battery. *American Journal of Alzheimer's Disease and Other Dementias, 26*(4), 326–333.

Hardman, R. J., Kennedy, G., Macpherson, H., Scholey, A. B., & Pipingas, A. (2016). Adherence to a Mediterranean-style diet and effects on cognition in adults: A qualitative evaluation and systematic review of longitudinal and prospective trials. *Frontiers in Nutrtion, 3,* 22.

Harmell, A. L., Chattillion, E. A., Roepke, S. K., & Mausbach, B. T. (2011). A review of the psychobiology of dementia caregiving: A focus on resilience factors. *Current Psychiatry Reports, 13,* 219–224.

Harrell, K. M., Wilkins, S. S., Connor, M. K., & Chodosh, J. (2014). Telemedicine and the evaluation of cognitive impairment: The additive value of neuropsychological assessment. *Journal of American Medical Directors Association, 15*(8), 600–606.

Harrell, L. E., Marson, D., Chatterjee, A., & Parrish, J. A. (2000). The Severe Mini-Mental State Examination: A new neuropsychologic instrument for the bedside assessment of severely impaired patients with Alzheimer disease. *Alzheimer Disease and Associated Disorders, 14*(3), 168–175.

Hartley, A. A. (1993). Evidence for the selective preservation of spatial selective attention in old age. *Psychology and Aging, 8*(3), 371–379.

Hartz, G. W. (1986). Adult grief and its interface with mood disorder: Proposal of a new diagnosis of complicated bereavement. *Comprehensive Psychiatry, 27*, 60–64.

Haslam, C., Morton, T. A., Haslam, S. A., Varnes, L., Graham, R., & Gamaz, L. (2012). "When the age is in, the wit is out": Age-related self-categorization and deficit expectations reduce performance on clinical tests used in dementia assessment. *Psychology and Aging, 27*(3), 778–784.

Hassiotis, A., Strydom, A., Allen, K., & Walker, Z. (2003). A memory clinic for older people with intellectual disabilities. *Aging and Mental Health, 7*(6), 418–423.

Haxby, J. V. (1989). Neuropsychological evaluation of adults with Down's syndrome: Patterns of selective impairment in non-demented old adults. *Journal of Mental Deficiency Research, 33*(3), 193–210.

Hayden, K. M., Norton, M. C., Darcey, D., Ostbye, T., Zandi, P. P., Breitner, J. C., & Welsh-Bohmer, K. A. (2010). Occupational exposure to pesticides increases the risk of incident AD: The Cache County study. *Neurology, 74*(19), 1524–1530.

Hayes, S. C., Strosahl, K., & Wilson, K. G. (2012). *Acceptance and commitment therapy: The process and practice of mindful change* (2nd ed.). New York: Guilford Press.

Hays, P. (1996). Culturally responsive assessment with diverse older clients. *Professional Psychology: Research and Practice, 27*, 188–193.

Heaton, R. K., Grant, I., & Matthews, C. G. (1991). *Comprehensive norms for an expanded Halstead-Reitan Battery: Demographic corrections, research findings and clinical applications.* Odessa, FL: Psychological Assessment Resources.

Heaton, R. K., Miller, S. W., Taylor, M. J., & Grant, I. (2004). *Revised comprehensive norms for an expanded Halstead-Reitan Battery: Demographically adjusted neuropsychological norms for African American and Caucasian adults scoring program.* Odessa, FL: Psychological Assessment Resources.

Heilbronner, R. L., Sweet, J. J., Attix, D. K., Krull, K. R., Henry, G. K., & Hart, R. P. (2010). Official position of the American Academy of Clinical Neuropsychology on serial neuropsychological assessments: The utility and challenges of repeat test administrations in clinical and forensic contexts. *The Clinical Neuropsychologist, 24*(8), 1267–1278.

Heisel, M. J., Talbot, N. L., King, D. A., Tu, X. M., & Duberstein, P. R. (2015). Adapting interpersonal psychotherapy for older adults at risk of suicide. *American Journal of Geriatric Psychiatry, 23*, 87–98.

Hendricks, G.-J. (2014). Therapeutics in late-life anxiety disorders: An update. *Current Treatment Options in Psychiatry, 1*, 27–36.

Herr, M., & Ankri, J. (2013). A critical review of the use of telephone tests to identify cognitive impairment in epidemiology and clinical research. *Journal of Telemedicine and Telecare, 19*(1), 45–54.

Hess, T. M., & Blanchard-Fields, F. (1999). *Social cognition and aging.* San Diego, CA: Academic Press.

Hildebrand, R., Chow, H., Williams, C., Nelson, M., & Wass, P. (2004). Feasibility of neuropsychological testing of older adults via videoconference: Implications for assessing the capacity for independent living. *Journal of Telemedicine and Telecare, 10*(3), 130–134.

Hill, J., McVay, J. M., Walter-Ginzburg, A., Mills, C. S., Lewis, J., Lewis, B. E., & Fillit, H. (2005). Validation of a Brief Screen for Cognitive Impairment (BSCI) administered by telephone for use in the Medicare population. *Disease Management, 8*(4), 223–234.

Hill, N. T. M., Mowszowski, L., Naismith, S. L., Chadwick, V. L., Valenzuela, M., & Lampit, A. (2017). Computerized cognitive training in older adults with mild cognitive impairment or dementia: A systematic review and meta-analysis. *American Journal of Psychiatry, 174*(4), 329–340.

Hinrichsen, G. A., & Clougherty, K. F. (2006). *Interpersonal psychotherapy for depressed older adults*. Washington, DC: American Psychological Association.

Hoelterhoff, M., & Chung, M. C. (2013). Death anxiety and well-being: Coping with life threatening events. *Traumatology, 19*, 280–291.

Hofer, S. M., & Alwin, D. F. (2008). *Handbook of cognitive aging: Interdisciplinary perspectives*. Thousand Oaks, CA: SAGE.

Hoffman, R., & Gerber, M. (2013). Evaluating and adapting the Mediterranean diet for non-Mediterranean populations: A critical appraisal. *Nutrition Reviews, 71*(9), 573–584.

Hofmann, S. G., Asnaan, A., Vonk, I. J. J., Sawyer, A. T., & Fang, A. (2012). The efficacy of cognitive behavioral therapy: A review of meta-analyses. *Cognitive Therapy and Research, 36*, 427–440.

Hofmann, S. G., Sawyer, A. T., Witt, A. A., & Oh, D. (2010). The effect of mindfulness-based therapy on anxiety and depression: A meta-analytic review. *Journal of Consulting and Clinical Psychology, 78*, 169–183.

Holland, A. J., Hon, J., Huppert, F. A., & Stevens, F. (2000). Incidence and course of dementia in people with Down's syndrome: Findings from a population-based study. *Journal of Intellectual Disability Research, 44*(2), 138–146.

Holland, J. M., & Gallagher-Thompson, D. (2014). Interventions for mental health problems in later life. In D. H. Barlow (Ed.), *The Oxford handbook of clinical psychology* (pp. 810–836). New York: Oxford University Press.

Holtzer, R., Goldin, Y., Zimmerman, M., Katz, M., Buschke, H., & Lipton, R. B. (2008). Robust norms for selected neuropsychological tests in older adults. *Archives of Clinical Neuropsychology, 23*(5), 531–541.

Horn, J. L. (1982). The aging of human abilities. In B. B. Wolman (Ed.), *Handbook of developmental psychology* (pp. 847–870). Englewood Cliffs, NJ: Prentice Hall.

Horowitz, M. J., Siegel, B., Holen, A., Bonnano, G. A., Milbrath, C., & Stinson, C. H. (1997). Diagnostic criteria for complicated grief disorder. *American Journal of Psychiatry, 154*, 904–910.

Hsu, B., Cumming, R. G., Waite, L. M., Blyth, F. M., Naganathan, V., Le Couteur, D. G., . . . Handelsman, D. J. (2015). Longitudinal relationships between reproductive hormones and cognitive decline in older men: The Concord Health and Ageing in Men Project. *Journal of Clinical Endocrinology Metabolism, 100*(6), 2223–2230.

Hsu, L. M. (1989). Reliable changes in psychotherapy: Taking into account regression toward the mean. *Behavioral Assessment, 11*(4), 459–467.

Hsu, L. M. (1999). A comparison of three methods of identifying reliable and clinically significant client changes: Commentary on Hageman and Arrindell. *Behaviour Research and Therapy, 37*(12), 1195–1202.

Hu, X., Weber, B., Kleinschmidt, H., & Jessen, F. (2014). Delay discounting in subjects with subjective cognitive decline, elderly controls. *Alzheimer's and Dementia, 10*(4, Suppl.), P721–P722.

Huckans, M., Hutson, L., Twamley, E., Jak, A., Kaye, J., & Storzbach, D. (2013). Efficacy of cognitive rehabilitation therapies for mild cognitive impairment (MCI) in older adults: Working toward a theoretical model and evidence-based interventions. *Neuropsychology Review, 23,* 63–80.

Huizenga, H., van Rentergem, J. A., Grasman, R. P. P. P., Muslimovic, D., & Schmand, B. (2016). Normative comparisons for large neuropsychological test batteries: User-friendly and sensitive solutions to minimize familywise false positives. *Journal of Clinical and Experimental Neuropsychology, 38*(6), 611–629.

Hultsch, D. F., Hertzog, C., Small, B. J., & Dixon, R. A. (1999). Use it or lose it: Engaged lifestyle as a buffer of cognitive decline in aging? *Psychology of Aging, 14*(2), 245–263.

Hultsch, D. F., Strauss, E., Hunter, M. A., & MacDonald, S. W. S. (2008). Intraindividual variability, cognition, and aging. In F. I. M. Craik & T. A. Salthouse (Eds.), *The handbook of aging and cognition* (3rd ed., pp. 491–556). New York: Psychology Press.

Ihle, A., Oris, M., Fagot, D., Baeriswyl, M., Guichard, E., & Kliegel, M. (2015). The association of leisure activities in middle adulthood with cognitive performance in old age: The moderating role of educational level. *Gerontology, 61*(6), 543–550.

Imtiaz, B., Tolppanen, A.-M., Kivipelto, M., & Soininen, H. (2014). Future directions in Alzheimer's disease from risk factors to prevention. *Biochemical Pharmacology, 88,* 661–670.

Inoue, M., Jimbo, D., Taniguchi, M., & Urakami, K. (2011). Touch Panel-type Dementia Assessment Scale: A new computer-based rating scale for Alzheimer's disease. *Psychogeriatrics, 11*(1), 28–33.

Irani, F., Kalkstein, S., Moberg, E. A., & Moberg, P. J. (2011). Neuropsychological performance in older patients with schizophrenia: A meta-analysis of cross-sectional and longitudinal studies. *Schizophrenia Bulletin, 37*(6), 1318–1326.

Iverson, G. L., Gardner, A. J., McCrory, P., Zafonte, R., & Castellani, R. J. (2015). A critical review of chronic traumatic encephalopathy. *Neuroscience and Biobehavioral Reviews, 56,* 276–293.

Ivnik, R. J., Malec, J. F., Smith, G. E., Tangalos, E. G., & Petersen, R. C. (1996). Neuropsychological tests' norms above age 55: COWAT, BNT, MAE Token, WRAT-R Reading, AMNART, Stroop, TMT, and JLO. *The Clinical Neuropsychologist, 10,* 262–278.

Ivnik, R. J., Smith, G. E., Lucas, J. A., Petersen, R. C., Boeve, B. F., Kokmen, E., & Tangalos, E. G. (1999). Testing normal older people three or four times at 1- to 2-year intervals: Defining normal variance. *Neuropsychology, 13*(1), 121–127.

Jackson, J. D., Rentz, D. M., Aghjayan, S. L., Buckley, R. F., Meneide, T.-F., Sperling, R. A., & Amariglio, R. (2016). Subjective cognitive concerns are associated with objective memory performance in older Caucasian but not African-American persons. *Alzheimer's and Dementia, 12*(7, Suppl.), P1173.

Jacobson, N. S., Follette, W. C., & Revenstorf, D. (1984). Psychotherapy outcome research: Methods for reporting variability and evaluating clinical significance. *Behavior Therapy, 15*(4), 336–352.

Jacobson, N. S., & Truax, P. (1991). Clinical significance: A statistical approach to defining meaningful change in psychotherapy research. *Journal of Consulting and Clinical Psychology, 59*(1), 12–19.

Jak, A. (2012). The impact of physical and mental activity on cognitive aging. *Current Topics in Behavioral Neurosciences, 10,* 273–291.

Jak, A. J., Bondi, M. W., Delano-Wood, L., Wierenga, C., Corey-Bloom, J., Salmon, D. P., . . . Delis, D. C. (2009). Quantification of five neuropsychological approaches to defining mild cognitive impairment. *American Journal of Geriatric Psychiatry, 17,* 368–375.

James, B. D., Bennett, D. A., Boyle, P. A., Leurgans, S., & Schneider, J. A. (2012). Dementia from Alzheimer disease and mixed pathologies in the oldest old. *Journal of the American Medical Association, 307,* 1798–1800.

James, I. A. (2014). The use of CBT for behaviors that challenge in dementia. In N. A. Pachana & K. Laidlaw (Eds.), *The Oxford handbook of clinical geropsychology* (pp. 753–775). New York: Oxford University Press.

James, W. (1890). *Principles of psychology.* New York: Henry Holt.

Janelsins, M. C., Kesler, S. R., Ahles, T. A., & Morrow, G. R. (2014). Prevalence, mechanisms, and management of cancer-related cognitive impairment. *International Review of Psychiatry, 26*(1), 102–113.

Janicki, M. P., & Dalton, A. J. (2000). Prevalence of dementia and impact on intellectual disability services. *Mental Retardation, 38*(3), 276–288.

Järvenpää, T., Rinne, J. O., Räihä, I., Koskenvuo, M., Löppönen, M., Hinkka, S., & Kaprio, J. (2002). Characteristics of two telephone screens for cognitive impairment. *Dementia and Geriatric Cognitive Disorders, 13*(3), 149–155.

Jefferson, A. L., Beiser, A. S., Himali, J. J., Seshadri, S., O'Donnell, C. J., Manning, W. J., . . . Benjamin, E. J. (2015). Low cardiac index is associated with incident dementia and Alzheimer disease: The Framingham Heart Study. *Circulation, 131*(15), 1333–1339.

Jellinger, K. A., & Attems, J. (2013). Neuropathological approaches to cerebral aging and neuroplasticity. *Dialogues in Clinical Neuroscience, 15,* 29–43.

Jeong, J. (2004). EEG dynamics in patients with Alzheimer's disease. *Clinical Neurophysiology, 115,* 1490–1505.

Jessen, F., Amariglio, R. E., van Boxtel, M., Breteler, M., Ceccaldi, M., Chételat, G., . . . the Subjective Cognitive Decline Initiative (SCD-I) Working Group. (2014). A conceptual framework for research on subjective cognitive decline in preclinical Alzheimer's disease. *Alzheimer's and Dementia, 10,* 844–852.

Jessen, F., Feyen, L., Freymann, K., Tepest, R., Maier, W., Heun, R., . . . Scheef, L. (2006). Volume reduction of the entorhinal cortex in subjective memory impairment. *Neurobiology of Aging, 27,* 1751–1756.

Jessen, F., Wiese, B., Bachmann, C., Eifflaender-Gorfer, S., Haller, F., Kölsch, H., . . . the German Study on Aging, Cognition and Dementia in Primary Care Patients Study Group. (2010). Prediction of dementia by subjective memory impairment: Effects of severity and temporal association with cognitive impairment. *Archives of General Psychiatry, 67,* 414–422.

Jessen, F., Wolfsgruber, S., Wiese, B., Bickel, H., Mösch, E., Kaduszkiewicz, H., . . . for the German Study on Aging, Cognition and Dementia in Primary Care Patients. (2013). AD dementia risk in late MCI, in early MCI, and in subjective memory impairment. *Alzheimer's and Dementia, 10,* 76–83.

Jeste, D. V., & Finkel, S. I. (2000). Psychosis of Alzheimer's disease and related dementias: Diagnostic criteria for a distinct syndrome. *American Journal of Geriatric Psychiatry, 8,* 29–34.

Jiang, T., Yu, J. T., & Tan, L. (2012). Novel disease-modifying therapies for Alzheimer's disease. *Journal of Alzheimer's Disease, 31,* 475–492.

Jiao, J., Li, Q., Chu, J., Zeng, W., Yang, M., & Zhu, S. (2014). Effect of n-3 PUFA supplementation on cognitive function throughout the life span from infancy to old age: A systematic review and meta-analysis of randomized controlled trials. *American Journal of Clinical Nutrition, 100*(6), 1422–1436.

Johansson, P. E., & Terenius, O. (2002). Development of an instrument for early detection of dementia in people with Down syndrome. *Journal of Intellectual and Developmental Disability, 27*(4), 325–345.

Jones, W. P., Loe, S. A., Krach, S. K., Rager, R. Y., & Jones, H. M. (2008). Automated Neuropsychological Assessment Metrics (ANAM) and Woodcock-Johnson III Tests of Cognitive Ability: A concurrent validity study. *The Clinical Neuropsychologist, 22*(2), 305–320.

Jonker, C., Geerlings, M. I., & Schmand, B. (2000). Are memory complaints predictive for dementia?: A review of clinical and population-based studies. *International Journal of Geriatric Psychiatry, 15*, 983–991.

Jordan, B. D. (2013). The clinical spectrum of sport-related traumatic brain injury. *Nature Reviews Neurology, 9*(4), 222–230.

Jorm, A. F. (2001). History of depression as a risk factor for dementia: An updated review. *Australian and New Zealand Journal of Psychiatry, 35*(6), 776–781.

Jorm, A. F. (2004). The Informant Questionnaire on Cognitive Decline in the Elderly (IQCODE): A review. *International Psychogeriatrics, 16*, 1–19.

Jorm, A. F., & Jacomb, P. A. (1989). The Informant Questionnaire on Cognitive Decline in the Elderly (IQCODE): Socio-demographic correlates, reliability, validity and some norms. *Psychological Medicine, 19*, 1015–1022.

Joshi, Y. B., & Pratico, D. (2013). Stress and HPA axis dysfunction in Alzheimer's disease. In D. Pratico & P. Mecocci (Eds.), *Studies on Alzheimer's disease* (pp. 159–165). New York: Springer.

Jozsvai, E., Kartakis, P., & Collings, A. (2002). Neuropsychological test battery to detect dementia in Down syndrome. *Journal on Developmental Disabilities, 9*(1), 27–34.

Judd, T. (1999). *Neuropsychotherapy and community integration: Brain illness, emotions and behaviour.* New York: Kluwer Academic/Plenum.

Jurica, P. J., Leitten, C. L., & Mattis, S. (2001). *Dementia Rating Scale-2: Professional manual.* Lutz, FL: Psychological Assessment Resources.

Kabat-Zinn, J. (1990). *Full catastrophe living: Using the wisdom of your body and mind to face stress, pain, and illness.* New York: Delta.

Kahl, K. G., Winter, L., & Schweiger, U. (2012). The third wave of cognitive behavioural therapies: What is new and what is effective? *Current Opinion in Psychiatry, 25*, 522—528.

Kalantarian, S., Stern, T. A., Mansour, M., & Ruskin, J. N. (2013). Cognitive impairment associated with atrial fibrillation: A meta-analysis. *Annal of Internal Medicine, 158*(5, Pt. 1), 338–346.

Kalbe, E., Salmon, E., Perani, D., Holthoff, V., Sorbi, S., Elsner, A., . . . Herholz, K. (2005). Anosognosia in very mild Alzheimer's disease but not in mild cognitive impairment. *Dementia and Geriatric Cognitive Disorders, 19*, 349–356.

Kalechstein, A. D., van Gorp, W. G., & Rapport, L. J. (1998). Variability in clinical classification of raw test scores across normative data sets. *The Clinical Neuropsychologist, 12*(3), 339–347.

Kales, H. C., Gitlin, L. N., & Lyketsos, C. G. (2015). State of the art review: Assessment and management of behavioral and psychological symptoms of dementia. *British Medical Journal, 350*, 369.

Kalsy-Lillico, S., Adams, D., & Oliver, C. (2012). Older adults with intellectual disabilities: Issues in ageing and dementia. In E. Emerson, C. Hatton, K. Dickson, R. Gone, A. Caine, & J. Bromley (Eds.), *Clinical psychology and people with intellectual disabilities* (2nd ed., pp. 359–392). Oxford, UK: Wiley-Blackwell.

Kane, R. L., Roebuck-Spencer, T., Short, P., Kabat, M., & Wilken, J. (2007). Identifying and monitoring cognitive deficits in clinical populations using Automated Neuropsychological Assessment Metrics (ANAM) tests. *Archives of Clinical Neuropsychology, 22*(Suppl.), S115–S126.

Kang, C., Lee, G. J., Yi, D., McPherson, S., Rogers, S., Tingus, K., & Lu, P. H. (2013). Normative data for healthy older adults and an abbreviated version of the Stroop test. *The Clinical Neuropsychologist, 27*(2), 276–289.

Karel, M. J., Molinari, V., Emery-Tiburcio, E. E., & Knight, B. G. (2015). Pikes Peak conference and competency-based training in professional geropsychology. In P. A. Lichtenberg, B. T. Mast, B. D. Carpenter, & J. Loebach Wetherell (Eds.), *APA handbook of clinical geropsychology: Vol. 1. History and status of the field and perspectives on aging* (pp. 19–43). Washington, DC: American Psychological Association.

Karp, A., Paillard-Borg, S., Wang, H. X., Silverstein, M., Winblad, B., & Fratiglioni, L. (2006). Mental, physical and social components in leisure activities equally contribute to decrease dementia risk. *Dementia and Geriatric Cognitive Disorders, 21*(2), 65–73.

Karr, J. E., Areshenkoff, C. N., Rast, P., & Garcia-Barrera, M. A. (2014). An empirical comparison of the therapeutic benefits of physical exercise and cognitive training on the executive functions of older adults: A meta-analysis of controlled trials. *Neuropsychology, 28*, 829–845.

Katz, S., Moskowitz, R. W., Jackson, B. A., & Jaffe, M. W. (1963). Studies of illness in the aged: The index of ADL: A standardized measure of biological and psychosocial function. *JAMA, 185*(12), 94–99.

Katzenschlager, R., & Evans, A. (2014). Impulse control and dopamine dysregulation syndrome. In K. R. Chaudhuri, E. Tolosa, A. H. V. Schapira, & W. Poewe (Eds.), *Non-motor symptoms of Parkinson's disease* (2nd ed., pp. 420–435). New York: Oxford University Press.

Kave, G., Eyal, N., Shorek, A., & Cohen-Mansfield, J. (2008). Multilingualism and cognitive state in the oldest old. *Psychology of Aging, 23*(1), 70–78.

Kawas, C., Karagiozis, H., Resau, L., Corrada, M., & Brookmeyer, R. (1995). Reliability of the Blessed Telephone Information-Memory-Concentration test. *Journal of Geriatric Psychiatry and Neurology, 8*(4), 238–242.

Kazdin, A. E. (2011). *Single-case research designs: Methods for clinical and applied settings.* New York: Oxford University Press.

Kelleher, M., Tolea, M. I., & Galvin, J. E. (2015). Anosognosia increases caregiver burden in mild cognitive impairment. *International Journal of Geriatric Psychiatry, 31*, 799–808.

Kennedy, R. E., Williams, C. P., Sawyer, P., Allman, R. M., & Crowe, M. (2014). Comparison of in-person and telephone administration of the Mini-Mental State Examination in the University of Alabama at Birmingham Study of Aging. *Journal of the American Geriatrics Society, 62*(10), 1928–1932.

Kennelly, S., & Collins, O. (2012). Walking the cognitive "minefield" between high and low blood pressure. *Journal of Alzheimer's Disease, 32*(3), 609–621.

Kensinger, E. A., Allard, E. R., & Krendl, A. C. (2014). The effects of age on memory for socioemotional material: An affective neuroscience perspective. In P. Verhaegen

& C. Hertzog (Eds.), *The Oxford handbook of emotion, social cognition, and problem-solving in adulthood* (pp. 26–46). New York: Oxford University Press.

Kensinger, E. A., & Gutchess, A. H. (2016). Cognitive aging in a social and affective context: Advances over the past 50 years. *Journals of Gerontology, Series B, Psychological Sciences, 72*(1), 61–70.

Kent, B. A., Oomen, C. A., Bekinschtein, P., Bussey, T. J., & Saksida, L. M. (2015). Cognitive enhancing effects of voluntary exercise, caloric restriction and environmental enrichment: A role for adult hippocampal neurogenesis and pattern separation? *Current Opinion in Behavioral Sciences, 4*, 179–185.

Kim, B., & Feldman, E. L. (2015). Insulin resistance as a key link for the increased risk of cognitive impairment in the metabolic syndrome. *Experimental and Molecular Medicine, 47*, e149.

Kinsella, G. J. (2010). Everyday memory for everyday tasks: Prospective memory as an outcome measure following TBI in older adults. *Brain Impairment, 11*(1), 37–41.

Kinsella, G. J., Olver, J., Ong, B., Gruen, R., & Hammersley, E. (2014). Mild traumatic brain injury in older adults: Early cognitive outcome. *Journal of International Neuropsychological Society, 20*(6), 663–671.

Kinsella, G. J., Olver, J., Ong, B., Hammersley, E., & Plowright, B. (2014). Traumatic brain injury in older adults: Does age matter? In H. S. Levin, D. H. K. Shum, & R. C. K. Chan (Eds.), *Understanding traumatic brain injury: Current research and future directions* (pp. 356–369). New York: Oxford University Press.

Kishita, N., Takei, Y., & Stewart, I. (2016). A meta-analysis of third wave mindfulness-based cognitive behavioral therapies for older persons. *International Journal of Geriatric Psychiatry, 32*(12), 1352–1361.

Kit, K. A., Tuokko, H. A., & Mateer, C. A. (2008). A review of the stereotype threat literature and its application in a neurological population. *Neuropsychology Review, 18*(2), 132–148.

Kleim, J. A., & Jones, T. A. (2008). Principles of experience-dependent neural plasticity: Implications for rehabilitation after brain damage. *Journal of Speech, Language, and Hearing Research, 51*, S225–S239.

Klerman, G. L., Weissman, M. M., Rounsaville, B. J., & Chevron, E. S. (1984). *Interpersonal psychotherapy of depression*. New York: Basic Books.

Kliegel, M., Martin, M., & Jäger, T. (2007). Development and validation of the Cognitive Telephone Screening Instrument (COGTEL) for the assessment of cognitive function across adulthood. *Journal of Psychology: Interdisciplinary and Applied, 141*(2), 147–170.

Knight, B. G., Karel, M. J., Hinrichsen, G. A., Qualls, S. H., & Duffy, M. (2009). Pikes Peak model for training in professional geropsychology. *American Psychologist, 64*(3), 205–214.

Knopman, D. S., Knudson, D., Yoes, M. E., & Weiss, D. J. (2000). Development and standardization of a new telephonic cognitive screening test: The Minnesota Cognitive Acuity Screen (MCAS). *Neuropsychiatry, Neuropsychology, and Behavioral Neurology, 13*(4), 286–296.

Knopman, D. S., Roberts, R. O., Geda, Y. E., Pankratz, V. S., Christianson, T. J. H., Petersen, R. C., & Rocca, W. A. (2010). Validation of the Telephone Interview for Cognitive Status modified in subjects with normal cognition, mild cognitive impairment, or dementia. *Neuroepidemiology, 34*(1), 34–42.

Kontos, P. C. (2012). Rethinking sociability in long-term care: An embodied dimension of selfhood. *Dementia: The International Journal of Social Research and Practice, 11*(3), 329–346.

Koocher, G. P., & Keith-Spiegel, P. (2008). *Ethics in psychology and the mental health professions: Standards and cases* (3rd ed.). New York: Oxford University Press.

Koppara, A., Frommann, I., Polcher, A., Parra, M. A., Maier, W., Jessen, F., . . . Wagner, M. (2015). Feature binding deficits in subjective cognitive decline and in mild cognitive impairment. *Journal of Alzheimer's Disease, 48*(Suppl. 1), S161–S170.

Korczyn, A. D., & Aharonson, V. (2007). Computerized methods in the assessment and prediction of dementia. *Current Alzheimer Research, 4*(4), 364–369.

Korner-Bitensky, N., Gélinas, I., Man-Son-Hing, M., & Marshall, S. (2005). Recommendations of the Canadian Consensus Conference on Driving Evaluation in Older Drivers. *Physical and Occupational Therapy in Geriatrics, 23*(2–3), 123–144.

Kowalski, K., Love, J., Tuokko, H., MacDonald, S., Hultsch, D., & Strauss, E. (2011). The influence of cognitive impairment with no dementia on driving restriction and cessation in older adults. *Accident Analysis and Prevention, 49,* 308–315.

Kral, V. A. (1962). Senescent forgetfulness: Benign and malignant. *Journal of the Canadian Medical Association, 86,* 257–260.

Kreuter, M. W., & Skinner, C. (2000). Tailoring: What's in a name? [Editorial]. *Health Education Research, 15,* 1–4.

Krinsky-McHale, S. J., & Silverman, W. (2013). Dementia and mild cognitive impairment in adults with intellectual disability: Issues of diagnosis. *Developmental Disabilities Research Reviews, 18*(1), 31–42.

Kroger, E., Verreault, R., Carmichael, P. H., Lindsay, J., Julien, P., Dewailly, E., . . . Laurin, D. (2009). Omega-3 fatty acids and risk of dementia: The Canadian Study of Health and Aging. *American Journal of Clinical Nutrition, 90*(1), 184–192.

Kshtriya, S., Barnstaple, R., Rabinovich, D. B., & DeSouza, J. F. X. (2015). Dance and aging: A critical review of findings in neuroscience. *American Journal of Dance Therapy, 37,* 81–112.

Kuiper, J. S., Zuidersma, M., Oude Voshaar, R. C., Zuidema, S. U., van den Heuvel, E. R., Stolk, R. P., & Smidt, N. (2015). Social relationships and risk of dementia: A systematic review and meta-analysis of longitudinal cohort studies. *Ageing Research and Review, 22,* 39–57.

Kuluski, K., Dow, C., Locock, L., Lyons, R. F., & Lasserson, D. (2014). Life interrupted and life regained?: Coping with stroke at a young age. *International Journal of Qualitative Studies on Health and Well-Being, 9,* 1–12.

Kuske, B., Wolff, C., Govert, U., & Muller, S. V. (2017). Early detection of dementia in people with an intellectual disability—A German pilot study. *Journal of Applied Research in Intellectual Disabilities, 30,* 49–57.

LaBar, K. S., & Cabeza, R. (2006). Cognitive neuroscience of emotional memory. *Nature Reviews Neuroscience, 7,* 54e64.

Lachman, M. E., Agrigoroaei, S., Tun, P. A., & Weaver, S. L. (2014). Monitoring cognitive functioning: Psychometric properties of the Brief Test of Adult Cognition by Telephone. *Assessment, 21*(4), 404–417.

Lahiri, D. K., Maloney, B., Basha, M. R., Ge, Y. W., & Zawia, N. H. (2007). How and when environmental agents and dietary factors affect the course of Alzheimer's disease: The "LEARn" model (latent early-life associated regulation) may explain the triggering of AD. *Current Alzheimer Research, 4*(2), 219–228.

Laidlaw, K. (2014). Cognitive-behavior therapy with older people. In N. A. Pachana & K. Laidlaw (Eds.), *The Oxford handbook of clinical geropsychology* (pp. 603–621). New York: Oxford University Press.

Lampit, A., Hallock, H., & Valenzuela, M. (2014). Computerized cognitive training in cognitively healthy older adults: A systematic review and meta-analysis of effect modifiers. *PLOS Medicine, 11,* e1001756.

Landa, Y., Mueser, K. T., Wyka, K. E., Shreck, E., Jespersen, R., Jacobs, M. A., . . . Walkup, J. T. (2016). Development of a group and family-based cognitive behavioral therapy program for youth at risk for psychosis. *Early Intervention Psychiatry, 10,* 511–521.

Lanska, D. J., Schmitt, F. A., Stewart, J. M., & Howe, J. N. (1993). Telephone-assessed mental state. *Dementia, 4*(2), 117–119.

Lauenroth, A., Ioannidis, A. E., & Teichmann, B. (2016). Influence of combined physical and cognitive training on cognition: A systematic review. *BioMed Central Geriatrics, 16,* 141.

Laurin, D., Verreault, R., Lindsay, J., MacPherson, K., & Rockwood, K. (2001). Physical activity and risk of cognitive impairment and dementia in elderly persons. *Archives of Neurology, 58*(3), 498–504.

Lawton, M. P., & Brody, E. M. (1969). Assessment of older people: Self-maintaining and instrumental activities of daily living. *The Gerontologist, 9,* 179–186.

Lawton, M. P., Moss, M. S., Fulcomer, M., & Kleban, M. H. (1982). A research and service oriented multilevel assessment instrument. *Journal of Gerontology, 37*(1), 91–99.

Le Carret, N., Lafont, S., Mayo, W., & Fabrigoule, C. (2003). The effect of education on cognitive performances and its implication for the constitution of the cognitive reserve. *Developmental Neuropsychology, 23*(3), 317–337.

Le Couter, D. G., & McLean, A. J. (1998). The aging liver: Drug clearance and oxygen diffusion barrier hypothesis. *Clinical Pharmacokinetics, 34,* 359–373.

Lecours, A., Sirois, M. J., Ouellet, M. C., Boivin, K., & Simard, J. F. (2012). Long-term functional outcome of older adults after a traumatic brain injury. *Journal of Head Trauma Rehabilitation, 27*(6), 379–390.

Lee, S., Buring, J. E., Cook, N. R., & Grodstein, F. (2006). The relation of education and income to cognitive function among professional women. *Neuroepidemiology, 26*(2), 93–101.

Lee, S. J., Ritchie, C. S., Yaffe, K., Stijacic Cenzer, I., & Barnes, D. E. (2014). A clinical index to predict progression from mild cognitive impairment to dementia due to Alzheimer's disease. *PLOS ONE, 9*(12), e113535.

Lehrer, J., Kogler, S., Lamm, C., Moser, D., Klug, S., Pusswald, G., . . . Auff, E. (2015). Awareness of memory deficits in subjective cognitive decline, mild cognitive impairment, Alzheimer's disease and Parkinson's disease. *International Psychogeriatrics, 27,* 357–366.

Lenze, E. J., Dew, M. A., Mazumdar, S., Begley, A. E., Cornes, C., Miller, M. D., . . . Reynolds, C. F., III. (2002). Combined pharmacotherapy and psychotherapy as maintenance treatment for late-life depression: Effects on social adjustment. *American Journal of Psychiatry, 159,* 466–468.

Leung, G. T. Y., & Lam, L. C. W. (2007). Leisure activities and cognitive impairment in late life—A selective literature review of longitudinal cohort studies. *Hong Kong Journal of Psychiatry, 17*(3), 91–100.

Levine, B., Stuss, D. T., Winocur, G., & Binns, M. A. (2007). Cognitive rehabilitation in the elderly: Effects on strategic behavior in relation to goal management. *Journal of the International Neuropsychological Society, 13,* 143–152.

Levinson, D., Reeves, D., Watson, J., & Harrison, M. (2005). Automated neuropsychological assessment metrics (ANAM) measures of cognitive effects of Alzheimer's disease. *Archives of Clinical Neuropsychology, 20*(3), 403–408.

Levy, R. (1994). Aging-associated cognitive decline: Working Party of the International Psychogeriatric Association in collaboration with the World Health Organization. *International Psychogeriatrics, 6,* 63–68.

Lezak, M. D., Howieson, D. B., Bigler, E. D., & Tranel, D. (2012). *Neuropsychological assessment* (5th ed.). New York: Oxford University Press.

Lezak, M. D., Howieson, D. B., Loring, D. W., Hannay, H. J., & Fischer, J. S. (2004). *Neuropsychological assessment* (4th ed.). New York: Oxford University Press.

Li, J., Wang, Y. J., Zhang, M., Xu, Z. Q., Gao, C. Y., Fang, C. Q., . . . Zhou, H. D. (2011). Vascular risk factors promote conversion from mild cognitive impairment to Alzheimer disease. *Neurology, 76*(17), 1485–1491.

Li, L., Wang, Y., Yan, J., Chen, Y., Zhou, R., Yi, X., . . . Zhou, H. (2012). Clinical predictors of cognitive decline in patients with mild cognitive impairment: The Chongqing aging study. *Journal of Neurology, 259*(7), 1303–1311.

Li, Y., Hai, S., Zhou, Y., & Dong, B. R. (2015). Cholinesterase inhibitors for rarer dementias associated with neurological conditions. *Cochrane Database of Systematic Reviews, 3,* CD009444.

Libon, D. J., Rascovsky, K., Powers, J., Irwin, D. J., Boller, A., Weinberg, D., . . . Grossman, M. (2013). Comparative semantic profiles in semantic dementia and Alzheimer's disease. *Brain: A Journal of Neurology, 136*(8), 2497–2509.

Light, L. L. (2012). Dual-process theories of memory in old age: An update. In M. Naveh-Benjamin & N. Ohta (Eds.), *Memory and aging: Current issues and future directions* (pp. 97–124). New York: Psychology Press.

Lim, Y. Y., Ellis, K., Harrington, K., Ames, D., Martins, R., Masters, C., . . . Maruff, P. (2012). Use of the CogState Brief Battery in the assessment of Alzheimer's disease related cognitive impairment in the Australian Imaging, Biomarkers and Lifestyle (AIBL) study. *Journal of Clinical and Experimental Neuropsychology, 34*(4), 345–358.

Lim, Y. Y., Jaeger, J., Harrington, K., Ashwood, T., Ellis, K. A., Stöffler, A., . . . Maruff, P. (2013). Three-month stability of the CogState brief battery in healthy older adults, mild cognitive impairment, and Alzheimer's disease: Results from the Australian Imaging, Biomarkers, and Lifestyle-Rate of Change Substudy (AIBL-ROCS). *Archives of Clinical Neuropsychology, 28*(4), 320–330.

Lin, J.-D., Wu, C.-L., Lin, P.-Y., Lin, L.-P., & Chu, C. M. (2011). Early onset ageing and service preparation in people with intellectual disabilities: Institutional managers' perspective. *Research in Developmental Disabilities, 32*(1), 188–193.

Lindbergh, C., Dishman, R. K., & Miller, S. L. (2016). Functional disability in mild cognitive impairment: A systematic review and meta-analysis. *Neuropsychology Review, 26,* 129–159.

Lindsay, J., Laurin, D., Verreault, R., Hebert, R., Helliwell, B., Hill, G. B., & McDowell, I. (2002). Risk factors for Alzheimer's disease: A prospective analysis from the Canadian Study of Health and Aging. *American Journal of Epidemiology, 156*(5), 445–453.

Linehan, M. M. (2015). *DBT skills training manual* (2nd ed.). New York: Guilford Press.

Lipton, R. B., Katz, M. J., Kuslansky, G., Sliwinski, M. J., Stewart, W. F., Verghese, J., . . . Buschke, H. (2003). Screening for dementia by telephone using the memory impairment screen. *Journal of American Geriatrics Society, 51*(10), 1382–1390.

Litvan, I., Goldman, J. G., Tröster, A. I., Schmand, B. A., Weintraub, D., Petersen, R. C., . . . Emre, M. (2012). Diagnostic criteria for mild cognitive impairment in

Parkinson's disease: Movement Disorder Society Task Force guidelines. *Movement Disorders, 27,* 349–356.

Liu, Y. C., Yip, P. K., Fan, Y. M., & Meguro, K. (2012). A potential protective effect in multilingual patients with semantic dementia: Two case reports of patients speaking Taiwanese and Japanese. *Acta Neurologica Taiwan, 21*(1), 25–30.

Locke, D. E. C., Dassel, K. B., Hall, G., Baxter, L. C., Woodruff, B. K., Snyder, C. H., . . . Caselli, R. J. (2009). Assessment of patient and caregiver experiences of dementia-related symptoms: Development of the Multidimensional Assessment of Neurodegenerative Symptoms Questionnaire. *Dementia and Geriatric Cognitive Disorders, 27*(3), 260–272.

Lockwood, K. A., Alexopoulos, G. S., Kakuma, T., & Van Gorp, W. G. (2000). Subtypes of cognitive impairment in depressed older adults. *American Journal of Geriatric Psychiatry, 8*(3), 201–208.

Loewenstein, D., & Acevedo, A. (2009). The relationship between instrumental activities of daily living and neuropsychological performance. In T. D. Marcotte & I. Grant (Eds.), *Neuropsychology of everyday functioning* (pp. 93–112). New York: Guilford Press.

Loewenstein, D. A., Acevedo, A., Small, B. J., Agron, J., Crocco, E., & Duara, R. (2009). Stability of different subtypes of mild cognitive impairment among the elderly over a 2- to 3- year follow-up period. *Dementia and Geriatric Cognitive Disorders, 27,* 418–423.

Lopez, S. J., Edwards, L. M., Floyd, R. K., Magyar-Moe, J., Rehfeldt, J. D., & Ryder, J. A. (2001). Note on comparability of MicroCog test forms. *Perceptual and Motor Skills, 93*(3), 825–828.

Loring, D. W., & Bauer, R. M. (2010). Testing the limits: Cautions and concerns regarding the new Wechsler IQ and memory scales. *Neurology, 74,* 685–690.

Lott, I. T., & Dierssen, M. (2010). Cognitive deficits and associated neurological complications in individuals with Down's syndrome. *The Lancet Neurology, 9*(6), 623–633.

Lott, I. T., Doran, E., Nguyen, V. Q., Tournay, A., Movsesyan, N., & Gillen, D. L. (2012). Down syndrome and dementia: Seizures and cognitive decline. *Journal of Alzheimer's Disease, 29*(1), 177–185.

Lourida, I., Soni, M., Thompson-Coon, J., Purandare, N., Lang, I. A., Ukoumunne, O. C., & Llewellyn, D. J. (2013). Mediterranean diet, cognitive function, and dementia: A systematic review. *Epidemiology, 24*(4), 479–489.

Love, J., & Tuokko, H. (2015). Older driver safety: A survey of psychologists' attitudes, knowledge, and practices. *Canadian Journal on Aging, 35,* 393–404.

Low, L. F., Harrison, F., & Lackersteen, S. M. (2013). Does personality affect risk for dementia?: A systematic review and meta-analysis. *American Journal of Geriatric Psychiatry, 21*(8), 713–728.

Lowe, C., & Rabbitt, P. (1998). Test/re-test reliability of the CANTAB and ISPOCD neuropsychological batteries: Theoretical and practical issues: Cambridge Neuropsychological Test Automated Battery, International Study of Post-Operative Cognitive Dysfunction. *Neuropsychologia, 36*(9), 915–923.

Lowe, P. A., & Reynolds, C. R. (2006). Examination of the psychometric properties of the Adult Manifest Anxiety Scale-Elderly Version scores. *Educational and Psychological Measurement, 66,* 93–115.

Lucas, J. A., Ivnik, R. J., Smith, G. E., Bohac, D. L., Tangalos, E. G., Graff-Radford, N. R., & Petersen, R. C. (1998). Mayo's older Americans normative studies: Category fluency norms. *Journal of Clinical and Experimental Neuropsychology, 20,* 194–200.

Luders, E. (2014). Exploring age-related brain degeneration in meditation practitioners. *Annals of the New York Academy of Sciences, 1307,* 82–88.

Luppa, M., Sikorski, C., Luck, T., Ehreke, L., Konnopka, A., Wiese, B., . . . Riedel-Heller, S. G. (2012). Age- and gender-specific prevalence of depression in latest life—Systematic review and meta-analysis. *Journal of Affective Disorders, 136,* 212–221.

Lüscher, C., Nicoll, R. A., Malenka, R. C., & Muller, D. (2000). Synaptic plasticity and dynamic modulation of the postsynaptic membrane. *Nature Neuroscience, 3,* 545–550.

Lustig, C., Shah, P., Seidler, R., & Reuter-Lorenz, P. (2009). Aging, training, and the brain: A review and future directions. *Neuropsychology Review, 19,* 504–522.

Lutz, A., Slagter, H. A., Dunne, J. D., & Davidson, R. J. (2008). Attention regulation and monitoring in meditation. *Trends in Cognitive Sciences, 12,* 163–169.

Maassen, G. H. (2000). Principles of defining reliable change indices. *Journal of Clinical and Experimental Neuropsychology, 22*(5), 622–632.

Maassen, G. H., Bossema, E., & Brand, N. (2008). Reliable change and practice effects: Outcomes of various indices compared. *Journal of Clinical and Experimental Neuropsychology, 31*(3), 339–352.

MacCallum, F., & Bryant, R. A. (2013). A cognitive attachment model of prolonged grief: Integrating attachments, memory, and identity. *Clinical Psychology Review, 33,* 713–727.

MacDonald, S. W., DeCarlo, C. A., & Dixon, R. A. (2011). Linking biological and cognitive aging: Toward improving characterizations of developmental time. *Journals of Gerontology Series B, Psychological Sciences and Social Sciences, 66*(Suppl. 1), i59–i70.

MacDonald, S. W., Dixon, R. A., Cohen, A. L., & Hazlitt, J. E. (2004). Biological age and 12-year cognitive change in older adults: Findings from the Victoria Longitudinal Study. *Gerontology, 50*(2), 64–81.

MacKnight, C., Rockwood, K., Awalt, E., & McDowell, I. (2002). Diabetes mellitus and the risk of dementia, Alzheimer's disease and vascular cognitive impairment in the Canadian Study of Health and Aging. *Dementis Geriatric Cognitive Disorders, 14*(2), 77–83.

MacLean, K. A., Ferrer, E., Aichele, S. R., Bridwell, D. A., Zanesco, A. P., Jacobs, T. L., . . . Saron, C. D. (2010). Intensive meditation training improves perceptual discrimination and sustained attention. *Psychological Science, 21,* 829–839.

Maki, P. M. (2012). Minireview: Effects of different HT formulations on cognition. *Endocrinology, 153*(8), 3564–3570.

Maki, Y., Amari, M., Yamaguchi, T., Nakaaki, S., & Yamaguchi, H. (2012). Anosognosia: Patients' distress and self-awareness of deficits in Alzheimer's disease. *American Journal of Alzheimer's Disease and Other Dementias, 27,* 339–345.

Malkinson, R., & Bar-Tur, L. (2014). Cognitive grief therapy: Coping with the inevitability of loss and grief in later life. In N. A. Pachana & K. Laidlaw (Eds.), *The Oxford handbook of clinical geropsychology* (pp. 837–855). New York: Oxford University Press.

Malloy, P., Tremont, G., Grace, J., & Frakey, L. (2007). The Frontal Systems Behavior Scale discriminates frontotemporal dementia from Alzheimer's disease. *Alzheimer's and Dementia, 3,* 200–203.

Manly, J. J. (2006). Cultural issues. In D. K. Attix & K. A. Welsh-Bohmer (Eds.),

Geriatric neuropsychology: Assessment and intervention (pp. 198–222). New York: Guilford Press.

Manly, J. J., Byrd, D., Touradji, P., Sanchez, D., & Stern, Y. (2004). Literacy and cognitive change among ethnically diverse elders. *International Journal of Psychology, 39*(1), 47–60.

Manly, J. J., & Mungas, D. (2015). JGPS special series on race, ethnicity, life experiences, and cognitive aging. *Journals of Gerontology: Series B: Psychological Sciences and Social Sciences, 70*(4), 509–511.

Markowitz, J. C., & Weissman, M. M. (2004). Interpersonal psychotherapy: Principles and applications. *World Psychiatry, 3*, 136–139.

Márquez-González, M. O., Losada, A., & Romero-Moreno, R. (2014). Acceptance and commitment therapy with dementia caregivers. In N. A. Pachana & K. Laidlaw (Eds.), *The Oxford handbook of clinical geropsychology* (pp. 658–674). New York: Oxford University Press.

Martin, M., & Hofer, S. M. (2004). Intraindividual variability, change, and aging: Conceptual and analytical issues. *Gerontology, 50*(1), 7–11.

Mastellos, N., Gunn, L. H., Felix, L. M., Car, J., & Majeed, A. (2014). Transtheoretical model stages of change for dietary and physical exercise modification in weight loss management for overweight and obese adults. *Cochrane Database of Systematic Reviews, 2*, CD008066.

Mateer, C. A., & Smart, C. M. (2013). Cognitive rehabilitation—Innovation, application and evidence. In S. Koffler, J. Morgan, I. S. Baron, & M. F. Griffenstein (Eds.), *Neuropsychology: Science and practice: I* (pp. 222–255). New York: Oxford University Press.

Mather, M. (2012). The emotion paradox in the brain. *Annals of the New York Academy of Sciences, 1251*, 33–49.

Mather, M. (2016). The affective neuroscience of aging. *Annual Review of Psychology, 67*, 213–238.

Matthews, B. R. (2010). Alzheimer disease update. *Continuum (Minneapolis, MN), 16*(2), 15–30.

Mattis, S. (1988). *Dementia Rating Scale: Professional manual*. Odessa, FL: Psychological Assessment Resources.

Mauri, M., Sinforiani, E., Bono, G., Cittadella, R., Quattrone, A., Boller, F., & Nappi, G. (2006). Interaction between apolipoprotein epsilon 4 and traumatic brain injury in patients with Alzheimer's disease and mild cognitive impairment. *Functional Neurology, 21*(4), 223–228.

McCabe, D. P., & Loaiza, V. M. (2012). Working memory. In S. K. Whitbourne & M. J. Sliwinski (Eds.), *The Wiley-Blackwell handbook of adulthood and aging* (pp. 154–173). Oxford, UK: Wiley-Blackwell.

McCarron, M., McCallion, P., Reilly, E., & Mulryan, N. (2014). A prospective 14-year longitudinal follow-up of dementia in persons with Down syndrome. *Journal of Intellectual Disability Research, 58*(1), 61–70.

McComb, E., Tuokko, H., Brewster, P., Chou, P. H. B., Kolitz, K., Crossley, M., & Simard, M. (2011). Mental Alternation Test: Administration mode, age, and practice effects. *Journal of Clinical and Experimental Neuropsychology, 33*(2), 234–241.

McConnell, H. (2014). Laboratory testing in neuropsychology. In M. W. Parsons & T. A. Hammeke (Eds.), *Clinical neuropsychology: A pocket handbook for assessment* (3rd ed., pp. 53–73). Washington, DC: American Psychiatric Association.

McCurry, S. M., Gibbons, L. E., Uomoto, J. M., Thompson, M. L., Graves, A. B.,

Edland, S. D., . . . Larson, E. B. (2001). Neuropsychological test performance in a cognitively intact sample of older Japanese American adults. *Archives of Clinical Neuropsychology, 16*(5), 447–459.

McDonough, I., Haber, S., Bischof, S., & Park, D. C. (2015). The Synapse Project: Engagement in mentally challenging activities enhances neural efficiency. *Restorative Neurology and Neuroscience, 33*, 865–882.

McDowell, I., Xi, G., Lindsay, J., & Tierney, M. (2007). Mapping the connections between education and dementia. *Journal of Clinical and Experimental Neuropsychology, 29*(2), 127–141.

McGlinchey, J. B., & Jacobson, N. S. (1999). Clinically significant but impractical?: A response to Hageman and Arrindell. *Behaviour Research and Therapy, 37*(12), 1211–1217.

McGrath, J. C. (2008). Post-acute in-patient rehabilitation. In A. Tyerman & N. S. King (Eds.), *Psychological approaches to rehabilitation after traumatic brain injury* (pp. 39–64). Malden, MA: Blackwell.

McGuire, J. (2009). Ethical considerations when working with older adults in psychology. *Ethics and Behavior, 19*(2), 112–128.

McKhann, G. M., Knopman, D. S., Chertkow, H., Hyman, B. T., Jack, C. R., Jr., Kawas, C. H., . . . Phelps, C. H. (2011). The diagnosis of dementia due to Alzheimer's disease: Recommendations from the National Institute on Aging-Alzheimer's Association workgroups on diagnostic guidelines for Alzheimer's disease. *Alzheimer's and Dementia, 7*(3), 263–269.

McShane, R., Areosa Sastre, A., & Minakaran, N. (2006). Memantine for dementia. *Cochrane Database Systematic Review*, CD003154.

McSweeney, A. J., Naugle, R. I., Chelune, G. J., & Luders, H. (1993). "T scores for change": An illustration of a regression approach to depicting change in clinical neuropsychology. *The Clinical Neuropsychologist, 7*, 300–312.

Meagher, D., O'Regan, N., Ryan, D., Connolly, W., Boland, E., O'Caoimhe, R., . . . Timmons, S. (2014). Frequency of delirium and subsyndromal delirium in an adult acute hospital population. *British Journal of Psychiatry, 205*(6), 478–485.

Medley, A. R., & Powell, T. (2010). Motivational interviewing to promote self-awareness and engagement in rehabilitation following acquired brain injury: A conceptual review. *Neuropsychological Rehabilitation, 20*, 481–508.

Meiberth, D., Scheef, L., Wolfsgruber, S., Boecker, H., Block, W., Träber, F., . . . Jessen, F. (2015). Cortical thinning in individuals with subjective memory impairment. *Journal of Alzheimer's Disease, 45*, 139–146.

Melby-Lervåg, M., & Hulme, C. (2013). Is working memory training effective?: A meta-analytic review. *Developmental Psychology, 49*, 270–291.

Melby-Lervåg, M., Redick, T. S., & Hulme, C. (2016). Working memory training does not improve performance on measures of intelligence or other measures of "far transfer": Evidence from a meta-analytic review. *Perspectives on Psychological Science, 11*, 512–534.

Meng, X., & D'Arcy, C. (2012). Education and dementia in the context of the cognitive reserve hypothesis: A systematic review with meta-analyses and qualitative analyses. *PLOS ONE, 7*(6), e38268.

Metternich, B., Kosch, D., Kriston, L., Härter, M., & Hüll, M. (2010). The effects of nonpharmacological interventions on subjective memory complaints: A systematic review and meta-analysis. *Psychotherapy and Psychosomatics, 79*, 6–19.

Meyer, A. N. D., & Logan, J. M. (2013). Taking the testing effect beyond the college freshman: Benefits for lifelong learning. *Psychology and Aging, 28*, 142–147.

Middleton, L. E., Barnes, D. E., Lui, L. Y., & Yaffe, K. (2010). Physical activity over the life course and its association with cognitive performance and impairment in old age. *Journal of the American Geriatrics Society, 58*(7), 1322–1326.

Miller, D. I., Taler, V., Davidson, P. S. R., & Messier, C. (2012). Measuring the impact of exercise on cognitive aging: Methodological issues. *Neurobiology of Aging, 33*(3), e29–e43.

Miller, G. E., Chen, E., & Parker, K. J. (2011). Psychological stress in childhood and susceptibility to the chronic diseases of aging: Moving toward a model of behavioral and biological mechanisms. *Psychological Bulletin, 137,* 959–997.

Miller, W. R., & Rollnick, S. (2002). *Motivational interviewing: Preparing people for change* (2nd ed.). New York: Guilford Press.

Miller, W. R., & Rollnick, S. (2009). Ten things that motivational interviewing is not. *Behavioural and Cognitive Psychotherapy, 37,* 129–140.

Miller, W. R., & Rose, G. S. (2009). Toward a theory of motivational interviewing. *American Psychologist, 64,* 527–537.

Mistridis, P., Egli, S. C., Iverson, G. L., Berres, M., Willmes, K., Welsh-Bohmer, K. A., & Monsch, A. U. (2015). Considering the base rates of low performance in cognitively healthy older adults improves the accuracy to identify neurocognitive impairment with the Consortium to Establish a Registry for Alzheimer's Disease—Neuropsychological Assessment Battery (CERAD-NAB). *European Archives of Psychiatry and Clinical Neuroscience, 265*(5), 407–417.

Mitchell, A. J., Beaumont, H., Ferguson, D., Yadegarfar, M., & Stubbs, B. (2014). Risk of dementia and mild cognitive impairment in older people with subjective memory complaints: Meta-analysis. *Acta Psychiatrica Scandinavica, 130,* 439–451.

Mitnitski, A., Song, X., & Rockwood, K. (2012). Trajectories of changes over twelve years in the health status of Canadians from late middle age. *Experimental Gerontology, 47*(12), 893–899.

Mitnitski, A., Song, X., & Rockwood, K. (2013). Assessing biological aging: The origin of deficit accumulation. *Biogerontology, 14*(6), 709–717.

Mitrushina, M., & Satz, P. (1991). Stability of cognitive functions in young–old versus old–old individuals. *Brain Dysfunction, 4*(4), 174–181.

Mitsis, E. M., Jacobs, D., Luo, X., Andrews, H., Andrews, K., & Sano, M. (2010). Evaluating cognition in an elderly cohort via telephone assessment. *International Journal of Geriatric Psychiatry, 25*(5), 531–539.

Möhler, H. (2013). The GABA system in anxiety and depression and its therapeutic potential. *Neuropsychopharmacology, 62,* 42–53.

Mohlman, J. (2008). More power to the executive?: A preliminary test of CBT plus Executive Skills Training for treatment of late-life GAD. *Cognitive and Behavioral Practice, 15,* 306–316.

Mohlman, J., & Gorman, J. M. (2005). The role of executive functioning in CBT: A pilot study with older adults. *Behaviour Research and Therapy, 43,* 447–465.

Molinuevo, J. L., Rabin, L. A., Amariglio, R., Buckley, R., Dubois, B., Ellis, K. A., . . . the Subjective Cognitive Decline Initiative (SCD-I) Working Group. (2017). Implementation of subjective cognitive decline criteria in research studies. *Alzheimer's and Dementia, 13*(3), 296–311.

Moniz-Cook, E. D., Swift, K., James, I., Malouf, R., De Vugt, M., & Verhey, F. (2012). Functional analysis-based interventions for challenging behavior in dementia. *Cochrane Database Systematic Reviews, 2* CD006929.

Monsell, S. (2003). Task switching. *Trends in Cognitive Sciences, 7*(3), 134–140.

Montenigro, P. H., Baugh, C. M., Daneshvar, D. H., Mez, J., Budson, A. E., Au, R.,

... Stern, R. A. (2014). Clinical subtypes of chronic traumatic encephalopathy: Literature review and proposed research diagnostic criteria for traumatic encephalopathy syndrome. *Alzheimers Research and Therapy, 6*(5), 68.

Moriarty, O., McGuire, B. E., & Finn, D. P. (2011). The effect of pain on cognitive function: A review of clinical and preclinical research. *Progress in Neurobiology, 93*(3), 385–404.

Moroney, A. C. (July 2013a). Overview of pharmacodynamics. Retrieved October 15, 2016, from *www.merckmanuals.com/professional/clinical-pharmacology/pharmacodynamics/overview-of-pharmacodynamics*.

Moroney, A. C. (July 2013b). Dose–response relationship. Retrieved October 15, 2016, from *www.merckmanuals.com/professional/clinical-pharmacology/pharmacodynamics/dose-response-relationships*.

Morris, J. C. (2012). Revised criteria for mild cognitive impairment may compromise the diagnosis of Alzheimer disease dementia. *Archives of Neurology, 69*, 700–708.

Morris, M. C., Tangney, C. C., Wang, Y., Sacks, F. M., Bennett, D. A., & Aggarwal, N. T. (2015). MIND diet associated with reduced incidence of Alzheimer's disease. *Alzheimer's and Dementia, 11*(9), 1007–1014.

Morris, J. K., Vidoni, E. D., Honea, R. A., & Burns, J. M. (2014). Impaired glycemia increases disease progression in mild cognitive impairment. *Neurobiology of Aging, 35*(3), 585–589.

Mosconi, L., De Santi, S., Brys, M., Tsui, W. H., Pirraglia, E., Glodzik-Sobanska, L., ... de Leon, M. J. (2008). Hypometabolism and altered cerebrospinal fluid markers in normal apolipoprotein E E4 carriers with subjective memory complaints. *Biological Psychiatry, 63*, 609–618.

Mowszowski, L., Lampit, A., Walton, C. C., & Naismith, S. L. (2016). Strategy-based cognitive training for improving executive functions in older adults: A systematic review. *Neuropsychology Review, 26*, 252–270.

Mulligan, B. P., Smart, C. M., & Ali, J. I. (2016). Relationship of subjective and objective performance indicators in subjective cognitive decline. *Psychology and Neuroscience, 9*, 362–378.

Mundt, J. C., Kinoshita, L. M., Hsu, S., Yesavage, J. A., & Greist, J. H. (2007). Telephonic Remote Evaluation of Neuropsychological Deficits (TREND): Longitudinal monitoring of elderly community-dwelling volunteers using touch-tone telephones. *Alzheimer Disease and Associated Disorders, 21*(3), 218–224.

Mungas, D., Beckett, L., Harvey, D., Tomaszewski Farias, S., Reed, B., Carmichael, O., ... DeCarli, C. (2010). Heterogeneity of cognitive trajectories in diverse older persons. *Psychology and Aging, 25*(3), 606–619.

Murray, A. M., Bell, E. J., Tupper, D. E., Davey, C. S., Pederson, S. L., Amiot, E. M., ... Knopman, D. S. (2016). The Brain in Kidney Disease (BRINK) Cohort Study: Design and baseline cognitive function. *American Journal of Kidney Disease, 67*(4), 593–600.

Napoles, A. M., Chadiha, L., Eversley, R., & Moreno-John, G. (2010). Reviews: Developing culturally sensitive dementia caregiver interventions: Are we there yet? *American Journal of Alzheimer's Disease and Other Dementias, 25*, 389–406.

National Task Group on Intellectual Disabilities and Dementia Practices. (2012). Early Detection Screen for Dementia (NTG-EDSD). Retrieved from *https://aadmd.org/index.php?q=ntg/screening*.

Nesselroade, J. R., Stigler, S. M., & Baltes, P. B. (1980). Regression toward the mean and the study of change. *Psychological Bulletin, 88*, 622–637.

Nestor, P. J., Graham, K. S., Bozeat, S., Simons, J. S., & Hodges, J. R. (2002). Memory consolidation and the hippocampus: Further evidence from studies of autobiographical memory in semantic dementia and frontal variant frontotemporal dementia. *Neuropsychologia, 40*(6), 633–654.

Newkirk, L. A., Kim, J. M., Thompson, J. M., Tinklenberg, J. R., Yesavage, J. A., & Taylor, J. L. (2004). Validation of a 26-point telephone version of the Mini-Mental State Examination. *Journal of Geriatric Psychiatry Neurology, 17*(2), 81–87.

Newson, R. S., & Kemps, E. B. (2005). General lifestyle activities as a predictor of current cognition and cognitive change in older adults: A cross-sectional and longitudinal examination. *Journal of Gerontology Series B: Psychology Sciences and Social Sciences, 60*(3), 113–120.

Nicolia, V., Lucarelli, M., & Fuso, A. (2015). Environment, epigenetics and neurodegeneration: Focus on nutrition in Alzheimer's disease. *Experimental Gerontology, 68*, 8–12.

Nieuwenhuis-Mark, R. E. (2009). Diagnosing Alzheimer's dementia in Down syndrome: Problems and possible solutions. *Research in Developmental Disabilities, 30*(5), 827–838.

Nishimura, K., Yokoyama, K., Yamauchi, N., Koizumi, M., Harasawa, N., Yasuda, T., . . . Ishigooka, J. (2016). Sensitivity and specificity of the Confusion Assessment Method for the Intensive Care Unit (CAM-ICU) and the Intensive Care Delirium Screening Checklist (ICDSC) for detecting post-cardiac surgery delirium: A single-center study in Japan. *Heart Lung, 45*(1), 15–20.

Noggle, C. A., Dean, R. S., Bush, S. S., & Anderson, S. W. (2015). *The neuropsychology of cortical dementias.* New York: Springer.

Nooyens, A. C., Milder, I. E., van Gelder, B. M., Bueno-de-Mesquita, H. B., van Boxtel, M. P., & Verschuren, W. M. (2015). Diet and cognitive decline at middle age: The role of antioxidants. *British Journal of Nutrition, 113*(9), 1410–1417.

Norton, M. C., Dew, J., Smith, H., Fauth, E., Piercy, K. W., Breitner, J. C., . . . Welsh-Bohmer, K. (2012). Lifestyle behavior pattern is associated with different levels of risk for incident dementia and Alzheimer's disease: The Cache County study. *Journal of American Geriatric Society, 60*(3), 405–412.

Norton, M. C., Tschanz, J. A. T., Fan, X., Plassman, B. L., Welsh-Bohmer, K. A., West, N., . . . Breitner, J. C. S. (1999). Telephone adaptation of the Modified Mini-Mental State Exam. *Neuropsychiatry, Neuropsychology, and Behavioral Neurology, 12*(4), 270–276.

Novakovic-Agopian, T., Chen, A. J.-W., Rome, S., Abrams, G., Castelli, H., Rossi, A., . . . D'Esposito, M. (2010). Rehabilitation of executive functioning with training in attention regulation applied to individually defined goals: A pilot study bridging theory, assessment, and treatment. *Journal of Head Trauma Rehabilitation, 26*, 325–338.

Nunnemann, S., Kurz, A., Leucht, S., & Diehl-Schmid, J. (2012). Caregivers of patients with frontotemporal lobar degeneration: A review of burden, problems, needs, and interventions. *International Psychogeriatrics, 24*, 1368.

Nygaard, H. A., Naik, M., & Geitung, J. T. (2009). The Informant Questionnaire on Cognitive Decline in the Elderly (IQCODE) is associated with informant stress. *International Journal of Geriatric Psychiatry, 24*(11), 1185–1191.

O'Brien, J. T., & Thomas, A. (2015). Vascular dementia. *The Lancet, 386*, 1698–1706.

O'Connell, M. E., & Tuokko, H. (2010). Age corrections and dementia classification accuracy. *Archives of Clinical Neuropsychology, 25*(2), 126–138.

Office of Human Research Protections, U.S. Department of Health and Human

Services, Policy and Guidance (2018). Retrieved March 1, 2018, from *www.hhs.gov/ohrp/regulations-and-policy/index.html*.

Okai, D., Askey-Jones, S., Samuel, M., O'Sullivan, S. S., Chaudhuri, K., Martin, A., . . . David, A. S. (2013). Trial of CBT for impulse control behaviors affecting Parkinson patients and their caregivers. *Neurology, 80,* 792–799.

Olichney, J. M., & Hillert, D. G. (2004). Clinical applications of cognitive event-related potentials in Alzheimer's disease. *Physical Medicine and Rehabilitation Clinics of North America, 15,* 205–233.

Onyike, C. U. (2006). Cerebrovascular disease and dementia. *International Review of Psychiatry, 18*(5), 423–431.

Orellano, E., Colon, W. I., & Arbesman, M. (2012). Effect of occupation and activity-based interventions on instrumental activities of daily living performance among community dwelling older adults: A systematic review. *American Journal of Occupational Therapy, 66,* 292–300.

Oslin, D., Ten Have, T. R., Streim, J. E., Datto, C. J., Weintraub, D., DiFilippo, S., & Katz, I. R. (2003). Probing the safety of medications in the frail elderly: Evidence from a randomized clinical trial of sertraline and venlafaxine in depressed nursing home residents. *Journal of Clinical Psychiatry, 64,* 875–882.

Ossher, L., Bialystok, E., Craik, F. I., Murphy, K. J., & Troyer, A. K. (2013). The effect of bilingualism on amnestic mild cognitive impairment. *Journal of Gerontology Series B: Psychology Sciences Social Sciences, 68*(1), 8–12.

Owen, A. M., Hampshire, A., Grahn, J. A., Stenton, R., Dajani, S., Burns, A. S., . . . Ballard, C. G. (2010). Putting brain training to the test. *Nature, 465,* 775–778.

Ownby, R. L., Crocco, E., Acevedo, A., John, V., & Loewenstein, D. (2006). Depression and risk for Alzheimer disease: Systematic review, meta-analysis, and metaregression analysis. *Archives of General Psychiatry, 63*(5), 530–538.

Padilla, C., & Isaacson, R. S. (2011). Genetics of dementia. *CONTINUUM: Lifelong Learning in Neurology, 17*(2), 326–342.

Pagano, G., Rengo, G., Pasqualetti, G., Femminella, G. D., Monzani, F., Ferrara, N., & Tagliati, M. (2015). Cholinesterase inhibitors for Parkinson's disease: A systematic review and meta-analysis. *Journal of Neurology Neurosurgery and Psychiatry, 86,* 767–773.

Palmer, B. W., Boone, K. B., Lesser, I. M., & Wohl, M. A. (1998). Base rates of "impaired" neuropsychological test performance among healthy older adults. *Archives of Clinical Neuropsychology, 13,* 503–511.

Papa, L., Mendes, M. E., & Braga, C. F. (2012). Mild traumatic brain injury among the geriatric population. *Current Translational Geriatrics Experimental Gerontology Reports, 1*(3), 135–142.

Parikh, M., Grosch, M. C., Graham, L. L., Hynan, L. S., Weiner, M., Shore, J. H., & Cullum, C. M. (2013). Consumer acceptability of brief videoconference-based neuropsychological assessment in older individuals with and without cognitive impairment. *The Clinical Neuropsychologist, 27*(5), 808–817.

Park, D. C., Lodi-Smith, J., Drew, L., Haber, S., Hebrank, A., Bischof, G. N., & Aamodt, W. (2013). The impact of sustained engagement on cognitive function in older adults: The Synapse Project. *Psychological Science, 25,* 103–112.

Park, D. C., & McDonough, I. M. (2013). The dynamic aging mind: Revelations from functional neuroimaging research. *Perspectives on Psychological Sciences, 8,* 62–67.

Park, D. C., & Reuter-Lorenz, P. (2009). The adaptive brain: Aging and neurocognitive scaffolding. *Annual Review of Psychology, 60,* 173–196.

Park, D. C., & Schwarz, N. (2000). *Cognitive aging: A primer.* New York: Psychology Press.

Park, L. Q., Harvey, D., Johnson, J., & Farias, S. T. (2015). Deficits in everyday function differ in AD and FTD. *Alzheimer Disease and Associated Disorders, 29*(4), 301–306.

Parks, R. W., Zec, R. F., & Wilson, R. S. (1993). *Neuropsychology of Alzheimer's disease and other dementias.* New York: Oxford University Press.

Patja, K., Iivanainen, M., Vesala, H., Oksanen, H., & Ruoppila, I. (2000). Life expectancy of people with intellectual disability: A 35-year follow-up study. *Journal of Intellectual Disability Research, 44*(5), 591–599.

Patterson, C., Feightner, J., Garcia, A., & MacKnight, C. (2007). General risk factors for dementia: A systematic evidence review. *Alzheimer's and Dementia, 3*(4), 341–347.

Pauker, J. D. (1988). Constructing overlapping cell tables to maximize the clinical usefulness of normative test data: Rationale and an example from neuropsychology. *Journal of Clinical Psychology, 44*(6), 526–534.

Paukert, A. L., Calleo, J., Kraus-Schuman, C., Snow, L., Wilson, N., Petersen, N. J., . . . Stanley, M. A. (2010). Peaceful mind: An open trial of cognitive-behavioral therapy for anxiety in persons with dementia. *International Psychogeriatrics, 22,* 1012–1021.

Paukert, A. L., Kraus-Schuman, C., Wilson, N., Snow, L., Calleo, J., Kunik, M. E., & Stanley, M. A. (2013). The Peaceful Mind manual: A protocol for treating anxiety in persons with dementia. *Behavior Modification, 37,* 631–634.

Payne, R. W., & Jones, H. G. (1957). Statistics for the investigation of individual cases. *Journal of Clinical Psychology, 13,* 115–121.

Peavy, G. M., Salmon, D. P., Rice, V. A., Galasko, D., Samuel, W., Taylor, K. I., . . . Thal, L. (1996). Neuropsychological assessment of severely demeted elderly: The severe cognitive impairment profile. *Archives of Neurology, 53*(4), 367–372.

Pedraza, O., Lucas, J. A., Smith, G. E., Petersen, R. C., Graff-Radford, N. R., & Ivnik, R. J. (2010). Robust and expanded norms for the Dementia Rating Scale. *Archives of Clinical Neuropsychology, 25*(5), 347–358.

Pedraza, O., & Mungas, D. (2008). Measurement in cross-cultural neuropsychology. *Neuropsychology Review, 18*(3), 184–193.

Pendlebury, S. T., Welch, S. J., Cuthbertson, F. C., Mariz, J., Mehta, Z., & Rothwell, P. M. (2013). Telephone assessment of cognition after transient ischemic attack and stroke: Modified telephone interview of cognitive status and telephone Montreal Cognitive Assessment versus face-to-face Montreal Cognitive Assessment and neuropsychological battery. *Stroke, 44*(1), 227–229.

Perkins, E. A., & Moran, J. A. (2010). Aging adults with intellectual disabilities. *JAMA, 304*(1), 91–92.

Perquin, M., Schuller, A. M., Vaillant, M., Diederich, N., Bisdorff, A., Leners, J. C., . . . Lair, M. L. (2012). The epidemiology of mild cognitive impairment (MCI) and Alzheimer's disease (AD) in community-living seniors: Protocol of the MemoVie cohort study, Luxembourg. *BioMed Central Public Health, 12,* 519.

Perquin, M., Vaillant, M., Schuller, A. M., Pastore, J., Dartigues, J. F., Lair, M. L., & Diederich, N. (2013). Lifelong exposure to multilingualism: New evidence to support cognitive reserve hypothesis. *PLOS ONE, 8*(4), e62030.

Perrotin, A., de Flores, R., Lamberton, F., Poisnel, G., La Joie, R., de la Sayette, V., . . . Chételat, G. (2015). Hippocampal subfield volumetry and 3D surface mapping in subjective cognitive decline. *Journal of Alzheimer's Disease, 48*(Suppl. 1), S141–S150.

Perrotin, A., Mormino, E. C., Madison, C. M., Hayenga, A. O., & Jagust, W. J. (2012). Subjective cognition and amyloid deposition imaging: A Pittsburgh Compound B positron emission tomography study in normal elderly individuals. *Archives of Neurology, 69,* 223–229.

Perry, D. C., Sturm, V. E., Peterson, M. J., Pieper, C. F., Bullock, T., Boeve, B. F., . . . Welsh-Bohmer, K. A. (2016). Association of traumatic brain injury with subsequent neurological and psychiatric disease: A meta-analysis. *Journal of Neurosurgery, 124*(2), 511–526.

Perusini, G. (1910). Uber klinisch und histologisch eigenartige psychische Erkrankungen des spateren Lebensalters. In F. Nissl & A. Alzheimer (Eds.), *Histologische und Histopathologische Arbeiten Über die Grosshirnrinde: Mit Besonderer Berüocksichtigung der Pathologischen Anatomie der Geistekrankheiten* (pp. 297–352). Jena, Germany: Fischer.

Peter, J., Scheef, L., Abdulkadir, A., Boecker, H., Heneka, M., Wagner, M., . . . the Alzheimer's Disease Neuroimaging Initiative. (2014). Gray matter atrophy pattern in elderly with subjective memory impairment. *Alzheimer's and Dementia, 10,* 99–108.

Peters, E., Hess, T. M., Västfjäll, D., & Auman, C. (2007). Adult age differences in dual information processes: Implications for the role of affective and deliberative processes in older adults' decision making. *Perspectives on Psychological Science, 2,* 1–23.

Peters, R., Poulter, R., Warner, J., Beckett, N., Burch, L., & Bulpitt, C. (2008). Smoking, dementia and cognitive decline in the elderly: A systematic review. *BMC Geriatrics, 8,* 36.

Petersen, R. C. (2004). Mild cognitive impairment as a diagnostic entity. *Journal of Internal Medicine, 256,* 183–194.

Petersen, R. C., Caracciolo, B., Brayne, C., Gauthier, S., Jelic, V., & Fratiglioni, L. (2014). Mild cognitive impairment: A concept in evolution. *Journal of Internal Medicine, 275,* 214–228.

Petersen, R. C., & Morris, J. C. (2005). Mild cognitive impairment as a clinical entity and treatment target. *Archives of Neurology, 62,* 1160–1163.

Petersen, R. C., Smith, G. E., Waring, S. C., Ivnik, R. J., Tangalos, E. G., & Kokmen, E. (1999). Mild cognitive impairment: Clinical characterization and outcome. *Archives of Neurology, 56,* 303–308.

Petkus, A. J., & Wetherell, J. L. (2013). Acceptance and commitment therapy with older adults: Rationale and considerations. *Cognitive and Behavioral Practice, 20,* 47–56.

Petrova, M., Pavlova, R., Zhelev, Y., Mehrabian, S., Raycheva, M., & Traykov, L. (2016). Investigation of neuropsychological characteristics of very mild and mild dementia with Lewy bodies. *Journal of Clinical and Experimental Neuropsychology, 38*(3), 354–360.

Pfeffer, R. I., Kurosaki, T. T., Harrah, C. H., Jr., Chance, J. M., & Filos, S. (1982). Measurement of functional activities in older adults in the community. *Journals of Gerontology, 37,* 323–329.

Pharr, J. R., Francis, C. D., Terry, C., & Clark, M. C. (2014). Culture, caregiving, and health: Exploring the influence of culture on family caregiver experiences. *International Scholarly Research Notices, Public Health,* 689826.

Piccinin, A. M., & Hofer, S. M. (2008). Integrative analysis of longitudinal studies on aging: Collaborative research networks, meta-analysis, and optimizing future studies. In S. M. Hofer & D. F. Alwin (Eds.), *Handbook of cognitive aging: Interdisciplinary perspectives* (pp. 446–476). Thousand Oaks, CA: SAGE.

Pickering, G., & Lussier, D. (2015). Pharmacological pain management: For better or for worse? In G. Pickering & S. Gibson (Eds.), *Pain, emotion and cognition: A complex nexus* (pp. 137–151). New York: Springer.

Pietrzak, R. H., Lim, Y. Y., Ames, D., Harrington, K., Restrepo, C., Martins, R. N., . . . the Australian Imaging, Biomarkers, and Lifestyle (AIBL) Research Group. (2015b). Trajectories of memory decline in preclinical Alzheimer's disease: Results from the Australian Imaging, Biomarkers and Lifestyle Flagship Study of Ageing. *Neurobiology of Aging, 36,* 1231–1238.

Pietrzak, R. H., Lim, Y. Y., Neumeister, A., Ames, D., Ellis, K. A., Harrington, K., . . . the Australian Imaging, Biomarkers, and Lifestyle (AIBL) Research Group. (2015a). Amyloid-β, anxiety, and cognitive decline in preclinical Alzheimer disease. *JAMA Psychiatry, 72,* 284–291.

Pillai, J. A., & Verghese, J. (2009). Social networks and their role in preventing dementia. *Indian Journal of Psychiatry, 51*(Suppl. 1), S22–S28.

Pinquart, M., & Duberstein, P. R. (2007). Treatment of anxiety disorders in older adults: A meta-analytic comparison of behavioral and pharmacological interventions. *American Journal of Geriatric Psychiatry, 15,* 639–651.

Plassman, B. L., Havlik, R. J., Steffens, D. C., Helms, M. J., Newman, T. N., Drosdick, D., . . . Breitner, J. C. (2000). Documented head injury in early adulthood and risk of Alzheimer's disease and other dementias. *Neurology, 55*(8), 1158–1166.

Polich, J. (2004). Clinical application of the P300 event-related brain potential. *Physical Medicine and Rehabilitation Clinics of North America, 15,* 133–161.

Poortinga, W. (2007). The prevalence and clustering of four major lifestyle risk factors in an English adult population. *Preventive Medicine, 44*(2), 124–128.

Postal, K., & Armstrong, K. (2013). *Feedback that sticks: The art of communicating neuropsychological assessment results.* New York: Oxford University Press.

Potter, G. G., & Attix, D. K. (2006). An integrated model for geriatric neuropsychological assessment. In D. K. Attix & K. A. Welsh-Bohmer (Eds.), *Geriatric neuropsychology: Assessment and intervention* (pp. 5–26). New York: Guilford Press.

Pouryamout, L., Dams, J., Wasem, J., Dodel, R., & Neumann, A. (2012). Economic evaluation of treatment options in patients with Alzheimer's disease: A systematic review of cost-effectiveness analyses. *Drugs, 72,* 789–802.

Power, M. C., Weuve, J., Gagne, J. J., McQueen, M. B., Viswanathan, A., & Blacker, D. (2011). The association between blood pressure and incident Alzheimer disease: A systematic review and meta-analysis. *Epidemiology, 22*(5), 646–659.

Preston, J. D., O'Neal, J. H., & Talaga, M. C. (2013). *Handbook of clinical psychopharmacology for therapists* (8th ed.). Oakland, CA: New Harbinger.

Prochaska, J. O., & DiClemente, C. C. (1983). Stages and processes of self-change of smoking: Toward an integrative model of change. *Journal of Consulting and Clinical Psychology, 51,* 390–395.

Prochaska, J. O., DiClemente, C. C., & Norcross, J. C. (1992). In search of how people change: Applications to the addictive behaviors. *The American Psychologist, 47,* 1102–1114.

Pryor, K. (2006). *Don't shoot the dog!: The new art of teaching and training.* Lydney, UK: Ringpress Books.

Puente, A. E., & McCaffrey, R. J., III. (1992). *Handbook of neuropsychological assessment: A biopsychosocial perspective.* New York: Plenum Press.

Pyo, G., Kripakaran, K., Curtis, K., Curtis, R., & Markwell, S. (2007). A preliminary study of the validity of memory tests recommended by the Working Group for individuals with moderate to severe intellectual disability. *Journal of Intellectual Disability Research, 51*(5), 377–386.

Qina, T., Sanjo, N., Hizume, M., Higuma, M., Tomita, M., Atarashi, R., . . . Mizusawa, H. (2014). Clinical features of genetic Creutzfeldt–Jakob disease with V180I mutation in the prion protein gene. *BMJ Open, 4*(5), e004968.

Qiu, C., & Fratiglioni, L. (2015). A major role for cardiovascular burden in age-related cognitive decline. *Nature Reviews Cardiology, 12,* 267–277.

Qiu, C., von Strauss, E., Fastbom, J., Winblad, B., & Fratiglioni, L. (2003). Low blood pressure and risk of dementia in the Kungsholmen project: A 6-year follow-up study. *Archives of Neurology, 60*(2), 223–228.

Qiu, C., Winblad, B., & Fratiglioni, L. (2005). The age-dependent relation of blood pressure to cognitive function and dementia. *The Lancet of Neurology, 4*(8), 487–499.

Qualls, S. H. (2014). Family therapy with ageing families. In N. A. Pachana & K. Laidlaw (Eds.), *The Oxford handbook of clinical geropsychology* (pp. 710–732). New York: Oxford University Press.

Rabin, L. A., Borgos, M. J., Saykin, A. J., Wishart, H. A., Crane, P. K., Nutter-Upham, K. E., & Flashman, L. A. (2007). Judgment in older adults: Development and psychometric evaluation of the Test of Practical Judgment (TOP-J). *Journal of Clinical and Experimental Neuropsychology, 29,* 752–767.

Rabin, L. A., Burton, L. A., & Barr, W. B. (2007). Utilization rates of ecologically oriented instruments among clinical neuropsychologists. *The Clinical Neuropsychologist, 21,* 727–743.

Rabin, L. A., Chi, S. Y., Wang, C., Fogel, J., Kann, S. J., & Aronov, A. (2014). Prospective memory on a novel clinical task in older adults with mild cognitive impairment and subjective cognitive decline. *Neuropsychological Rehabilitation, 24,* 868–893.

Rabin, L. A., Saykin, A. J., Wishart, H. A., Nutter-Upham, K. E., Flashman, L. A., Pare, N., & Santulli, R. B. (2007). The Memory and Aging Telephone Screen: Development and preliminary validation. *Alzheimer's and Dementia, 3*(2), 109–121.

Rabin, L. A., Smart, C. M., & Amariglio, R. E. (2017). Subjective cognitive decline in preclinical Alzheimer's disease. *Annual Review of Clinical Psychology, 13,* 369–396.

Rabin, L. A., Smart, C. M., Crane, P. K., Amariglio, R. E., Berman, L. M., Boada M., . . . the Subjective Cognitive Decline Initiative (SCD-I) Working Group. (2015). Subjective cognitive decline in older adults: An overview of self-report measures used across 19 international research studies. *Journal of Alzheimer's Disease, 48*(Suppl. 1), S63–S86.

Rabin, L. A., Wang, C., Katz, M. J., Derby, C. A., Buschke, H., & Lipton, R. B. (2012). Predicting Alzheimer's disease: Neuropsychological tests, self reports, and informant reports of cognitive difficulties. *Journal of the American Geriatric Society, 60,* 1128–1134.

Rabinovici, G. D., & Miller, B. L. (2010). Frontotemporal lobar degeneration: Epidemiology, pathophysiology, diagnosis and management. *CNS Drugs, 24*(5), 375–398.

Rafii, M., Taylor, C., Coutinho, A., Kim, K., & Galasko, D. (2011). Comparison of the memory performance index with standard neuropsychological measures of cognition. *American Journal of Alzheimer's Disease and Other Dementias, 26*(3), 235–239.

Rajji, T. K., Miranda, D., & Mulsant, B. H. (2014). Cognition, function, and disability in patients with schizophrenia: A review of longitudinal studies. *Canadian Journal of Psychiatry, 59*(1), 13–17.

Rajji, T. K., & Mulsant, B. H. (2008). Nature and course of cognitive function in late-life schizophrenia: A systematic review. *Schizophrenia Research, 102*(1–3), 122–140.

Rajji, T. K., Voineskos, A. N., Butters, M. A., Miranda, D., Arenovich, T., Menon, M., . . . Mulsant, B. H. (2013). Cognitive performance of individuals with schizophrenia across seven decades: A study using the MATRICS consensus cognitive battery. *American Journal of Geriatric Psychiatry, 21*(2), 108–118.

Rapoport, M., Wolf, U., Herrmann, N., Kiss, A., Shammi, P., Reis, M., . . . Feinstein, A. (2008). Traumatic brain injury, apolipoprotein E-epsilon4, and cognition in older adults: A two-year longitudinal study. *Journal of Neuropsychiatry and Clinical Neurosciences, 20*(1), 68–73.

Rapp, S. R., Legault, C., Espeland, M. A., Resnick, S. M., Hogan, P. E., Coker, L. H., . . . Shumaker, S. A. (2012). Validation of a Cognitive Assessment Battery administered over the telephone. *Journal of the American Geriatrics Society, 60*(9), 1616–1623.

Raskin, S., & Buckheit, C. (2010). *Memory for Intentions Test.* Lutz, FL: Psychological Assessment Resources.

Rathlev, N. K., Medzon, R., Lowery, D., Pollack, C., Bracken, M., Barest, G., . . . Mower, W. R. (2006). Intracranial pathology in elders with blunt head trauma. *Academic Emergency Medicine, 13*(3), 302–307.

Raz, N., & Rodrigue, K. M. (2006). Differential aging of the brain: Patterns, cognitive correlates and modifiers. *Neuroscience and Biobehavioral Reviews, 30*(6), 730–748.

Raz, N., Rodrigue, K. M., Kennedy, K. M., & Acker, J. D. (2007). Vascular health and longitudinal changes in brain and cognition in middle-aged and older adults. *Neuropsychology, 21*(2), 149–157.

Razay, G., Williams, J., King, E., Smith, A. D., & Wilcock, G. (2009). Blood pressure, dementia and Alzheimer's disease: The OPTIMA longitudinal study. *Dementia and Geriatric Cognitive Disorders, 28*(1), 70–74.

Rebok, G. W., Ball, K., Guey, L. T., Jones, R. N., Kim, H.-Y., King, J. W., . . . Willis, S. L. for the ACTIVE Study Group. (2014). Ten-year effects of the Advanced Cognitive Training for Independent and Vital Elderly cognitive training trial on cognition and everyday functioning in older adults. *Journal of the American Geriatrics Society, 62,* 16–24.

Rediess, S., & Caine, E. D. (1996). Aging, cognition, and DSM-IV. *Aging, Neuropsychology, and Cognition, 3,* 105–117.

Reed, A. E., Chan, L., & Mikels, J. A. (2014). Meta-analysis of the age-related positivity effect: Age differences in preferences for positive over negative information. *Psychology and Aging, 29,* 1–15.

Reed, B. R., Dowling, M., Tomaszewski Farias, S., Sonnen, J., Strauss, M., Schneider, J. A., . . . Mungas, D. (2011). Cognitive activities during adulthood are more important than education in building reserve. *Journal of the International Neuropsychological Society, 17*(4), 615–624.

Reinhardt, M. M., & Cohen, C. I. (2015). Late-life psychosis: Diagnosis and treatment. *Current Psychiatry Reports, 17,* 1.

Reisberg, B., & Gauthier, S. (2008). Current evidence for subjective cognitive impairment (SCI) as the pre-mild cognitive impairment (MCI) stage of subsequently manifest Alzheimer's disease. *International Psychogeriatrics, 20,* 1–16.

Reisberg, B., Monteiro, I., Torossian, C., Auer, S., Shulman, M. B., Ghimire, S., . . . Xu, J. (2014). The BEHAVE-AD Assessment System: A perspective, a commentary on new findings, and a historical review. *Dementia and Geriatric Cognitive Disorders, 38*(1–2), 89–146.

Reisberg, B., Prichep, L., Mosconi, L., John, E. R., Glodzik-Sobanska, L., Boksay, I., . . . de Leon, M. J. (2008). The pre-mild cognitive impairment, subjective cognitive impairment stage of Alzheimer's disease. *Alzheimer's and Dementia, 4*, S98–S108.

Reisberg, B., Shulman, M. B., Torossian, C., Leng, L., & Zhu, W. (2010). Outcome over seven years of healthy adults with and without subjective cognitive impairment. *Alzheimer's and Dementia, 6*(1), 11–24.

Reisberg, B., Wegiel, J., Franssen, E., Kadiyala, S., Auer, S., Souren, L., . . . Golomb, J. (2006). Clinical features of severe dementia: Staging. In A. Burns & B. Winblad (Eds.), *Severe dementia* (pp. 83–115). New York: Wiley.

Rentz, D. M., Calvo, V. L., Scinto, L. F. M., Sperling, R. A., Budson, A. E., & Daffner, K. R. (2000). Detecting early cognitive decline in high-functioning elders. *Journal of Geriatric Psychiatry, 33*(1), 27–49.

Rentz, D. M., Huh, T. J., Faust, R. R., Budson, A. E., Scinto, L. F. M., Sperling, R. A., & Daffner, K. R. (2004). Use of IQ-adjusted norms to predict progressive cognitive decline in highly intelligent older individuals. *Neuropsychology, 18*, 38–49.

Resnik, D. B. (2009). The clinical investigator–subject relationship: A contextual approach. *Philosophy, Ethics, and Humanities in Medicine, 4*, 16.

Reuter-Lorenz, P. (2013). Aging and cognitive neuroimaging: A fertile union. *Perspectives on Psychological Sciences, 8*, 68–71.

Reuter-Lorenz, P. A., & Park, D. C. (2014). How does it STAC up?: Revisiting the Scaffolding Theory of Aging and Cognition. *Neuropsychology Review, 24*(3), 355–370.

Reynolds, C. F., III, Dew, M. A., Pollock, B. G., Mulsant, B. H., Frank, E., Miller, M. D., . . . Kupfer, D. J. (2006). Maintenance treatment of major depression in old age. *New England Journal of Medicine, 354*, 1130–1138.

Reynolds, C. F., III, Frank, E., Perel, J. M., Imber, S. D., Cornes, C., Miller, M. D., . . . Kupfer, D. J. (1999). Nortriptyline and interpersonal psychotherapy as maintenance therapies for recurrent major depression: A randomized controlled trial in patients older than 59 years. *Journal of the American Medical Association, 281*, 39–45.

Richardson, T. J., Lee, S. J., Berg-Weger, M., & Grossberg, G. T. (2013). Caregiver health: Health of caregivers of Alzheimer's and other dementia patients. *Current Psychiatry Reports, 15*, 1–7.

Riley, K. P., Snowdon, D. A., Desrosiers, M. F., & Markesbery, W. R. (2005). Early life linguistic ability, late life cognitive function, and neuropathology: Findings from the Nun Study. *Neurobiology of Aging, 26*(3), 341–347.

Ritchie, L. J., Frerichs, R. J., & Tuokko, H. (2007). Effective normative samples for the detection of cognitive impairment in older adults. *The Clinical Neuropsychologist, 21*(6), 863–874.

Rizzo, M., & Kellison, I. L. (2010). The brain on the road. In T. D. Marcotte & I. Grant (Eds.), *Neuropsychology of everyday functioning* (pp. 168–208). New York: Guilford Press.

Roberts, R. O., Cerhan, J. R., Geda, Y. E., Knopman, D. S., Cha, R. H., Christianson, T. J., . . . Petersen, R. C. (2010). Polyunsaturated fatty acids and reduced odds of MCI: The Mayo Clinic Study of Aging. *Journal of Alzheimers Disease, 21*(3), 853–865.

Robertson, J. H., Ward, A., Ridgeway, V., & Nimmo-Smith, I. (1996). Test of everyday attention. *Journal of the International Neurological Society, 2*, 525–534.

Roccaforte, W. H., Burke, W. J., Bayer, B. L., & Wengel, S. P. (1992). Validation of a telephone version of the Mini-Mental State Examination. *Journal of American Geriatrics Society, 40*(7), 697–702.

Roccaforte, W. H., Burke, W. J., Bayer, B. L., & Wengel, S. P. (1994). Reliability and validity of the Short Portable Mental Status Questionnaire administered by telephone. *Journal of Geriatric Psychiatry and Neurology, 7*(1), 33–38.

Rodda, J., Okello, A., Edison, P., Dannhauser, T., Brooks, D. J., & Walker, Z. (2010). (11)C-PIB PET in subjective cognitive impairment. *European Psychiatry, 25,* 123–125.

Rodríguez-Aranda, C., & Sundet, K. (2006). The frontal hypothesis of cognitive aging: Factor structure and age effects on four frontal tests among healthy individuals. *Journal of Genetic Psychology: Research and Theory on Human Development, 167*(3), 269–287.

Roebuck-Spencer, T., Sun, W., Cernich, A. N., Farmer, K., & Bleiberg, J. (2007). Assessing change with the Automated Neuropsychological Assessment Metrics (ANAM): Issues and challenges. *Archives of Clinical Neuropsychology, 22*(Suppl.), S79–S87.

Rohrer, J. D., Guerreiro, R., Vandrovcova, J., Uphill, J., Reiman, D., Beck, J., . . . Rossor, M. N. (2009). The heritability and genetics of frontotemporal lobar degeneration. *Neurology, 73*(18), 1451–1456.

Rolinski, M., Fox, C., Maidment, I., & McShane, R. (2012). Cholinesterase inhibitors for dementia with Lewy bodies, Parkinson's disease dementia and cognitive impairment in Parkinson's disease. *Cochrane Database Systematic Review, 14,* CD006504.

Rönnberg, L., & Ericsson, K. (1994). Reliability and validity of the Hierarchic Dementia Scale. *International Psychogeriatrics, 6*(1), 87–94.

Rosenblatt, P. C. (2012). Family grief in cross-cultural perspective. *Family Science, 4,* 12–19.

Rossato-Bennett, M. (2014). *Alive inside* [Motion picture].

Rovio, S., Kareholt, I., Helkala, E. L., Viitanen, M., Winblad, B., Tuomilehto, J., . . . Kivipelto, M. (2005). Leisure-time physical activity at midlife and the risk of dementia and Alzheimer's disease. *The Lancet Neurology, 4*(11), 705–711.

Rueda, A. D., Lau, K. M., Saito, N., Harvey, D., Risacher, S. L., Aisen, P. S., . . . the Alzheimer's Disease Neuroimaging Initiative. (2015). Self-rated and informant-rated everyday function in comparison to objective markers of Alzheimer's disease. *Alzheimer's and Dementia, 11,* 1080–1089.

Ruscin, J. M., & Linnebaur, S. A. (2014). Pharmacodynamics in the elderly. Retrieved October 15, 2016, from *www.merckmanuals.com/professional/geriatrics/drug-therapy-in-the-elderly/pharmacodynamics-in-the-elderly#v1132595.*

Russ, T. C., & Morling, J. R. (2012). Cholinesterase inhibitors for mild cognitive impairment. *Cochrane Database of Systematic Reviews 9,* CD009132.

Russo, A. C., Bush, S. S., & Rasin-Waters, D. (2013a). Ethical considerations in the neuropsychological assessment of older adults. In L. D. Ravdin & H. L. Katzen (Eds.), *Handbook on the neuropsychology of aging and dementia* (pp. 225–235). New York: Springer Science + Business Media.

Russo, A. C., Bush, S. S., & Rasin-Waters, D. (2013b). Professional competence as the foundation for ethical neuropsychological practice with older adults. In L. D. Ravdin & H. L. Katzen (Eds.), *Handbook on the neuropsychology of aging and dementia* (pp. 217–223). New York: Springer Science + Business Media.

Ryan, J. J., Paolo, A. M., & Brungardt, T. M. (1992). WAIS–R test-retest stability in normal persons 75 years and older. *The Clinical Neuropsychologist, 6*(1), 3–8.

Sabat, S. R., & Lee, J. M. (2012). Relatedness among people diagnosed with dementia: Social cognition and the possibility of friendship. *Dementia: The International Journal of Social Research and Practice, 11*(3), 315–327.

Sabbagh, M. N., Malek-Ahmadi, M., Kataria, R., Belden, C. M., Connor, D. J., Pearson, C., . . . Singh, U. (2010). The Alzheimer's Questionnaire: A proof of concept study for a new informant-based dementia assessment. *Journal of Alzheimer's Disease, 22*(3), 1015–1021.

Saczynski, J. S., Pfeifer, L. A., Masaki, K., Korf, E. S., Laurin, D., White, L., & Launer, L. J. (2006). The effect of social engagement on incident dementia: The Honolulu–Asia Aging Study. *American Journal of Epidemiology, 163*(5), 433–440.

Sahakian, B. J., & Owen, A. M. (1992). Computerized assessment in neuropsychiatry using CANTAB: Discussion paper. *Journal of the Royal Society of Medicine, 85*(7), 399–402.

Sahathevan, R., Brodtmann, A., & Donnan, G. A. (2011). Dementia, stroke, and vascular risk factors: A review. *International Journal of Stroke, 7,* 61–73.

Salive, M. E. (2013). Multimorbidity in older adults. *Epidemiological Reviews, 35,* 75–83.

Salthouse, T. A. (1992). Shifting levels of analysis in the investigation of cognitive aging. *Human Development, 35,* 321–342.

Salthouse, T. A. (1996). Constraints on theories of cognitive aging. *Psychnomic Bulletin and Review, 3*(3), 287–299.

Salthouse, T. A. (1997). The processing speed theory of adult age differences in cognition. *Psychological Review, 103,* 403–429.

Sambati, L., Calandra-Buonaura, G., Poda, R., Guaraldi, P., & Cortelli, P. (2014). Orthostatic hypotension and cognitive impairment: A dangerous association? *Neurological Sciences, 35*(6), 951–957.

Sattler, C., Toro, P., Schönknecht, P., & Schröder, J. (2012). Cognitive activity, education and socioeconomic status as preventive factors for mild cognitive impairment and Alzheimer's disease. *Psychiatry Research, 196*(1), 90–95.

Saunders, N. L., & Summers, M. J. (2011). Longitudinal deficits to attention, executive, and working memory in subtypes of mild cognitive impairment. *Neuropsychology, 25*(2), 237–248.

Saxton, J., Kastango, K. B., Hugonot-Diener, L., Boller, F., Verny, M., Sarles, C. E., . . . DeKosky, S. T. (2005). Development of a short form of the Severe Impairment Battery. *American Journal of Geriatric Psychiatry, 13*(11), 999–1005.

Saxton, J., McGonigle-Gibson, K. L., Swihart, A. A., Miller, V. J., & Boller, F. (1990). Assessment of the severely impaired patient: Description and validation of a new neuropsychological test battery. *Psychological Assessment: A Journal of Consulting and Clinical Psychology, 2*(3), 298–303.

Saxton, J., Morrow, L., Eschman, A., Archer, G., Luther, J., & Zuccolotto, A. (2009). Computer assessment of mild cognitive impairment. *Postgraduate Medical, 121*(2), 177–185.

Saxton, J., Ratcliff, G., Munro, C. A., Coffey, C. E., Becker, J. T., Fried, L., & Kuller, L. (2000). Normative data on the Boston Naming Test and two equivalent 30-item short forms. *The Clinical Neuropsychologist, 14*(4), 526–534.

Saykin, A. J., Wishart, H. A., Rabin, L. A., Santulli, R. B., Flashman, L. A., West, J. D., . . . Mamourian, A. C. (2006). Older adults with cognitive complaints show brain atrophy similar to that of amnestic MCI. *Neurology, 67,* 834–842.

Scarmeas, N., Levy, G., Tang, M. X., Manly, J., & Stern, Y. (2001). Influence of leisure activity on the incidence of Alzheimer's disease. *Neurology, 57*(12), 2236–2242.

Schatzberg, A., & Roose, S. A. (2006). A double-blind, placebo-controlled study of venlafaxine and fluoxetine in geriatric outpatients with major depression. *American Journal of Geriatric Psychiatry, 14,* 361–370.

Scheef, L., Spottke, A., Daerr, M., Joe, A., Striepens, N., Kölsch, H., . . . Jessen, F. (2012). Glucose metabolism, gray matter structure, and memory decline in subjective memory impairment. *Neurology, 79,* 1332–1339.

Schicktanz, S., Schweda, M., Ballenger, J. F., Fox, P. J., Halpern, J., Kramer, J. H., . . . Jagust, W. J. (2014). Before it is too late: Professional responsibilities in late-onset Alzheimer's research and pre-symptomatic prediction. *Frontiers in Human Neuroscience, 8,* 921.

Schmucker, D. L. (2001). Liver function and phase I metabolism in the elderly: A paradox. *Drugs and Aging, 18,* 837–851.

Schneider, J. A., Arvanitakis, Z., Bang, W., & Bennett, D. A. (2007). Mixed brain pathologies account for most dementia cases in community-dwelling older persons. *Neurology, 69,* 2197–2204.

Schooler, C., Mulatu, M. S., & Oates, G. (2004). Occupational self-direction, intellectual functioning, and self-directed orientation in older workers: Findings and implications for individuals and societies. *American Journal of Sociology, 110*(1), 161–197.

Schroder, J., Kratz, B., Pantel, J., Minnemann, E., Lehr, U., & Sauer, H. (1998). Prevalence of mild cognitive impairment in an elderly community sample. *Journal of Neural Transmissions Supplementa, 54,* 51–59.

Schwarz, N., Strack, F., Hippler, H.-J., & Bishop, G. (1991). The impact of administration mode on response effects in survey measurement. *Applied Cognitive Psychology, 5*(3), 193–212.

Schweizer, T. A., Ware, J., Fischer, C. E., Craik, F. I., & Bialystok, E. (2012). Bilingualism as a contributor to cognitive reserve: Evidence from brain atrophy in Alzheimer's disease. *Cortex, 48*(8), 991–996.

Sclan, S. G., Foster, J. R., Reisberg, B., & Franssen, E. (1990). Application of Piagetian measures of cognition in severe Alzheimer's disease. *Psychiatric Journal of the University of Ottawa, 15*(4), 221–226.

Sclan, S. G., & Reisberg, B. (1992). Functional Assessment Staging (FAST) in Alzheimer's disease: Reliability, validity, and ordinality. *International Psychogeriatrics, 4*(Suppl. 1), 55–69.

Scogin, F., Welsh, D., Hanson, A., Stump, J., & Coates, A. (2005). Evidence-based psychotherapies for depression in older adults. *Clinical Psychology: Science and Practice 12,* 222–237.

Seeman, T. E., Lusignolo, T. M., Albert, M., & Berkman, L. (2001). Social relationships, social support, and patterns of cognitive aging in healthy, high-functioning older adults: MacArthur studies of successful aging. *Health Psychology, 20*(4), 243–255.

Seetharaman, S., Andel, R., McEvoy, C., Aslan, A. K. D., Finkel, D., & Pedersen, N. L. (2015). Blood glucose, diet-based glycemic load and cognitive aging among dementia-free older adults. *Journals of Gerontology: Series A: Biological Sciences and Medical Sciences, 70A*(4), 471–479.

Segal, D. L., June, A., Payne, M., Coolidge, F. L., & Yochim, B. (2010). Development and initial validation of a self-report assessment tool for anxiety among older adults: The Geriatric Anxiety Scale. *Journal of Anxiety Disorders, 24*(7), 709–714.

Segal, Z., Williams, M., & Teasdale, J. (2012). *Mindfulness-based cognitive therapy for depression* (2nd ed.). New York: Guilford Press.

Seidler, R. D., Bo, J., & Anguera, J. A. (2012). Neurocognitive contributions to motor skill learning: The role of working memory. *Journal of Motor Behavior, 44*, 445–453.

Seliger, S. L., Wendell, C. R., Waldstein, S. R., Ferrucci, L., & Zonderman, A. B. (2015). Renal function and long-term decline in cognitive function: The Baltimore Longitudinal Study of Aging. *American Journal of Nephrology, 41*(4–5), 305–312.

Seppi, K., Weintraub, D., Coelho, M., Perez-Lloret, S., Fox, S. H., Katzenschlager, R., . . . Sampaio, C. (2011). The Movement Disorder Society Evidence-Based Medicine Review update: Treatments for the non-motor symptoms of Parkinson's disease. *Movement Disorders, 26*(Suppl. 3), S42–S50.

Sexton, C. E., McKay, C. E., & Ebmeier, K. P. (2013). A systematic review and meta-analysis of magnetic resonance imaging studies in late-life depression. *American Journal of Geriatric Psychiatry, 21*, 184–195.

Shah, J. N., Qureshi, S. U., Jawaid, A., & Schulz, P. E. (2012). Is there evidence for late cognitive decline in chronic schizophrenia? *Psychiatric Quarterly, 83*(2), 127–144.

Shaik, M. A., Xu, X., Chan, Q. L., Hui, R. J. Y., Chong, S. S. T., Chen, C. L.-H., & Dong, Y. (2015). The reliability and validity of the informant ad8 by comparison with a series of cognitive assessment tools in primary healthcare. *International Psychogeriatrics, 28*(3), 443–452.

Shankle, W. R., Mangrola, T., Chan, T., & Hara, J. (2009). Development and validation of the Memory Performance Index: Reducing measurement error in recall tests. *Alzheimer's and Dementia, 5*(4), 295–306.

Sharp, E. S., & Gatz, M. (2011). Relationship between education and dementia: An updated systematic review. *Alzheimer Disease and Associated Disorders, 25*(4), 289–304.

Shea, T. B., & Remington, R. (2015). Nutritional supplementation for Alzheimer's disease? *Current Opinion in Psychiatry, 28*(2), 141–147.

Shear, M. K. (2015). Complicated grief. *New England Journal of Medicine, 372*, 153–160.

Shear, M. K., Wang, Y., Skritskaya, N., Duan, N., Mauro, C., & Ghesquiere, A. (2014). Treatment of complicated grief in elderly persons: A randomized clinical trial. *JAMA Psychiatry, 71*, 1287–1295.

Short, P., Cernich, A., Wilken, J. A., & Kane, R. L. (2007). Initial construct validation of frequently employed ANAM measures through structural equation modeling. *Archives of Clinical Neuropsychology, 22*(Suppl.), S63–S77.

Shultz, J., Aman, M., Kelbley, T., LeClear Wallace, C., Burt, D. B., Primeaux-Hart, S., . . . Tsiouris, J. (2004). Evaluation of screening tools for dementia in older adults with mental retardation. *American Journal on Mental Retardation, 109*(2), 98–110.

Sikkes, S. A. M., Crane, P., Jones, R., Rabin. L., & the Subjective Cognitive Decline Initiative (SCD-I) Working Group. (2017). Subjective cognitive decline and preclinical Alzheimer's disease: Harmonization of measurement instruments. *Journal of the International Neuropsychological Society.*

Sikkes, S. A. M., Knol, D. L., van den Berg, M. T., de Lange-de Klerk, E. S. M., Scheltens, P., Klein, M., . . . Uitdehaag, B. M. J. (2011). An informant questionnaire for detecting Alzheimer's disease: Are some items better than others? *Journal of the International Neuropsychological Society, 17*(4), 674–681.

Silveri, M. C., Reali, G., Jenner, C., & Puopolo, M. (2007). Attention and memory in the preclinical stage of dementia. *Journal of Geriatric Psychiatry and Neurology, 20*(2), 67–75.

Simmons, B. B., Hartmann, B., & DeJoseph, D. (2011). Evaluation of suspected dementia. *American Family Physician, 84,* 895–902.

Simons, D. J., Boot, W. R., Charness, N., Gathercole, S. E., Chabris, C. F., Hambrick, D. Z., & Stine-Morrow, E. A. L. (2016). Do "brain training" programs work? *Psychological Science in the Public Interest, 17,* 103–186.

Sitzer, D. I., Twamley, E. W., & Jeste, D. V. (2006). Cognitive training in Alzheimer's disease: A meta-analysis of the literature. *Acta Psychiatrica Scandinavica, 114,* 75–90.

Skrobot, O. A., O'Brien, J., Black, S., Chen, C., DeCarli, C., Erkinjuntti, T., . . . Kehoe, P. G. (2017). The ascular Impairment of Cognition Classification Consensus Study. *Alzheimer's and Dementia, 13*(6), 624–633.

Slavin, M. J., Brodaty, H., Kochan, N. A., Crawford, J. D., Trollor, J. N., Draper, B., & Sachdev, P. S. (2010). Prevalence and predictors of "subjective cognitive complaints" in the Sydney Memory and Ageing Study. *American Journal of Geriatric Psychiatry, 18,* 701–710.

Slavin, M. J., Sachdev, P. S., Kochan, N. A., Woolf, C., Crawford, J. D., Giskes, K., . . . Brodaty, H. (2015). Predicting cognitive, functional, and diagnostic change over 4 years using baseline subjective cognitive complaints in the Sydney Memory and Ageing Study. *American Journal of Geriatric Psychiatry, 23,* 906–914.

Sliwinski, M., Buschke, H., Stewart, W. F., Masur, D., & Lipton, R. B. (1997). The effect of dementia risk factors on comparative and diagnostic selective reminding norms. *Journal of the International Neuropsychological Society, 3*(4), 317–326.

Sliwinski, M., Lipton, R., Buschke, H., & Wasylyshyn, C. (2003). Optimizing cognitive test norms for detection. In R. C. Petersen (Ed.), *Mild cognitive impairment: Aging to Alzheimer's disease* (pp. 89–104). New York: Oxford University Press.

Slot, R. E. R., Sikkes, S. A. M., Verfaillie, S. C. J., Wolfsgruber, S., Brodaty, H., Buckley, R. F., . . . van der Flier, W. M. (2016). Subjective cognitive decline and progression to dementia due to AD and non-AD in memory clinic and community-based cohorts. *Alzheimer's and Dementia, 12*(Suppl.), 1073.

Smart, C. M., Karr, J. E., Areshenkoff, C. N., Rabin, L. A., Hudon, C., Gates, N., . . . the Subjective Cognitive Decline Initiative (SCD-I) Working Group. (2017). Nonpharmacologic interventions for older adults with subjective cognitive decline: Systematic review, meta-analysis, and preliminary recommendations. *Neuropsychology Review, 27*(3), 245–257.

Smart, C. M., Koudys, J., & Mulligan, B. P. (2015). Examining conscientiousness in older adults with subjective cognitive decline: Are we really measuring personality? *Alzheimer's and Dementia, 11*(Suppl. 7), 583.

Smart, C. M., & Krawitz, A. (2015). The impact of subjective cognitive decline on Iowa gambling task performance. *Neuropsychology, 29,* 971–987.

Smart, C. M., & Segalowitz, S. J. (2017). Respond, don't react: The influence of mindfulness training on performance monitoring in older adults. *Cognitive, Affective, and Behavioral Neuroscience, 17,* 1151–1163.

Smart, C. M., Segalowitz, S. J., Mulligan, B. P., Koudys, J., & Gawryluk, J. (2016). Mindfulness training for older adults with subjective cognitive decline: Results from a pilot randomized controlled trial. *Journal of Alzheimer's Disease, 52,* 757–774.

Smart, C. M., Segalowitz, S. J., Mulligan, B. P., & MacDonald, S. W. S. (2014a). Attention capacity and self-report of subjective cognitive decline: A P300 ERP study. *Biological Psychology, 103,* 144–151.

Smart, C. M., Spulber, G., & Garcia-Barrera, M. A. (2014b). Structural brain changes evident in default mode network areas in older adults with subjective cognitive decline compared to healthy peers. *Alzheimer's and Dementia, 10*(4, Suppl.), 608.

Smith, M. M., Tremont, G., & Ott, B. R. (2009). A review of telephone-administered screening tests for dementia diagnosis. *American Journal of Alzheimer's Disease and Other Dementias, 24*(1), 58–69.

Smits, L. L., van Harten, A. C., Pijnenburg, Y. A. L., Koedam, E. L. G. E., Bouwman, F. H., Sistermans, N., . . . van der Flier, W. M. (2015). Trajectories of cognitive decline in different types of dementia. *Psychological Medicine, 45*(5), 1051–1059.

Smoski, M. J., McClintock, A., & Keeling, L. (2016). Mindfulness training for emotional and cognitive health in late life. *Current Behavioral Neuroscience Reports, 3,* 301–307.

Snowden, M. B., Atkins, D. C., Steinman, L. E., Bell, J. F., Bryant, L. L., Copeland, C., & Fitzpatrick, A. L. (2015). Longitudinal association of dementia and depression. *American Journal of Geriatric Psychiatry, 23*(9), 897–905.

Snyder, H. M., Corriveau, R. A., Craft, S., Faber, J. E., Greenberg, S. M., Knopman, D., . . . Carrillo, M. C. (2015). Vascular contributions to cognitive impairment and dementia including Alzheimer's disease. *Alzheimer's and Dementia, 11*(6), 710–717.

Sofi, F., Abbate, R., Gensini, G. F., & Casini, A. (2010). Accruing evidence on benefits of adherence to the Mediterranean diet on health: An updated systematic review and meta-analysis. *American Journal of Clinical Nutrition, 92*(5), 1189–1196.

Sohlberg, M. M., & Mateer, C. A. (2001). *Cognitive rehabilitation: An integrative neuropsychological approach* (2nd ed.). New York: Guilford Press.

Song, X., Mitnitski, A., & Rockwood, K. (2010). Prevalence and 10-year outcomes of frailty in older adults in relation to deficit accumulation. *Journal of the American Geriatrics Society, 58*(4), 681–687.

Song, X., Mitnitski, A., & Rockwood, K. (2011). Nontraditional risk factors combine to predict Alzheimer disease and dementia. *Neurology, 77*(3), 227–234.

Speer, D. C. (1992). Clinically significant change: Jacobson and Truax (1991) revisited. *Journal of Consulting and Clinical Psychology, 60*(3), 402–408.

Sperling, R. A., Aisen, P. S., Beckett, L. A., Bennett, D. A., Craft, S., Fagan, A. M., . . . Phelps, C. H. (2011). Toward defining the preclinical stages of Alzheimer's disease: Recommendations from the National Institute on Aging and the Alzheimer's Association workgroup. *Alzheimer's and Dementia, 7,* 280–292.

Starkstein, S. E., & Jorge, R. (2005). Dementia after traumatic brain injury. *International Psychogeriatrics, 17*(Suppl. 1), S93–S107.

Steffens, D. C., & Potter, G. G. (2008). Geriatric depression and cognitive impairment. *Psychological Medicine, 38,* 163–175.

Stein, J., Luppa, M., Brähler, E., König, H.-H., & Riedel-Heller, S. G. (2010). The assessment of changes in cognitive functioning: Reliable change indices for neuropsychological instruments in the elderly—A systematic review. *Dementia and Geriatric Cognitive Disorders, 29*(3), 275–286.

Stephan, B. C., Hunter, S., Harris, D., Llewellyn, D. J., Siervo, M., Matthews, F. E., & Brayne, C. (2012). The neuropathological profile of mild cognitive impairment (MCI): A systematic review. *Molecular Psychiatry, 17,* 1056–1076.

Stern, C., & Munn, Z. (2010). Cognitive leisure activities and their role in preventing dementia: A systematic review. *International Journal of Evidence-Based Healthcare, 8*(1), 2–17.

Stern, R. A., Daneshvar, D. H., Baugh, C. M., Seichepine, D. R., Montenigro, P. H.,

Riley, D. O., . . . McKee, A. C. (2013). Clinical presentation of chronic traumatic encephalopathy. *Neurology, 81*(13), 1122–1129.

Stern, Y. (2002). What is cognitive reserve?: Theory and research application of the reserve concept. *Journal of the International Neuropsychological Society, 8*(3), 448–460.

Stern, Y. (2009). Cognitive reserve. *Neuropsychologia, 47,* 2015–2028.

Stern, Y. (2012). Cognitive reserve in ageing and Alzheimer's disease. *The Lancet Neurology, 11,* 1006–1012.

Stern, Y., Albert, S., Tang, M. X., & Tsai, W. Y. (1999). Rate of memory decline in AD is related to education and occupation: Cognitive reserve? *Neurology, 53*(9), 1942–1947.

Stern, Y., Alexander, G. E., Prohovnik, I., Stricks, L., Link, B., Lennon, M. C., & Mayeux, R. (1995). Relationship between lifetime occupation and parietal flow: Implications for a reserve against Alzheimer's disease pathology. *Neurology, 45*(1), 55–60.

St. John, P., & Montgomery, P. (2002). Are cognitively intact seniors with subjective memory loss more likely to develop dementia? *International Journal of Geriatric Psychiatry, 17,* 814–820.

Strauss, E., Sherman, E. M. S., & Spreen, O. (2006). *A compendium of neuropsychological tests: Administration, norms, and commentary* (3rd ed.). New York: Oxford University Press.

Stroebe, M., Schut, H., & van den Bout, J. (2013). *Complicated grief: Scientific foundations for health care professionals.* New York: Routledge.

Strydom, A., Chan, T., Fenton, C., Jamieson-Craig, R., Livingston, G., & Hassiotis, A. (2013). Validity of criteria for dementia in older people with intellectual disability. *American Journal of Geriatric Psychiatry, 21*(3), 279–288.

Suhr, J. A., & Gunstad, J. (2002). "Diagnosis threat": The effect of negative expectations on cognitive performance in head injury. *Journal of Clinical and Experimental Neuropsychology, 24*(4), 448–457.

Suhr, J. A., & Gunstad, J. (2005). Further exploration of the effect of "diagnosis threat" on cognitive performance in individuals with mild head injury. *Journal of the International Neuropsychological Society, 11*(1), 23–29.

Suo, C., Singh, M. F., Gates, N., Wen, W., Sachdev, P., Brodaty, H., . . . Valenzuela, M. J. (2016). Therapeutically relevant structural and functional mechanisms triggered by physical and cognitive exercise. *Molecular Psychiatry, 21,* 1633–1642.

Supiano, K. P., & Luptak, M. (2014). Complicated grief in older adults: A randomized controlled trial of complicated grief group therapy. *The Gerontologist, 54,* 840–856.

Swan, G. E., & Lessov-Schlaggar, C. N. (2007). The effects of tobacco smoke and nicotine on cognition and the brain. *Neuropsychology Review, 17*(3), 259–273.

Szeto, J. Y., Mowszowski, L., Gilat, M., Walton, C. C., Naismith, S. L., & Lewis, S. J. (2015). Assessing the utility of the Movement Disorder Society Task Force Level 1 diagnostic criteria for mild cognitive impairment in Parkinson's disease. *Parkinsonism and Related Disorders, 21,* 31–35.

Tales, A., Jessen, F., Butler, C., Wilcock, G., Phillips, J., & Bayer, T. (2015). Subjective cognitive decline. *Journal of Alzheimer's Disease, 48*(Suppl. 1), S1–S3.

Tan, C.-C., Yu, J.-T., Wang, H.-F., Tan, M.-S., Meng, Z.-F., Wang, C., . . . Tan, L. (2014). Efficacy and safety of donepezil, galantamine, rivastigmine, and memantine for the treatment of Alzheimer's disease: A systematic review and meta-analysis. *Journal of Alzheimer's Disease, 41,* 615–631.

Tangney, C. C. (2014). DASH and Mediterranean-type dietary patterns to maintain cognitive health. *Current Nutrition Reports, 3*(1), 51–61.

Tanwani, P., Fernie, B. A., Nikčević, A. V., & Spada, M. M. (2015). A systematic review of treatments for impulse control disorders and related behaviors in Parkinson's disease. *Psychiatry Research, 225,* 402–406.

Tarter, R. E., Butters, M., & Beers, S. R. (2001). *Medical neuropsychology* (2nd ed.). Dordrecht, The Netherlands: Kluwer.

Tate, R. L., Perdices, M., Rosenkoetter, U., Shadish, W., Vohra, S., Barlow, D. H., . . . Wilson, B. (2016). The Single-Case Reporting guideline In BEehavioural interventions (SCRIBE) 2016 statement. *Journal of School Psychology, 56,* 133–142.

Taulbee, L. R., & Folsom, J. C. (1966). Reality orientation for geriatric patients. *Hospital and Community Psychiatry, 17,* 133–135.

Taylor, W. D. (2014). Depression in the elderly. *New England Journal of Medicine, 371,* 1228–1236.

Temkin, N. R., Heaton, R. K., Grant, I., & Dikmen, S. S. (1999). Detecting significant change in neuropsychological test performance: A comparison of four models. *Journal of the International Neuropsychological Society, 5*(4), 357–369.

Teng, E., Becker, B. W., Woo, E., Knopman, D. S., Cummings, J. L., & Lu, P. H. (2010). Utility of the Functional Activities Questionnaire for distinguishing mild cognitive impairment from very mild Alzheimer's disease. *Alzheimer's Disease and Associated Disorders, 24,* 348–353.

Teri, L., McCurry, S. M., Edland, S. D., Kukull, W. A., & Larson, E. B. (1995). Cognitive decline in Alzheimer's disease: A longitudinal investigation of risk factors for accelerated decline. *Journals of Gerontology Series A: Biological Sciences and Medical Sciences, 50*(1), M49–M55.

Teri, L., Truax, P., Logsdon, R., Uomoto, J., Zarit, S., & Vitaliano, P. P. (1992). Assessment of behavioral problems in dementia: The Revised Memory and Behavior Problems Checklist. *Psychology and Aging, 7*(4), 622–631.

Terry, R. D. (2006). Alzheimer's disease and the aging brain. *Journal of Geriatric Psychiatry and Neurology, 19*(3), 125–128.

Terry, R. D. (2007). Alzheimer's disease and the aging brain. In T. Sunderland, D. V. Jeste, O. Baiyewu, P. J. Sirovatka, & D. A. Regier (Eds.), *Diagnostic issues in dementia: Advancing the research agenda for DSM-V* (pp. 1–7). Arlington, VA: American Psychiatric Association.

Testa, J. A., Malec, J. F., Moessner, A. M., & Brown, A. W. (2005). Outcome after traumatic brain injury: Effects of aging on recovery. *Archives of Physical Medicines and Rehabilitation, 86*(9), 1815–1823.

Thal, L. J. (2006). Prevention of Alzheimer disease. *Alzheimer Disease and Associated Disorders, 20,* S97–S99.

The Economist. (2013, August 10). Commercialising neuroscience: Brain sells. Retrieved December 27, 2016, from *www.economist.com/news/business/21583260-cognitive-training-may-be-moneyspinner-despite-scientists-doubts-brain-sells.*

The FTD Disorders. (2016). Retrieved from *www.theaftd.org/understandingftd/disorders.*

Theisen, M. E., Rapport, L. J., Axelrod, B. N., & Brines, D. B. (1998). Effects of practice in repeated administrations of the Wechsler Memory Scale—Revised in normal adults. *Assessment, 5*(1), 85–92.

Thompson, L. W., Dick-Siskin, L., Coon, D. W., Powers, D. V., & Gallagher-Thompson, D. (2010). *Treating late-life depression: A cognitive behavioral therapy approach workbook.* New York: Oxford University Press.

Thorvaldsson, V., Macdonald, S. W., Fratiglioni, L., Winblad, B., Kivipelto, M., Laukka, E. J., . . . Backman, L. (2011). Onset and rate of cognitive change before dementia diagnosis: Findings from two Swedish population-based longitudinal studies. *Journal of the International Neuropsychological Society, 17*(1), 154–162.

Tierney, M. C., & Lermer, M. A. (2010). Computerized cognitive assessment in primary care to identify patients with suspected cognitive impairment. *Journal of Alzheimer's Disease, 20*(3), 823–832.

Tornatore, J. B., Hill, E., Laboff, J. A., & McGann, M. E. (2005). Self-administered screening for mild cognitive impairment: Initial validation of a computerized test battery. *Journal of Neuropsychiatry and Clinical Neurosciences, 17*(1), 98–105.

Toro, P., Degen, C., Pierer, M., Gustafson, D., Schroder, J., & Schonknecht, P. (2014). Cholesterol in mild cognitive impairment and Alzheimer's disease in a birth cohort over 14 years. *European Archives of Psychiatry and Clinical Neurosciences, 264*(6), 485–492.

Trenkle, D. L., Shankle, W. R., & Azen, S. P. (2007). Detecting cognitive impairment in primary care: Performance assessment of three screening instruments. *Journal of Alzheimer's Disease, 11*(3), 323–335.

Troyer, A. (2001). Improving memory knowledge, satisfaction, and functioning via an education and intervention program for older adults. *Aging, Neuropsychology, and Cognition, 8,* 256–268.

Trustram Eve, C., & de Jager, C. A. (2014). Piloting and validation of a novel self-administered online cognitive screening tool in normal older persons: The Cognitive Function Test. *International Journal of Geriatric Psychiatry, 29*(2), 198–206.

Trzepacz, P. T., Mittal, D., Torres, R., Kanary, K., Norton, J., & Jimerson, N. (2001). Validation of the Delirium Rating Scale–Revised–98: Comparison with the Delirium Rating Scale and the Cognitive Test for Delirium. *Journal Neuropsychiatry and Clinical Neurosciences, 13*(2), 229–242.

Tschanz, J. T., Norton, M. C., Zandi, P. P., & Lyketsos, C. G. (2013). The Cache County Study on Memory in Aging: Factors affecting risk of Alzheimer's disease and its progression after onset. *International Review of Psychiatry, 25*(6), 673–685.

Tsuboi, K., Harada, T., Ishii, T., Morishita, H., Ohtani, H., & Ishizaki, F. (2009). Evaluation of the usefulness of a simple touch-panel method for the screening of dementia. *Hiroshima Journal of Medical Sciences, 58*(2–3), 49–53.

Tun, P. A., & Lachman, M. E. (2006). Telephone assessment of cognitive function in adulthood: The Brief Test of Adult Cognition by Telephone. *Age and Ageing, 35*(6), 629–632.

Tuokko, H. A., Chou, P. H. B., Bowden, S. C., Simard, M., Ska, B., & Crossley, M. (2009). Partial measurement equivalence of French and English versions of the Canadian Study of Health and Aging neuropsychological battery. *Journal of the International Neuropsychological Society, 15*(3), 416–425.

Tuokko, H., Crockett, D., Holliday, S., & Coval, M. (1987). The relationship between performance on the Multi-focus Assessment Scale and functional status. *Canadian Journal on Aging, 6*(1), 33–45.

Tuokko, H., & Hadjistavropoulos, T. (1998). *An assessment guide to geriatric neuropsychology.* Mahwah, NJ: Erlbaum.

Tuokko, H. A., & Hultsch, D. F. (2006a). *Mild cognitive impairment: International perspectives.* Philadelphia: Taylor & Francis.

Tuokko, H. A., & Hultsch, D. F. (2006b). The future of mild cognitive impairment. In H. A. Tuokko & D. F. Hultsch (Eds.), *Mild cognitive impairment: International perspectives* (pp. 291–304). Philadelphia: Taylor & Francis.

Tuokko, H. A., & McDowell, I. (2006). An overview of mild cognitive impairment. In H. A. Tuokko & D. F. Hultsch (Eds.), *Mild cognitive impairment* (pp. 3–28). New York: Taylor & Francis.

Tuokko, H., & Ritchie, L. (2016). Impairment in the geriatric population. In S. Goldstein & J. A. Naglieri (Eds.), *Assessing impairment: From theory to practice* (2nd ed., pp. 91–122). New York: Springer Science + Business Media.

Tuokko, H. A., & Smart, C. M. (2014). Functional sequelae of cognitive decline in later life. In N. A. Pachana & K. Laidlaw (Eds.), *The Oxford handbook of clinical geropsychology* (pp. 306–334). New York: Oxford University Press.

Tuokko, H. A., & Woodward, T. S. (1996). Development and validation of a demographic correction system for neuropsychological measures used in the Canadian Study of Health and Aging. *Journal of Clinical and Experimental Neuropsychology, 18*(4), 479–616.

Turner, R. C., Lucke-Wold, B. P., Robson, M. J., Lee, J. M., & Bailes, J. E. (2016). Alzheimer's disease and chronic traumatic encephalopathy: Distinct but possibly overlapping disease entities. *Brain Injury, 30*(11), 1279–1292.

Turvey, C., Coleman, M., Dennison, O., Drude, K., Goldenson, M., Hirsch, P., . . . Bernard, J. (2013). ATA practice guidelines for video-based online mental health services. *Telemedicine and e-Health, 19*(9), 722–731.

Tyas, S. L., Manfreda, J., Strain, L. A., & Montgomery, P. R. (2001). Risk factors for Alzheimer's disease: A population-based, longitudinal study in Manitoba, Canada. *International Journal of Epidemiology, 30*(3), 590–597.

United Nations. (2013). World Population Ageing 2013. Retrieved from *www.un.org/en/development/desa/population/publications/pdf/ageing/WorldPopulationAgeing2013.pdf.*

Valkanova, V., Rodriguez, R. E., & Ebmeier, K. P. (2014). Mind over matter—what do we know about neuroplasticity in adults? *International Psychogeriatrics, 26,* 891–909.

van de Rest, O., Berendsen, A. A., Haveman-Nies, A., & de Groot, L. C. (2015). Dietary patterns, cognitive decline, and dementia: A systematic review. *Advances in Nutrition, 6*(2), 154–168.

van den Berg, E., Kant, N., & Postma, A. (2012). Remember to buy milk on the way home!: A meta-analytic review of prospective memory in mild cognitive impairment and dementia. *Journal of the International Neuropsychological Society, 18,* 706–716.

van den Berg, N., Schumann, M., Kraft, K., & Hoffmann, W. (2012). Telemedicine and telecare for older patients—A systematic review. *Maturitas, 73,* 94–114.

van der Flier, W. M., van Buchem, M. A., Weverling-Rijnsburger, A. W., Mutsaers, E. R., Bollen, E. L., Admiraal-Behloul, F., . . . Middelkoop, H. A. (2004). Memory complaints in patients with normal cognition are associated with smaller hippocampal volumes. *Journal of Neurology, 251,* 671–675.

van Gelder, B. M., Tijhuis, M. A., Kalmijn, S., Giampaoli, S., Nissinen, A., & Kromhout, D. (2004). Physical activity in relation to cognitive decline in elderly men: The FINE Study. *Neurology, 63*(12), 2316–2321.

van Harten, A. C., Visser, P. J., Pijnenburg, Y. A., Teunissen, C. E., Blankenstein, M. A., Scheltens, P., & van der Flier, W. (2013). Cerebrospinal fluid Aβ42 is the best predictor of clinical progression in patients with subjective complaints. *Alzheimer's and Dementia, 9,* 481–487.

Van Hooren, S. A. H., Valentijn, S. A. M., Bosma, H., Ponds, R. W. H. M., van Boxtel, M. P. J., . . . Jolles, J. (2007). Effect of a structured course involving goal management training in older adults: A randomized controlled trial. *Patient Education and Counseling, 65,* 205–213.

van Oijen, M., de Jong, F. J., Hofman, A., Koudstaal, P. J., & Breteler, M. M. (2007). Subjective memory complaints, education, and risk of Alzheimer's disease. *Alzheimer's and Dementia, 3,* 92–97.

Van Petten, C., Plante, E., Davidson, P. S. R., Kuo, T. Y., Bajuscak, L., & Glisky, E. L. (2004). Memory and executive function in older adults: Relationships with temporal and prefrontal gray matter volumes and white matter hyperintensities. *Neuropsychologia, 42*(10), 1313–1335.

Vandermorris, S., Davidson, S., Au, A., Sue, J., Fallah, S., & Troyer, A. K. (2016). "Accepting where I'm at"—a qualitative study of the mechanisms, benefits, and impact of a behavioral memory intervention for community-dwelling older adults. *Aging and Mental Health, 4,* 1–7.

Verdoux, H., Lagnaoui, R., & Begaud, B. (2005). Is benzodiazepine use a risk factor for cognitive decline and dementia?: A literature review of epidemiological studies. *Psychological Medicine, 35*(3), 307–315.

Verghese, J., LeValley, A., Derby, C., Kuslansky, G., Katz, M., Hall, C., . . . Lipton, R. B. (2006). Leisure activities and the risk of amnestic mild cognitive impairment in the elderly. *Neurology, 66*(6), 821–827.

Verghese, J., Lipton, R. B., Katz, M. J., Hall, C. B., Derby, C. A., Kuslansky, G., . . . Buschke, H. (2003). Leisure activities and the risk of dementia in the elderly. *New England Journal of Medicine, 348*(25), 2508–2516.

Verhaeghen, P. (2013). *The elements of cognitive aging: Meta-analyses of age-related differences in processing speed and their consequences.* New York: Oxford University Press.

Veroff, A. E., Bodick, N. C., Offen, W. W., Sramek, J. J., & Cutler, N. R. (1998). Efficacy of xanomeline in Alzheimer disease: Cognitive improvement measured using the Computerized Neuropsychological Test Battery (CNTB). *Alzheimer Disease and Associated Disorders, 12*(4), 304–312.

Veroff, A. E., Cutler, N. R., Sramek, J. J., Prior, P. L., Mickelson, W., & Hartman, J. K. (1991). A new assessment tool for neuropsychopharmacologic research: The Computerized Neuropsychological Test Battery. *Journal of Geriatric Psychiatry and Neurology, 4*(4), 211–217.

Versijpt, J. (2014). Effectiveness and cost-effectiveness of pharmacological treatment for Alzheimer's disease and vascular dementia. *Journal of Alzheimer's Disease, 42,* S19–S25.

Victoroff, J. (2013). Traumatic encephalopathy: Review and provisional research diagnostic criteria. *NeuroRehabilitation, 32*(2), 211–224.

Visser, P. J., Verhey, F., Knol, D. L., Scheltens, P., Wahlund, L. O., Freund-Levi, Y., . . . Blenow, K. (2009). Prevalence and prognostic value of CSF markers of Alzheimer's disease pathology in patients with subjective cognitive impairment or mild cognitive impairment in the DESCRIPA study: A prospective cohort study. *The Lancet Neurology, 8,* 619–627.

Voelcker-Rehage, C. (2008). Motor-skill learning in older adults—a review of age-related differences. *European Review of Aging and Physical Activity, 5,* 5–16.

Volkert, J., Schulz, H., Härter, M., Wlodarczyk, O., & Andreas, S. (2013). The prevalence of mental disorders in older people in Western countries: A meta-analysis. *Ageing Research Reviews, 12,* 339–353.

Wang, H. X., Karp, A., Winblad, B., & Fratiglioni, L. (2002). Late-life engagement in social and leisure activities is associated with a decreased risk of dementia: A longitudinal study from the Kungsholmen project. *American Journal of Epidemiology, 155*(12), 1081–1087.

Wang, J. Y., Zhou, D. H., Li, J., Zhang, M., Deng, J., Tang, M., . . . Chen, M. (2006). Leisure activity and risk of cognitive impairment: The Chongqing Aging Study. *Neurology, 66*(6), 911–913.

Wang, P. N., Wang, S. J., Fuh, J. L., Teng, E. L., Liu, C. H., Lin, C. H., . . . Liu, H. C. (2000). Subjective memory complaint in relation to cognitive performance and depression: A longitudinal study of a rural Chinese population. *Journal of the American Geriatrics Society, 48*(3), 295–299.

Ward, A., Arrighi, H. M., Michels, S., & Cedarbaum, J. M. (2012). Mild cognitive impairment: Disparity of incidence and prevalence estimates. *Alzheimer's and Dementia, 8*, 14–21.

Wechsler, D. (1987). *Wechsler Memory Scale—Revised*. San Antonio, TX: Pearson Assessments.

Wechsler, D. (1997). *Wechsler Memory Scale* (3rd ed.). San Antonio, TX: Pearson Assessments.

Wechsler, D. (2008). *Wechsler Adult Intelligence Scale* (4th ed.). San Antonio, TX: Pearson Assessments.

Wechsler, D. (2009). *Wechsler Memory Scale* (4th ed.). San Antonio, TX: Pearson Assessments.

Weller, F. (2015). *The wild edge of sorrow: Rituals of renewal and the sacred work of grief*. Berkeley, CA: North Atlantic Books.

Wengreen, H., Munger, R. G., Cutler, A., Quach, A., Bowles, A., Corcoran, C., . . . Welsh-Bohmer, K. A. (2013). Prospective study of Dietary Approaches to Stop Hypertension- and Mediterranean-style dietary patterns and age-related cognitive change: The Cache County Study on Memory, Health and Aging. *American Journal of Clinical Nutrition, 98*(5), 1263–1271.

Werner, P., & Korczyn, A. D. (2008). Mild cognitive impairment: Conceptual, assessment, ethical, and social issues. *Clinical Interventions in Aging, 3*(3), 413–420.

Werner, P., & Korczyn, A. D. (2012). Willingness to use computerized systems for the diagnosis of dementia: Testing a theoretical model in an Israeli sample. *Alzheimer Disease and Associated Disorders, 26*(2), 171–178.

West, R. L. (1996). An application of prefrontal cortex function theory to cognitive aging. *Psychological Bulletin, 120*(2), 272–292.

Westerhof, G. J., Bohlmeijer, E., & Webster, J. D. (2010). Reminiscence and mental health: A review of recent progress in theory, research and interventions. *Ageing and Society, 30*, 697–721.

Weuve, J., Kang, J. H., Manson, J. E., Breteler, M. M., Ware, J. H., & Grodstein, F. (2004). Physical activity, including walking, and cognitive function in older women. *JAMA, 292*(12), 1454–1461.

Whitbourne, S. K., Whitbourne, S. B., & Konnert, C. (2015). *Adult development and aging: Biopsychosocial perspectives* (Canadian ed.). Toronto, Ontario: Wiley & Sons Canada.

White, L., Katzman, R., Losonczy, K., Salive, M., Wallace, R., Berkman, L., . . . Havlik, R. (1994). Association of education with incidence of cognitive impairment in three established populations for epidemiologic studies of the elderly. *Journal of Clinical Epidemiology, 47*(4), 363–374.

Whitmer, R. A., Sidney, S., Selby, J., Johnston, S. C., & Yaffe, K. (2005). Midlife cardiovascular risk factors and risk of dementia in late life. *Neurology, 64*(2), 277–281.

Wiegand, M. A., Troyer, A. K., Gojmerac, C., & Murphy, K. J. (2013). Facilitating change in health-related behaviours and intentions: A randomized controlled trial of a multidimensional memory program for older adults. *Aging and Mental Health, 17,* 806–815.

Wild, K., Howieson, D., Webbe, F., Seelye, A., & Kaye, J. (2008). Status of computerized cognitive testing in aging: A systematic review. *Alzheimer's and Dementia, 4*(6), 428–437.

Willis, S. L. (1996). Assessing everyday competence in the cognitively challenged elderly. In M. A. Smyer, K. W. Schaie, & M. B. Kapp (Eds.), *Older adults' decision-making and the law* (pp. 87–127). New York: Springer.

Wilson, B. A., Baddeley, A., Evans, J. J., & Shiel, A. J. (1994). Errorless learning in the rehabilitation of memory impaired people. *Neuropsychological Rehabilitation, 4,* 307–326.

Wilson, B. A., Watson, P. C., Baddeley, A. D., Emslie, H., & Evans, J. J. (2000). Improvement or simply practice?: The effects of twenty repeated assessments on people with and without brain injury. *Journal of the International Neuropsychological Society, 6,* 469–479.

Wilson, R. S., Bennett, D. A., Bienias, J. L., Aggarwal, N. T., Mendes De Leon, C. F., Morris, M. C., . . . Evans, D. A. (2002). Cognitive activity and incident AD in a population-based sample of older persons. *Neurology, 59*(12), 1910–1914.

Wilson, R. S., Boyle, P. A., Capuano, A. W., Shah, R. C., Hoganson, G. M., Nag, S., & Bennett, D. A. (2016). Late-life depression is not associated with dementia-related pathology. *Neuropsychology, 30*(2), 135–142.

Wilson, R. S., Boyle, P. A., Yu, L., Barnes, L. L., Schneider, J. A., & Bennett, D. A. (2013). Life-span cognitive activity, neuropathologic burden, and cognitive aging. *Neurology, 81*(4), 314–321.

Wilson, R. S., Hebert, L. E., Scherr, P. A., Barnes, L. L., Mendes de Leon, C. F., & Evans, D. A. (2009). Educational attainment and cognitive decline in old age. *Neurology, 72*(5), 460–465.

Wilson, R. S., Li, Y., Aggarwal, N. T., Barnes, L. L., McCann, J. J., Gilley, D. W., & Evans, D. A. (2004). Education and the course of cognitive decline in Alzheimer disease. *Neurology, 63*(7), 1198–1202.

Winblad B., Palmer, K., Kivipelto, M., Jelic, V., Fratiglioni, L., Wahlund, L. O., . . . Petersen, R. C. (2004). Mild cognitive impairment—beyond controversies, towards a consensus: Report of the International Working Group on Mild Cognitive Impairment. *Journal of Internal Medicine, 256,* 240–246.

Winner, B., Kohl, Z., & Gage, F. H. (2011). Neurodegenerative disease and adult neurogenesis. *European Journal of Neuroscience, 33,* 1139–1151.

Winslow, B. T., Onysko, M. K., Stob, C. M., & Hazlewood, K. A. (2011). Treatment of Alzheimer disease. *American Family Physician, 83,* 1403–1412.

Wolfsgruber, S., Kleineidam, L., Wagner, M., Mösch, E., Bickel, H., Lühmann, D., . . . AgeCoDe Study Group. (2016). Differential risk of incident Alzheimer's disease dementia in stable versus unstable patterns of subjective cognitive decline. *Journal of Alzheimer's Disease, 54,* 1135–1146.

Wolfson, C., Kirkland, S. A., Raina, P. S., Uniat, J., Roberts, K., Bergman, H., . . . Meneok, K. S. (2009). Telephone-administered cognitive tests as tools for the identification of eligible study participants for population-based research in aging. *Canadian Journal on Aging, 28*(3), 251–259.

Wolitzky-Taylor, K. B., Castriotta, N., Lenze, E. J., Stanley, M. A., & Craske, M. G. (2010). Anxiety disorders in older adults: A comprehensive review. *Depression and Anxiety, 27,* 190–211.

Woods, B., Aguirre, E., Spector, A. E., & Orrell, M. (2012). Cognitive stimulation to improve cognitive functioning in people with dementia. *Cochrane Database of Systematic Reviews, 2,* CD005562.

Woolcott, J. C., Richardson, K. J., Wiens, M. O., Patel, B., Marin, J., Khan, K. M., & Marra, C. A. (2009). Meta-analysis of the impact of 9 medication classes on falls in elderly. *Archives of Internal Medicine, 169,* 1952–1960.

World Health Organization. (1993). *International classification of diseases and related health problems* (10th ed.). Geneva, Switzerland: Author.

World Health Organization. (2001). *International classification of functioning, disability and health: ICF.* Geneva, Switzerland: Author.

World Health Organization. (2015). *International classification of diseases—10th edition—Clinical modification.* Geneva, Switzerland: Author. Retrieved from *www.icd10data.com.*

Worthy, D. A., Gorlick, M. A., Pacheco, J. L., Schyner, D. M., & Maddox, W. T. (2011). With age comes wisdom: Decision-making in younger and older adults. *Psychological Science, 22,* 1375–1380.

Wykes, T., Steel, C., Everitt, B., & Tarrier, N. (2008). Cognitive behavior therapy for schizophrenia: Effect sizes, clinical models, and methodological rigor. *Schizophrenia Bulletin, 34,* 523–537.

Wylie, S. A., Ridderinkhof, K. R., Eckerle, M. K., & Manning, C. A. (2007). Inefficient response inhibition in individuals with mild cognitive impairment. *Neuropsychologia, 45*(7), 1408–1419.

Wynne, H. A., Cope, L. H., Mutch, E., Rawlins, M. D., Woodhouse, K. W., & James, O. F. (1989). The effect of age upon liver volume and apparent liver blood flow in healthy man. *Hepatology, 9,* 297–301.

Xing, Y., Qin, W., Li, F., Jia, X. F., & Jia, J. (2013). Associations between sex hormones and cognitive and neuropsychiatric manifestations in vascular dementia (VaD). *Archives of Gerontology and Geriatrics, 56*(1), 85–90.

Xu, W., Caracciolo, B., Wang, H. X., Winblad, B., Backman, L., Qiu, C., & Fratiglioni, L. (2010). Accelerated progression from mild cognitive impairment to dementia in people with diabetes. *Diabetes, 59*(11), 2928–2935.

Yaffe, K., Vittinghoff, E., Lindquist, K., Barnes, D., Covinsky, K. E., Neylan, T., . . . Marmar, C. (2010). Posttraumatic stress disorder and risk of dementia among US veterans. *Archives of General Psychiatry, 67*(6), 608–613.

Yakovenko, I., Quigley, L., Hemmelgarn, B. R., Hodgins, D. C., & Ronksley, P. (2015). The efficacy of motivational interviewing for disordered gambling: Systematic review and meta-analysis. *Addictive Behaviors, 43,* 72–82.

Yau, S., Gil-Mohapel, J., Christie, B. R., & So, K. (2014). Physical exercise-induced adult neurogenesis: A good strategy to prevent cognitive decline in neurodegenerative diseases? *BioMed Research International, 2014,* 403120.

Yesavage, J. A., Brink, T., Rose, T., Lum, O., Huang, V., Adey, M., & Leirer, V. O. (1983). Development and validation of a geriatric depression screening scale: A preliminary report. *Journal of Psychiatric Research, 17,* 37–49.

Young, R., Camic, P. M., & Tischler, V. (2016). The impact of community-based arts and health interventions on cognition in people with dementia: A systematic literature review. *Aging and Mental Health, 20,* 337–351.

Zahodne, L. B., Schofield, P. W., Farrell, M. T., Stern, Y., & Manly, J. J. (2014). Bilingualism does not alter cognitive decline or dementia risk among Spanish-speaking immigrants. *Neuropsychology, 28*(2), 238–246.

Zaudig, M. (1992). A new systematic method of measurement and diagnosis of "mild cognitive impairment" and dementia according to ICD-10 and DSM-III-R criteria. *International Psychogeriatrics, 4,* 203–219.

Zeilinger, E. L., Stiehl, K. A. M., & Weber, G. (2013). A systematic review on assessment instruments for dementia in persons with intellectual disabilities. *Research in Developmental Disabilities, 34*(11), 3962–3977.

Zhou, X., Zhang, J., Chen, Y., Ma, T., Wang, Y., Wang, J., & Zhang, Z. (2014). Aggravated cognitive and brain functional impairment in mild cognitive impairment patients with type 2 diabetes: A resting-state functional MRI study. *Journal of Alzheimer's Disease, 41*(3), 925–935.

Zigman, W. B., Schupf, N., Devenny, D. A., Miezejeski, C., Ryan, R., Urv, T. K., . . . Silverman, W. (2004). Incidence and prevalence of dementia in elderly adults with mental retardation without Down syndrome. *American Journal of Mental Retardation, 109*(2), 126–141.

Zunzunegui, M. V., Alvarado, B. E., Del Ser, T., & Otero, A. (2003). Social networks, social integration, and social engagement determine cognitive decline in community-dwelling Spanish older adults. *Journal of Gerontology Series B: Psychological Sciences and Social Sciences, 58*(2), S93–S100.

Zygouris, S., & Tsolaki, M. (2015). Computerized cognitive testing for older adults: A review. *American Journal of Alzheimer's Disorder and Other Dementias, 30*(1), 13–28.

Zylowska, L., Ackerman, D. L., Yang, M. H., Futrell, J. L., Horton, N. L., Hale, T. S., . . . Smalley, S. L. (2008). Mindfulness meditation training in adults and adolescents with ADHD: A feasibility study. *Journal of Attention Disorders, 11*(6), 737–746.

Index

Note. *f* or *t* following a page number indicates a figure or a table.